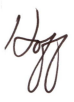

The Doctor in Literature

satisfaction or resentment?

Solomon Posen

**Foreword by
Edward J Huth**

Radcliffe Publishing
Oxford • Seattle

Radcliffe Publishing Ltd
18 Marcham Road
Abingdon
Oxon OX14 1AA
United Kingdom

<u>www.radcliffe-oxford.com</u>
Electronic catalog and worldwide online ordering facility.

British Library Cataloging in Publication Data

A catalog record for this book is available from the British Library.

ISBN 1 85775 609 6

Typeset by Anne Joshua & Associates, Oxford, UK
Printed and bound by TJ International Ltd, Padstow, Cornwall, UK

Contents

Cover design: The Doctor by Luke Fildes (1887). Francis Brett Young ridiculed this painting for what he considered its sentimentality. According to Young (himself a physician and author of medical novels), a doctor has no business to sit beside the bedside of his little patient contemplating the child's impending demise or recovery. His calling 'necessarily makes him a man of action rather than reflection' and, according to Young, he ought to be bustling about, doing something. (Introduction to the series, p. 15, Reference 56.) Picture reproduced by courtesy of the Tate Gallery, London.

Foreword

Oh wad some pow'r the giftie gie us
To see oursels as others see us!
It wad frae monie a blunder free us
An' foolish notion . . .

Robert Burns, *To a Louse*, 1786

Wise is the physician who takes to heart the advice of Robert Burns, to see, if possible, how others see us. The human race is a spectrum from saints to scoundrels. None of us in medicine is exempt from judgements of where we stand in the spectrum. But what, indeed, are the judgements of the world in which we work? And why are we thus seen?

Unspoken and unwritten judgements we will never know, whether they be those of the men and women who see us up close as our patients or of spectators quite detached. But through the millennia of the written word, novelists, playwrights and poets have worked us into their tapestries. Here is where Dr Posen has gone for this collection of judgements of what we have been and what we might be. He faced an intimidating task. Consider what Greek and Roman literature alone adds up to. He has had to pick widely and carefully. This he has done. What he offers is a full range of judgements; he has not hidden our critics and I think he finds a few halos. In my view, he has wisely drawn mostly from the literature of the past two or three centuries; this is literature most of us can readily find. It is legitimate to ask whether literary views of us are in fact an accurate picture of our profession. There is no clear answer. If we assume that writers draw on what they have seen, we can fairly conclude that at least some of what some writers put on paper about us is a correct picture, even if it is not a full picture.

Why should those of us who are physicians look at what Dr Posen has placed before us? Robert Burns' advice is cogent. If we know how we are seen by the rest of the world, we may be less prone to conduct ourselves in ways at odds with our professional values. We may be more likely to conduct ourselves so as to demonstrate the value of what we profess. No, Dr Posen's book will not purge our profession of scoundrels, professional cripples and incompetents. But those of us who keep an open mind about what we are and what we might do to be worthy of a place in our profession may profit.

What he shows us merits the attention not only of physicians. Among his readers should be physicians-to-be, medical students. Today's medical curriculum is stuffed to bulging not only with the necessary techniques in history taking and physical examination, in which they must show competence, but also with a far bigger intimidating bulk of complex science that may determine the nature of tomorrow's practice. There may be no place for yet another demand on it. And I am skeptical that students pay much attention to what is likely to be seen by them as peripheral to making their way through school. But some medical educators may be less skeptical; I hope so.

Dr Posen's book might be considered an informal social history of medicine from the past to the present. As such, it can speak to a much wider audience. Views of our profession have been and are now constantly of potential importance to many more persons than physicians: patients, parents, nurses, politicians, economists and historians. What is there about medicine that has remained unchanged for millennia? Why has there been no change in these aspects of care of the ill? What is there about medicine that through the same centuries has changed radically and may continue to change? Why? If society wishes to shape medicine and medical care to its advantage, it needs answers to these questions. What Dr Posen brings us may carry at least some answers.

Edward J Huth MD MACP FRCP
Emeritus Editor
Annals of Internal Medicine
August 2004

About the author

Solomon Posen majored in English before obtaining his medical degrees (MB, BS 1954, MD 1965) at the University of Adelaide, Australia. He is a Fellow of the Royal Australasian College of Physicians, a Fellow of the Royal College of Physicians, London, and a past president of the Endocrine Society of Australia.

Professor Posen taught General Medicine and Endocrinology at Sydney University for almost 30 years. He is the author of some 130 scientific papers (mainly in the field of calcium metabolism) and a co-author of a book on Alkaline Phosphatase. He has published a series of papers on the Doctor in Literature, some of which form the basis of this book. A second volume in this series entitled The Doctor's Private Life is planned for 2005.

Professor Posen is married with three grown up children and five grandchildren. He lives in Sydney, Australia.

Acknowledgements

My sincere thanks are due to Dr Carolyn Brimley Norris, who generously made available a full copy of her PhD dissertation (The Image of the Physician in Modern American Literature, University of Maryland, 1969) and who introduced me to the concept of 'earthy' physicians. In addition, Dr Norris corrected multiple stylistic and punctuation errors, she made many valuable suggestions concerning the organization of the material and she provided encouragement at times when no one else seemed interested in this work. Thank you, Carol.

Numerous authors, including the late Derek Lindsay (AE Ellis), Neil Ravin, Richard Selzer, Susan Cheever, Patricia Cornwell and Larry Schneiderman provided copies of their books, background information, encouragement or all three. I am grateful to all of them.

Dr Philippe Lanthony of Troyes, France, pointed out a number of important works not available in English, particularly Daudet's *Les Morticoles* and Malègue's *Augustin, ou, Le maître est là*. Marita Amm of Kiel, Germany, drew my attention to several fictional works relating to ophthalmologists.

The staff of the Douglas Piper Library, Royal North Shore Hospital, Sydney, particularly Helen Giltrap and Agnes Wroblewski, were most helpful in obtaining books from libraries all over Australia. Helen Pottie typed much of the material.

Most importantly, I thank my wife, Jean Katie Posen, for her love, her patience and her forbearance.

Reprint permissions for copyrighted material

Jonathan Cape/Vintage. Reprinted by permission of The Random House Group Ltd.

Tennessee Williams, *Suddenly Last Summer*. Copyright © 1971 Tennessee Williams. Reprinted by permission of Georges Borchardt, Inc., for The University of the South.

Tennessee Williams, *Summer and Smoke*. Copyright © 1971 Tennessee Williams. Reprinted by permission of Georges Borchardt, Inc., for The University of the South.

David Williamson, Taken from the play *Travelling North*. Copyright © 1980. First published by Currency Press, Pty Ltd, Sydney. Now available in Williamson's *Collected Plays, Volume 2*.

Every effort has been made to acknowledge correctly and to contact the copyright holders of citations considered in excess of 'fair use'. The author and the publishers apologize for any unintentional errors or omissions, which will be corrected in future reprints of this book.

Introduction

The aims of this work

This annotated anthology is intended to serve three purposes. It is a reference work bringing together, in an indexed form, some 1500 passages from approximately 600 works of literature describing physicians,* their attitudes and their activities. Second, it attempts to identify and analyze a number of themes that constantly recur in the portrayal of medical doctors, especially themes that seem unaffected by time, place or clinical training. Third, it is hoped that this work will provide some pleasure for readers who use it for browsing.

The book endeavors to correct an obvious deficiency – the lack of an index that will enable researchers, teachers or seekers of quotations to find fictional physicians or medical scenarios. While major medical characters such as Tertius Lydgate[1] and Martin Arrowsmith[2] appear in standard literary encyclopedias,[3] Cozzens' George Bull,[4] the archetypal 'earthy'[5] physician, and Roy Basch, the disillusioned, disgruntled, inadequate intern,[6] do not. Dictionaries of medical quotations[7,8] for the most part overlook or ignore important fictional passages, such as Proust's brilliant aphorism 'If . . . [non-organic disease] is capable of deceiving the doctor, how should it fail to deceive the patient?'[9] With the relevant material scattered through thousands of novels, short stories and plays, a full catalog is unlikely ever to be compiled. However, this book provides some assistance to readers in search of clinical settings in literature, by indexing major and minor fictional medical characters, vignettes and aphorisms. Hopefully, as well as filling an evident gap, it will form a basis for future, more comprehensive indices.

It is anticipated that this volume will be used as a companion – a junior companion – to Huth and Murray's magnificent *Medicine in Quotations*,[8] though it would be presumptuous to draw any comparisons between the breadth and erudition of that work and the more limited scope of *The Doctor in Literature*. I have tried to emulate their work in a number of ways. Like Huth and Murray, I have grouped together passages dealing with particular topics such as physicians' fees, degrees of detachment and career choices, regardless of historical or geographical considerations. I have used their system of indexing by author and subject. Page numbers are provided for specific events and sayings, but not for gradual developments, such as the decline in a doctor's practice.

Unlike Huth and Murray, who selected 'pithy, clear and compelling' quotations containing recognizable truths,[10] I have used citations from fiction, describing doctor–patient interactions and doctors' personal lives. These citations, which vary in length from a few words to several paragraphs, describe medical practice

---

* Throughout this book the term 'physician' refers to all medical doctors and not only to internists.

as it is portrayed, rather than as it should be. For instance, Huth and Murray list a number of aphorisms dealing with the importance of medical journals to a doctor's ongoing education.[11] The citations in this book tell of enthusiastic journal readers,[12,13] as well as piles of unopened periodicals,[14] doctors going to sleep trying to 'move with the times'[15] and doctors whose main interest in medical journals comes from advertisements[16] or the contents of the obituary columns.[17] There are sections on ward rounds, argumentative and flirtatious patients, dedicated and demotivated physicians, and interactions between doctors and nurses. Readers can find entries like 'Chemotherapy', 'Drug salesmen, visits by', 'Medical certificates', 'Ophthalmoscopy', 'White coats', and many other topics familiar to doctors and paramedical personnel.

The second objective of this work, which differentiates it from existing anthologies,[18-24] relates to the exploration of specific personality traits among fictional physicians. Such traits are particularly interesting if they recur in works written during different periods and seem unaffected by time, place or the changing social status of medical practitioners. How do writers perceive the attitudes of physicians and patients towards medical fees? Are fictional doctors good family men and loyal colleagues? What makes patients angry or resentful and how do fictional physicians react during a confrontation with a hostile patient? Do fictional doctors enjoy their work? Are they religious? How do they conduct themselves when a patient becomes amorous? Do they comply with demands for an abortion or euthanasia? How do they behave at the bedside, especially if the patient is very ill or dying? Is the doctor a versatile scholar or an ignorant boor? Why is it that although women have been practicing medicine for well over a hundred years, the conflict between women's traditional activities and a medical career appears unresolved? Why is the physician perceived as a poor politician? What makes a young man or woman choose medicine as a career and what determines the choice of a particular specialty? How do doctors' behavior patterns differ from those of nurses?

Obviously, works of fiction do not and cannot provide definitive answers to these questions and they certainly cannot furnish any statistical data. Literary representations of doctors and their activities are not historical or medical records. They reflect the authors' experiences and prejudices and they tend to stress the more unsatisfactory aspects of medical practice. They distort, omit and exaggerate, while the clinical details are often inaccurate. For instance, Denker's account of a child with corticosteroid-induced adrenal failure[25] inappropriately emphasizes the patient's skin pigmentation because the author and his medical advisors fail to distinguish two clinical conditions from each other. Sheldon's story of a patient with a peptic ulcer, who is kept in hospital for dietary treatment,[26] is clearly anachronistic in the last decade of the twentieth century. Nevertheless, scenes from novels, short stories and plays, even those of only slight literary merit, show how authors perceive doctors to behave in particular situations and may provide 'artistic truths' as well as insights into medical encounters not found in clinical journals or books.

> Many details relating to the character and to the life of physicians are gleaned only from secular authors . . . The satire of Molière, malicious though it be, has preserved for us phases of medical life in the seventeenth century for which we scan in vain the strictly medical writings of that period; and writers . . . like George Eliot have told for future generations . . . the little every-day details of the struggles and aspirations

of the profession of the nineteenth century of which we find no account whatever in the files of the *Lancet*.[27]

Some recognizable patterns emerge. The 'typical' doctor, usually a male, tends to be arrogant and paternalistic. He is a man of action rather than contemplation. He works hard but he is not a good family man. He is aggressively irreligious, though he has his own ethical standards. He frequently fights with his colleagues and he detests politics, politicians and administrators. He does not bear grudges against non-compliant patients. Most medical doctors enjoy their status, their power, their high incomes and the intrinsically interesting nature of their work, though some become disenchanted and a few join the ranks of the 'impaired' doctors who should not be allowed to practice medicine. Doctors patronize, belittle and insult nurses, some of whom deserve their lowly status. No attempts have been made to rectify 'incorrect' political attitudes. Patients are called 'patients' because no writer calls them 'clients'.[28] Where male nurses are portrayed as clowns or homosexuals or both,[29] such sentiments are recorded as they appear.

This aspect of the book will be of interest to physicians, medical students, paramedical personnel and the families of such individuals. It will provide source material for courses in medical ethics and sociology. Nurses and social workers will discover fictional doctors, admirable and reprehensible, who may help them understand the behavior of their own medical colleagues. Patients will be interested to find their doctors' mannerisms and witticisms reflected in works of literature written many years ago.

The third purpose of this work is to introduce the reader to particular passages in novels, short stories and plays which have not been given the attention they deserve. In particular, the works of Neil Ravin,[30–32] which provide some of the most realistic accounts of contemporary teaching hospitals, Wharton's *Dad*[33] and some French works,[34–36] are quoted at length. A moving passage describing an old-fashioned ward round[37] is cited in full.

Inclusion and exclusion criteria

The choice of material for a book of this nature is relatively easy when it involves works such as *Middlemarch*,[1] *Arrowsmith*[2] and other classics,[38–42] which portray doctors as heroes or at least as major characters. Well-known passages from such works appear in most anthologies, while the titles and main characters are cited in standard works of reference. The selection process becomes more complicated when the work in question is not of sufficient literary merit to be studied in colleges. The potential database is enormous. The bibliographies of Wilbanks,[43] Trautmann and Pollard,[44] Anne Hudson Jones,[45] Kalisch and Kalisch,[46] and Felice Aull[47] contain the titles of more than 1000 works of fiction in which a doctor is the principal character. Several PhD dissertations,[5,48–50] books[51–53] and journal articles[54–57] have attempted to bring some order into this vast collection of material.

The challenge is even greater when doctors appear as subsidiary figures. With some notable exceptions,[58–60] such minor medical characters are unlisted in bibliographies, dissertations and journal articles, despite the fact that many of them are involved in encounters of great significance. Even anonymous doctors who appear only briefly to administer emergency treatment, to diagnose pregnancy, to give a pregnant woman an expected date of confinement or to pronounce life extinct, may provide interesting glimpses of doctor–patient interactions that cannot be found in major works. The Arthurian physicians whose function consisted of 'searching wounds' and applying 'good salves' to injured knights[61] give some indication of the perception of the doctor in medieval times. Galsworthy's 'hastily sent for' anonymous doctor who 'after one look at the old face . . . announced that Miss Forsyte had passed away in her sleep'[62] contrasts sharply with the uncaring 'red-headed intern' at a hospital emergency room who 'filled out a DOA form . . . clipped his stylus to the outside pocket of his white jacket'[63] and impressed even a policeman with his callous attitude.

An exhaustive review of the relevant books would manifestly be impossible and some arbitrary omissions therefore had to be made so as to reduce this huge amount of potential material to manageable proportions. While almost all the medical characters in this book are educated in 'regular' medical establishments and possess documents attesting their status as 'legally qualified medical practitioners', the lack of a license to practice medicine has not, per se, been used as an exclusion criterion. Licensing bodies were introduced relatively recently whereas fictional physicians go back to classical times.[64] Even in twentieth-century literature geographically displaced[65,66] or isolated[67] physicians perform credibly despite the absence of the relevant piece of paper.

Inclusion and exclusion criteria did not comprise the authors' familiarity with or sympathy for medical practice. Many writers of medical fiction such as Chekhov, Conan Doyle, Georges Duhamel, Somerset Maugham, Francis Brett Young, William Carlos Williams, Archibald Joseph Cronin, Richard Gordon, Michael Crichton and Richard Selzer were themselves trained as physicians. Others, like Henry Handel Richardson, George Bernard Shaw, Marcel Proust, Sinclair Lewis, Francois Mauriac, John O'Hara, Roger Martin du Gard, Ernest Hemingway and Erich Segal either came from medical families or were sufficiently well acquainted with the medical profession to be able to represent the physician's point of view. A third group of authors (particularly women) scrutinize medicine from the outside. These writers evidently obtained their information while receiving disappointing treatment or during conversations with dissatisfied patients. Some members of this group, which includes Leo Tolstoy, Flannery O'Connor, Anne Sexton, Marjorie Piercy, Marylin French, Alison Lurie, Thomas Wolfe, Jean Stafford, Wilfred Sheed, William Wharton and Alan Lightman, represent the doctor–patient relationship as adversarial, they identify strongly with patients and they express considerable resentment towards individual physicians and the medical profession in general. So long as fictional physicians demonstrate some recognizable medical behavior, they have been included, regardless of the author's backgrounds or attitudes.

Clinical descriptions, whether impersonal case reports in Hippocrates' *Epidemics*[68] and in contemporary medical journals or extensive semi-philosophical narratives,[69] have been excluded even when they are of great literary or historical interest. Also, patients' accounts of their illnesses, their anguish, their denials, their frustrations and their ability or inability to cope, all powerfully illustrated in Mukand's anthology,[21] and vitally important in the practice of medicine, are included only if they describe encounters with recognizable physicians. Similarly, the interactions between sick people and their families are included only if they involve the intervention of a doctor. On the other hand, clinical inaccuracies or improbabilities are not used as exclusion criteria. One does not go to fiction for help with diagnostic or therapeutic problems.

Guessing games by contemporary physicians about diagnostic problems of historical or literary figures ('Did Goliath suffer from an endocrine problem?' or 'What was the organism in Philoctetes' wound?') are not within the scope of this work. Such exercises may be useful for the instruction or entertainment of medical students, but they tell us little about the attending doctors (if any).

Overt medical autobiographies have, with a few exceptions,[70,71] been avoided. Such works consist largely of self-serving, trivial anecdotes, which may be valuable from the anthropological or even historical points of view (a good deal of it is worthless trash) but give little insight into the perception of physicians by themselves, their clientele or the general public. With one exception, overt doctor–nurse romances have been excluded.

Also excluded are fictional physicians whose medical qualifications are relevant only as a plot device. Dr Jekyll, who was a medical practitioner during the day and a monster at night, might as well have had stock broking as his regular occupation.[72] Dr Watson, the unteachable disciple of Sherlock Holmes,[73,74] had a medical degree but could have played the confidant's role equally well had he been a theology student. Dr Aziz, the principal character in Forster's *A Passage to India*,[75] who is falsely accused of attempted rape, neither thinks nor behaves like a medical doctor. Lawrence Durrell's homosexual 'Bruce Drexel MD',[76] medical adviser to a British embassy, is seen on occasions taking his boyfriend's pulse,[77] but during most of his peregrinations around the globe, Drexel's medical degree is quite irrelevant. Stevenson's Dr Noel who helps Silas Scuddamore to conceal a corpse[78] is hardly acting in a recognizable 'medical' style. These and many similar 'non-medical' physicians are not listed and their activities are not discussed.

Similarly, Ibsen's Dr Rank in *A Doll's House*,[79] who is more concerned with his own illness than with taking care of patients, has been excluded. On the other hand, Relling, the cynical alcoholic in *The Wild Duck*, 'a doctor of sorts',[80,81] is mentioned because he at least exhibits some signs of medical behavior. He informs Hedvig Ekdal's parents of their daughter's death[81] and he points out, using a typical medical metaphor, that in some circumstances, chronic deception is preferable to absolute honesty: 'one can get through life in a wig'.[80]

Medical poltroons appear in works by Molière,[82,83] his contemporaries[84] and his successors[85] with the image of the outlandish and incompetent medical buffoon persisting well into the eighteenth and nineteenth centuries when fictional doctors bore names like Slop,[86] Nockemorf,[87] Fillgrave,[88] Cuticle[89] and Patella,[89] or French equivalents like Tuehomme[85] and Massacre.[85] Even some contemporary cartoonists depict physicians (particularly psychiatrists[90]) as mad, lecherous or sadistic. These medical clowns and caricatures are either not discussed at all or only at times when they cease acting like stage clowns and show a glimmer of medical behavior. Doctors, unlike insurance salesmen, policemen or real estate agents, are not intrinsically funny characters. They may be foolish or arrogant or both, but except in circumstances involving fake illnesses, the arrival of a doctor does not provide comic relief. Even doctors attending fancy dress balls[91] or noisy medical student functions[92,93] appear incongruous. The 'humorous' doctor using the Marx Brothers approach, wearing a false nose or a Santa Claus outfit and attempting to help his patients by making them laugh,[94] is inappropriate in most medical situations.

Some arbitrary decisions therefore had to be made concerning the inclusion, partial exclusion or total exclusion of eccentric and marginal physicians who display, in among their general clownishness, some recognizable medical traits. In Molière's *Love's The Best Doctor*,[82] the four physicians who act as stage buffoons around the bedside suddenly become very plausible characters when, in private, they boast to each other about their means of transportation, very much like present-day physicians discussing their BMW or Mercedes automobiles. Ivan Chebutykin, the ignorant, credulous and drunken government doctor in Chekhov's *Three Sisters*,[95] retains vestiges of medical traits. He still sees patients, he blames himself for an unfavorable outcome[96] and he is still used as a confidant by one of his friends.[97] These particular clowns are therefore included.

Likewise, Djuna Barnes' Dr Matthew O'Connor, to all appearances a most unpromising candidate for inclusion, is listed despite his clownish traits.[98] O'Connor, unlicensed gynecologist and abortionist,[99–101] cross-dresser,[102] drunkard[103] and thief,[101] spends his days (and nights) discussing topics such as the nature of darkness in semi-philosophical and semi-poetical terms, while his medical activities are confined to throwing water in the face of a woman who has fainted.[101] Even his attitude is non-medical. His claim that 'the doctor knows everything . . . because he's been everywhere at the wrong time'[102] turns the physician into a kind of voyeur whose experience derives from gruesome and disgusting events he has witnessed in the course of his professional life. 'Mighty' O'Connor, as he half-boastfully and half-sarcastically calls himself,[102] is nevertheless included, because he shows some familiarity with the practice of medicine. By contrast, Bellow's Dr Tamkin,[104] who provides bizarre accounts of his 'clinical' activities, is clearly a charlatan, whose medical 'expertise' is derived from public libraries and a fertile imagination. Similarly, the possessors of secret or semi-magical treatments (like those of Dr Raymond[105] which enable him to cure all forms of 'paralysis') are not ahead of their medical colleagues, but practice a different profession. 'Doctors' Tamkin, Raymond and less talented quacks are not included in this work.

Also excluded are fictional physicians who engage in criminal activities and who are discussed in some detail by Malmsheimer.[106] In classical literature such creatures appear as poisoners,[64,107] thieves[108] and violators of their patients' chastity.[109] Most of the doctors mentioned in Yearsley's *Doctors in Elizabethan Drama*[110] are clowns, felons or incompetents who declaim at length about what they are unable to do. The image of the physician as an evil alchemist persists into the nineteenth century,[111] and even in twentieth-century literature one can find a few medical delinquents.[112] Dorothy Sayers[113] describes a surgeon ('Dr Freke') whose behavior is motivated entirely by revenge, one of Graham Greene's doctors[114] organizes a spy network, while Pierre Ouellette's 'Doctor' David Vincent Muldane, a failed medical student with access to bacterial cultures, distributes pathogenic bacteria around restaurants and then visits his victims in hospital.[115] Henry Bellaman's *Kings Row* contains accounts of two criminal physicians.[116,117] One of these is revealed, after his death, to have been involved in an incestuous relationship with his daughter whom he poisons before he shoots himself,[116] while the other is unmasked, also after his death, as a vicious sadist who performs mutilating operations, sometimes without anesthesia, to punish what he considers moral misbehavior.[117] James Bridie's Dr Cyril Angelus, a poisoner and an outrageous hypocrite, is almost too clownish to qualify as an 'evil' physician.[118] Wycherley's doctor in *The Country*

Wife,[119] who spreads the false rumor that his patient is a eunuch, and Dickens' doctor in *Martin Chuzzlewit*,[120] who encourages his patient to invest unwisely, while not committing any overtly illegal acts, engage in activities which are generally considered incompatible with mainstream medicine and which make them accessories to felonies.

These medically qualified criminals, major or minor, ancient or modern, are discussed only when not engaged in 'felonious employment'. Dr Benjamin Phillips, who murders his wife but escapes detection, subsequently functions as a credible, aggressive surgeon[121] whose aphorisms include 'When in doubt, operate; you may save life, you are certain to acquire knowledge'. His medical activities are discussed; those of the concentration camp doctors[122] are not. Ariyoshi's Dr Seishu Hanaoka,[123] who experiments with new drugs and tries them out on his wife with disastrous results, would nowadays be considered a criminal. At the time, his behavior was evidently considered acceptable as the wife had 'volunteered' and he remains a credible medical figure. Abortion and euthanasia are or were considered criminal activities, but because of their particular links to medicine, fictional doctors who occupy themselves with these endeavors are discussed in detail in separate chapters.

Hidden meanings, symbolism, allegories and what is commonly described as the 'Poetry of Medicine',[124] are not, in general, explored in this book. For instance, two of the three short stories describing doctors lying in bed alongside their patients without lecherous intentions are obviously allegorical in intent and have little to do with clinical practice such as most physicians would experience or appreciate.[125,126] These two are excluded, even though the authors are major literary figures. The third, by a minor British writer, while set in unusual surroundings, involves an identifiable clinical scenario (a wet and cold doctor waiting to deliver a baby),[127] and is discussed in detail. For similar reasons, the interactions between psychiatrists and their patients plays a relatively minor role in this work. Psychiatrists deal with metaphors and imagery, while the 'enamel' doctors[128] are concerned with facts. Moreover there are several papers[129,130] relating to the portrayals of psychiatrists in fictional literature.

Scenes describing bizarre medical behavior are not used. Such descriptions include a sick intern taking his own temperature instead of the patient's,[92] a physician vomiting 'like a cat with a bone stuck in its throat' after inspecting an unusual skin lesion[131] or the pursuits of Strindberg's unnamed doctor,[132] who stores human limbs in his ice-chest and pulls them out for the edification of his visitors. This character also keeps a madman, whom he addresses as Caesar, locked up in his cellar; Caesar is allowed out at times and on these occasions the doctor tries to tame him. ' "Caesar, you must behave. Or I shall have to whip you." ' Science fiction doctors, with a few exceptions, are too far removed from generally recognized medical activities to warrant inclusion.

Place and time

Novels, plays and short stories unavailable in English have, with the exception of four important French works,[34-36,51] not been cited. This decision was based on linguistic rather than national considerations and no material was rejected on purely geographic grounds. Obviously, the prevalence rates of particular diseases, the available diagnostic and therapeutic measures, and many less important details of medical practice vary in different parts of the world. For instance, geographic differences determine to some extent whether sick individuals are seen by the doctor in their own homes, in a part of the doctor's residence especially set aside for the purpose (and referred to in Britain as a 'surgery'), in professional office buildings, in hospital clinics or even at a hotel.[133] While the dedicated office building was well established in the United States and Britain in the early part of the twentieth century,[134,135] in France the tradition of the doctors' home continued much longer[136–138] and even a prominent physician like Dr Paul Courrèges expresses a dislike of his office in the downtown Bordeaux area.[139] The displacement of general practitioners by an army of specialists, many of them employed by hospitals, universities or health maintenance organizations,[140] has 'progressed' further in some countries than in others. None of this alters the essential relationship between the sick person and the professional healer, and no attempt has therefore been made to draw any regional boundaries.

> Medicine is . . . [a] world-wide profession, following everywhere the same methods, actuated by the same ambitions and pursuing the same ends . . . While . . . we speak of German, French, English and American medicine, the differences are trifling in comparison with the general similarity.[141]

The same principles apply to historical considerations; the basic relationship between patients and trained expert helpers has remained essentially unchanged over two and a half millennia.[142] Clearly, numerous and profound changes have taken place over this long period. Even within the past hundred years, the settings of medical practice have altered almost beyond recognition, while physicians practicing in classical or Renaissance times were even further removed from their twenty-first-century counterparts. Surgical operations have gone in and out of fashion, while drug names (especially brand names) that were apparently household words a few decades ago are now totally unrecognizable. Modern private hospital rooms or intensive care units have replaced the 'Nightingale Hospital Wards' of the late nineteenth century. The stethoscope has changed its role from a French toy to a tool of trade to a status symbol. Peter Corris' account[143] of a visit to an impotence clinic, an alprostadil injection and the embarrassing result, could not possibly have been described 100 years ago, though the notion of drug-induced impotence and potency goes back at least 400 years.[144]

The selection and training methods of late-twentieth-century American medical students[145,146] were obviously drastically different from the apprenticeship system in vogue in Britain during the first half of the nineteenth century[147,148] while the 'education' provided for aspirants to membership of the medical fraternity in France in the seventeenth century and lampooned by Molière[83] differed even more profoundly. Dr Paul Courrèges, in a story published in 1925 but set in 1908, asks his examination candidates for the definition of hemoptysis,[149] making the contemporary medical reader wonder what sort of answer was expected. However, regardless of whether 'medical students' are boisterous apprentices using a mortar and pestle,[150] or intense college graduates stuffing themselves with useless anatomic facts,[145] one common denominator pertains to all of them: ultimately, they have to learn to look at patients objectively 'without pity and without contempt'. This attitude may be considered cynical,[71] but without it, clear-headed evaluation and intervention become impossible.

Clothing fashions such as the doctor's silk hat and frock coat of the late nineteenth century[151] or his smoking habits in the 1920s and 1930s[152,153] have altered in more recent times. The doctor's bag has become as old-fashioned as the house call so that, in a few decades, readers of Kornbluth's *The Little Black Bag*[154] may require a footnote to explain the term. The size of the fee has obviously changed. None of these trivialities has any bearing on the doctor's activities as a professional healer.

More importantly, quaint and archaic procedures employed in earlier historic periods are treated as part of mainstream medicine. The fact that some such practices are now known to be ineffective or harmful is considered irrelevant. Several recently popular procedures are becoming obsolete, and it is highly likely that some currently fashionable investigations, medications and surgical operations will be shown, at some future stage, to be as useless as urine casting, bloodletting and mustard plasters. The nineteenth-century transformation of the physician from a clownish and venal artisan into a self-respecting and esteemed bourgeois professional,[53] while important from the standpoint of the doctor's status and income, did no more to alter the basic nature of his work than did the changes in his means of transport or his office furniture. Although the citations in this book derive mainly from works written in the last two centuries, no material has been excluded because of differences between the outward trappings of contemporary doctors and their predecessors. Indeed, some of the medical characters dating from classical times conduct themselves in an almost contemporary style.[64] Plato's physician, who looks at his hypothetical patient's face and fingers and then asks him to disrobe,[142] is behaving in much the same way as a thoracic physician might in a modern setting. The resentment against the doctor's fee transcends time and place.

Sources

Primary material was obtained from four sources.

1 Generally known works such as *Madame Bovary*,[38] *Wives and Daughters*,[39] *Of Human Bondage*[40] and other classics[1,2] that feature doctors as main or major characters.
2 Fictional works listed in bibliographies such as those of Wilbanks,[43] Trautmann and Pollard,[44] and Aull.[47]
3 Novels, plays and short stories discussed or mentioned in books,[106] encyclopedias,[155] medical journals[54,55,156–161] and medical-literary magazines.[57] Some of these draw attention to a series of fictional doctors,[54,55,156] others confine themselves to doctors created by a single author,[157,158,161] while yet others concentrate on individual characters.[159,160] A few papers published in medical journals by well-known authors[162] provided further primary data.
4 Additional 'eclectic' material discovered incidentally or during searches of

library catalogs for titles containing terms such as 'doctor', 'medicine', 'medical' or 'hospital'.

Secondary material was obtained largely through searches of the 'Index Medicus' and 'Medline' under 'medicine in literature'. The relevant articles on the subject mostly appeared in well-known medical journals such as *JAMA*, the *New England Journal of Medicine*, the *Lancet* and the *Annals of Internal Medicine*, and as chapters of books on the sociology of medical practice.

The selected passages are illustrative rather than comprehensive. They do not necessarily represent historical 'firsts' (although many of them do). While every effort has been made to include works of genuine literary merit, many such works have, inevitably, been omitted. Moreover, a large number of quotations in this book are taken from novels and short stories, which, by no stretch of the imagination, can be described as literary masterpieces. Some crucial aspects of physicians' careers – how they decide to become doctors, how they are admitted into medical schools, how they choose a specialty – are barely mentioned or not discussed at all in serious literary works. There is therefore a disturbing juxtaposition of Nobel Laureates and very minor literary figures. Indeed, some of the quotations come from novels little better than airport literature.* No attempts have been made to perform statistical analyses.

This work is planned as a series of four volumes. This current book deals with doctor–patient interactions, particularly when these are unsatisfactory, with ensuing resentment, confrontation and litigation. The second concerns the doctor's personal life, his family, his job satisfaction, his colleagues and his health. The third involves career choices and the portrayal of different kinds of specialists, particularly surgeons and medical researchers. The fourth book takes in such topics as male and female doctors, doctors and nurses, the abortion and the abortionist, and sexual fantasies and encounters.

Satisfaction or resentment?

Dear David
Dead one, rest in peace.
Having been what all
Doctors should be, but few are.[163]

The entire discipline of clinical medicine depends on encounters between physicians and patients, as described by physicians. The body of collective clinical experience, which includes chapters in textbooks, articles in medical journals, and all the details

---

* Airport literature consists of works of fiction suitable for sale at international airports, for perusal during long flights and for abandonment at the point of destination. The authors use explicit sex and/or multiple acts of violence in an attempt to hold the readers' attention at times when various distractions make concentration difficult. The plots of such works are mostly unoriginal and the characters stereotyped.

relating to diagnosis, prognosis and treatment, ultimately derives from the observations, by doctors, of sick individuals. In this context the patients' opinions are, inevitably, de-emphasized or ignored. Hippocrates does not tell us what the young man, who died after a seven-days' illness, thought of his physician.[68] Present-day reports on clinical trials provide multiple details concerning subjective and objective findings including 'adverse events' or the subjects' 'quality of life', but not a hint about how these subjects perceive the personality or the behavior of the participating physicians.

In most instances, such perceptions are, in double-negative medical phraseology, 'not unfavorable'.[164] Millions of sufferers who seek advice from members of the profession on a daily basis, by and large, experience brief encounters that are satisfactory to both sides.[165] The patient, like Plato's carpenter,[166] obtains his 'rough and ready cure'* while the doctor receives an appropriate fee or salary and, at times, an additional gift of greater or lesser value.[167-8] In a minority of cases, however, this happy state of affairs is not achieved, and it is this minority which predominates in fictional accounts of doctors.[169] The patients are resentful about time, inadequate or inappropriate explanations, the doctors' perceived status and power, and their 'bedside manner'. They are disappointed with the information provided and angry at the way the message has been conveyed. They may come to believe that the fee is excessive, the doctor's effort inadequate and the treatment cruel, experimental or both.

Much of this seething discontent is represented as justified. The doctors' behavior may reflect insensitivity or insincerity. Their explanations strike the patients as fatuous, paternalistic or obscure. Inappropriate treatment may be employed in a particular case, because of the doctor's one-track mind. The patients' frustration may be so intense, that they regard the entire practice of medicine as a cruel joke. Remarkably, while the practice of medicine has changed profoundly over the years, the patients' grievances have not.

In a masterful and scholarly work, Rothfield[53] demonstrates that the evolution during the nineteenth century of newly established scientific disciplines and medical licensing bodies raised physicians to an eminent status, which their predecessors did not possess and did not deserve. Several recent works[170-1] purport to show that the golden age of medicine is over, and that the physician's status is once again on the decline. An entire genre of literature deals with the inadequacy of modern medical techniques and the disillusionment with physicians employing such techniques. As far as fictional literature is concerned, patients' accounts of their physicians' attitudes and activities seem largely unaffected by changes in the doctor's status.

Similarly, the revolution that has occurred in the practice of medicine over the last few centuries is reflected to only a minor extent in the patients' dissatisfaction. Obviously, Molière's doctors, who make house calls on mules, employ treatments that are different from those used by nineteenth-century doctors who arrive by horse and buggy. Twenty-first-century doctors, who make no house calls at all, practice a kind of medicine that is different again. The 'production line' treatment as seen in hospital emergency departments and operating rooms did not exist at the time of Molière except, possibly, under battlefield conditions. The doctors who wrote

---

* Plato was evidently aware that patient satisfaction does not provide a reliable guide to the quality of medical care.

'prescriptions' for alcohol during the days of Prohibition,[172–3] using fountain pens for the purpose, have been succeeded by more modern doctors who prescribe other semi-legal drugs and write with a ballpoint pen.

These trivial changes have done little to alter the fundamental relationship between a sick person and a physician practising rational medicine (as distinct from witchcraft and faith healing). At some point the two will be involved in a one-on-one encounter when the doctor says, like Plato's physician, 'take off your shirt and let me have a look at your chest'.[142] Similarly, there comes a moment when the expert healer (in contrast to a concerned family member or friend) will have to answer the pivotal questions: 'What is the matter with me?' and 'Can you do something?'

Owing to the circumstances surrounding the association between doctors and patients, some frustration with individual physicians, and with the medical profession in general, is almost inescapable. Resentment may simply reflect the dislike of the weak for the strong, the ignorant for the knowledgeable[170] and the horizontal for the vertical.[174] In this lop-sided relationship, everything pertaining to the doctor is liable to be subjected to critical analysis and comment. If he dresses well or clips his mustache, he is a fop. If his cuffs are frayed or his shoes scuffed, his medical skills, like his clothes, are obviously of poor quality. If he speaks well, he comes from a privileged background and cannot possibly understand the sufferings of ordinary folk. If his accent or syntax are less than impeccable, he is a continental fly-by-night whose credentials are suspect.[175]

When the patient suffers from an incurable disease, frustration may turn into hostility, with the doctor being blamed for the deplorable outcome. However, this discontent, which ranges from mild irritation to extreme animosity, tends to be expressed (if it is expressed at all) to family members, friends, doctors' receptionists, hospital clerks and nurses, with relatively few overt doctor–patient confrontations. The threat of litigation rarely becomes a reality in fiction. Occasional clues appear on how resentment and confrontational situations might have been averted. This book brings together a number of scenarios illustrating unsatisfactory doctor–patient encounters. Most of them come from twentieth-century fiction and almost all represent the point of view of the patients.

This book is not about the resolution of 'issues'. It is not a 'mission statement' concerning ideal medical practice. It does not provide a historical account of fashions in the doctor's clothing, his mode of transportation or whether he is paid in francs or dollars. On the contrary, it will be shown that changes in fashion or currency make little difference to the patient's satisfaction or discontent.

No conscious attempt is made to bring about changes in medical behavior. Unanswerable questions like whether works of fiction create or reflect attitudes[106] have been ignored. The book avoids problems of nomenclature such as the use of the word 'patient'.[176–7] Such petty issues, which seem to bother health administrators, do not worry physicians, sick people or writers. The use of the male gender reflects the fact that for centuries 'doctor' like 'soldier' implied a male person and a separate chapter in Book IV has been devoted to the female physician in literature. No attempt has been made to determine what proportion of fictional characters in a particular period declare themselves satisfied with their medical attendants.

The book brings together, in citations and quotations from fictional literature, the opinions of multiple authors, as expressed through their characters, of various aspects of interactions between doctors and patients. Where such perceptions differ from what happens in the real world, the differences are pointed out.

The 11 chapters describe various aspects of doctor–patient interactions. Chapter 1 discusses the ancient problem of the fee, which in recent times has been partially replaced by what health maintenance organizations will or will not cover (*see* Book II, Chapter 4). Chapter 2 covers the irreconcilable problems of time as seen from the patient's and the doctor's point of view. The behavior pattern of physicians towards their fictional patients, 'The bedside manner', is discussed in Chapter 3. History and physical examination, as perceived by patients, form the basis of Chapter 4, while Chapter 5 covers the debriefing process. Treatment is described in Chapter 6 but no attempt is made to provide detailed accounts of therapeutic fashions at different historical periods. Bloodletting in the eighteenth century,[178] calomel in the nineteenth,[179] and antibiotics in the twentieth[180] were all used by experienced physicians under the supposition that they might or would benefit the patient and in response to the request that the doctor 'do something'. The fact that some of the older treatment modalities are now known to be useless or even harmful is treated as irrelevant. The obsolescence of some 'modern' investigations[181] and the demonstration that therapeutic measures in recent use may not be efficacious[182] or safe[183] does not turn doctors practicing in the 1990s into charlatans.

Chapter 7 discusses the emotional barrier between doctors and patients, inherent in the practice of medicine. Chapter 8 lists some fictional characters, who decide, from their own experiences, that the entire discipline of medicine is a refined form of torture. A significant part of that chapter is devoted to three novels, Malègue's *Augustin, ou, Le maître est là*,[36] Ellis' *The Rack*,[184] and William Wharton's *Dad*,[33] all of which appear to draw that conclusion. 'The ward round in literature' forms the subject of Chapter 9. Remarkably, there appear to be almost no previous analyses of the subject. Chapter 10 is an attempt to analyze some of the factors that cause silent resentment to turn into an open doctor–patient confrontation. It is argued that despite statements to the contrary, the relative social status of the parties is a major factor in the doctor–patient relationship and that the problems of a physician taking care of rich and powerful patients are different from those of a prosperous doctor treating members of the 'lower orders'.[185] Chapter 11 discusses the ultimate expression of patient dissatisfaction (short of physical violence) – litigation against a former medical attendant. Malpractice suits are relatively rare in fictional literature, possibly because they have little to do with the realities of medical practice.

There is obviously some overlap between the subject matter discussed in the 11 chapters. Resentment over an exorbitant fee (Chapter 1) is likely to encompass a time element (Chapter 2). The divisions between 'The bedside manner' (Chapter 3), 'History and physical examination' (Chapter 4), 'Explanations' (Chapter 5) and 'Detachment' (Chapter 7) are, to some extent, arbitrary, so that the descriptions of particular events (such as Judge Clane's experiences at the Johns Hopkins Hospital[186]) appear in several chapters. However, despite their arbitrariness, these divisions make a vast topic more manageable. Hopefully, the subject and author indices will ensure that quotations and scenarios relating to particular topics are easily located.

Some of the material was first presented at the Annual Meeting of the American College of Physicians, New Orleans, April 1991. Parts were subsequently published as a series of papers in the *Journal of the Royal Society of Medicine*, London, 1992–4, in the *Australian and New Zealand Journal of Surgery*, 1996, and in the *Medical Journal of Australia*, 1997. They are here reproduced with the permission of the editors and publishers of these journals.

References

1 Eliot G (1871–2) *Middlemarch*. Penguin, London, 1988.

2 Lewis S (1924) *Arrowsmith*. Signet Books, New York, 1961.

3 *Merriam Webster's Encyclopedia of Literature* (1995) Merriam Webster Inc., Springfield, MA.

4 Cozzens JG (1933) *The Last Adam*. Harcourt Brace and Company, New York.

5 Norris CB (1969) The Image of the Physician in Modern American Literature. PhD dissertation, University of Maryland.

6 Shem S (1978) *The House of God*. Richard Marek, New York.

7 Strauss MB (1968) *Familiar Medical Quotations*. Little Brown and Company, Boston, MA.

8 Huth EJ and Murray TJ (2000) *Medicine in Quotations*, American College of Physicians, Philadelphia, PA.

9 Proust M (1913–22) *Remembrance of Things Past*, vol. 2. Translated by Scott Moncrieff CK and Kilmartin T, Penguin, Harmondsworth, 1987.

10 Huth EJ and Murray TJ, op. cit., Introduction, p. xi.

11 Ibid., pp. 208–9.

12 Martineau H (1839) *Deerbrook*. Virago Press, London, 1983, p. 209.

13 Mauriac F (1925) *The Desert of Love*. Translated by Hopkins G. Eyre and Spottiswoode, London, 1949, p. 11.

14 Hemingway E (1924) The Doctor and The Doctor's Wife. In: *The Complete Short Stories of Ernest Hemingway*, Scribner Paperback Edition. Simon and Schuster, New York, 1998, pp. 73–6.

15 Flaubert G (1857) *Madame Bovary*. Translated by Steegmuller F. Modern Library, New York, 1982, pp. 68–9.

16 Chekhov AP (1892) Ward Number Six. In: *The Oxford Chekhov*, vol. 6. Translated by Hingley R. Oxford University Press, London, 1971, p. 134.

17 Russell R (1985) *While You're Here, Doctor*. Souvenir Press, London, p. 66.

18 Cole H (ed.) (1963) *Under the Doctor*. Heinemann, London.

19 Ceccio J (ed.) (1978) *Medicine in Literature*. Longmans, New York.

20 Cousins N (ed.) (1982) *The Physician in Literature*. Saunders, Philadelphia, PA.

21 Mukand J (ed.) (1990) *Vital Lines*. St Martin's Press, New York.

22 Reynolds R and Stone J (eds) (1991) *On Doctoring: stories, poems, essays*. Simon and Schuster, New York.

23 Gordon R (ed.) (1993) *The Literary Companion To Medicine*. St Martin's Press, New York, 1996.

24 Ballantyne J (ed.) (1995) *Bedside Manners*. Virgin, London.

25 Denker H (1992) *Doctor on Trial*. William Morrow, New York, p. 38.

26 Sheldon S (1994) *Nothing Lasts Forever*. HarperCollins, London, p. 78.

27 Osler W (1893) Physic and Physicians as Depicted in Plato. In: Osler W (1920) *Aequanimitas*. HK Lewis and Co, London, pp. 47–76.

28 Walters H (1995) The meaning of words in the New Health Service. *J Roy Soc Med.* **88**: 365–6.

29 White P (1961) *Riders in the Chariot*. Penguin, Harmondsworth, 1986, pp. 348–56.

30 Ravin N (1981) *MD*. Delacorte Press/Seymour Lawrence, New York.

31 Ravin N (1983) *Informed Consent*. GP Putnam's Sons, New York.

32 Ravin N (1985) *Seven North*. EP Dutton/Seymour Lawrence, New York.

33 Wharton W (1981) *Dad*. Alfred A Knopf, New York.

34 Daudet LA (1894) *Les Morticoles*. Fasquelle, Paris, 1956.

35 Duhamel G (1928) *Les Sept Dernières Plaies*. Mercure de France, Paris.

36 Malègue J (1932) *Augustin, ou, Le maître est là*. Spes, Paris, 1935, 2 vols.

37 Sobel IP (1973) *The Hospital Makers*. Doubleday, Garden City, NY, pp. 20–26.

38 Flaubert G (1857) *Madame Bovary*. Translated by Steegmuller F. Modern Library, New York, 1982.

39 Gaskell E (1864–6) *Wives and Daughters*. Oxford University Press, Oxford, 1987.

40 Maugham WS (1915) *Of Human Bondage*. Signet Classics, New York, 1991.

41 Woolf V (1925) *Mrs Dalloway*. Zodiac Press, London, 1947.

42 Fitzgerald FS (1934) *Tender is the Night*. Penguin, Harmondsworth, 1998.

43 Wilbanks ER (1958) The physician in the American novel, 1870–1955. *Bull. Bibliog.* **22**: 164–8.

44 Trautmann J and Pollard C (1982) *Literature and Medicine, An Annotated Bibliography*. University of Pittsburgh Press, Pittsburgh, PA.

45 Jones AH (1989) Medicine and The Physician. In: Inge MT (ed.) *Handbook of American Popular Culture* (2e). Greenwood Press, New York, pp. 722–43.

46 Kalisch PA and Kalisch BJ (1987) *The Changing Image of the Nurse*. Addison Wesley, Menlo Park, CA.

47 Aull F (2001) Arts and Medicine. Database at New York University School of Medicine. http://endeavor.med.nyu.edu/lit-med/lit-med-db/descrips.html

48 De Bakey LF (1963) The Physician Scientist as Character in 19th Century American Literature. PhD dissertation, Tulane University.

49 Cameron AJ (1973) The Image of the Physician in the American Novel. PhD dissertation, University of Notre Dame.

50 Kochanek L (1999) Difficult Doctoring: figuring female physicians in Victorian and Edwardian England. PhD dissertation, University of Delaware.

51 Salières F (1948) *Écrivains contre Médecins*. Denoël, Paris.

52 Peschel ER (ed.) (1980) *Medicine and Literature*. Neale Watson Academic Publications, New York.

53 Rothfield L (1992) *Vital Signs: medical realism in nineteenth century fiction.* Princeton University Press, Princeton, NJ.

54 McDonald SF (1931) Medicine in fiction in the last hundred years. *Med J Aust.* **1**: 709–21.

55 Miller CJ (1931) The doctors of fiction. *Surg Gynecol Obstet.* **52**: 493–7.

56 Young FB (1936) The Doctor in Literature. In: Walpole H (ed.) *Essays by Divers Hands*, vol. 15. H Mulford, Oxford University Press, London, pp. 17–35.

57 Hill J (1987) The doctor as hero in nineteenth century British fiction. *The Pharos of Alpha Omega Alpha.* **50**: 31–3.

58 Shakespeare W (1606) *The Tragedy of Macbeth.* Wright LB and LaMar VA (eds) Washington Square Press, New York, 1969, pp. 78–9.

59 Proust M, op. cit., vol. 2, p. 333.

60 Mann T (1924) *The Magic Mountain.* Translated by Lowe-Porter HT. Penguin, Harmondsworth, 1960, pp. 203–19.

61 Malory T (1485) *Le Morte D'Arthur.* Dent, London, 1938, pp. 40–2.

62 Galsworthy J (1906) *The Man of Property.* Penguin, Harmondsworth, 1951, p. 101.

63 Chandler R (1949) *The Little Sister.* Houghton Mifflin, Boston, MA, p. 53.

64 Amundsen DW (1977) Image of physicians in classical times. *J Popular Culture.* **11**: 643–55.

65 Baum V (1939) *Nanking Road.* Translated by Creighton B. Geoffrey Bles, London.

66 Remarque EM (1945) *Arch of Triumph.* Translated by Sorell W and Lindley D. Appleton Century, New York.

67 Bernières L de (1994) *Captain Corelli's Mandolin.* Vintage, London, 1998.

68 Hippocrates (5th century BC) Epidemics III, Case VIII. Translated by Jones WHS. In: *Loeb's Classical Library*, vol. 1. Heinemann, London, 1923, p. 233.

69 Sacks O (1985) *The Man who Mistook his Wife for a Hat and Other Clinical Tales.* Simon and Schuster, New York, 1998.

70 Warren S (1832) *Diary of a Late Physician.* Blackwood, Edinburgh, 2 vols.

71 Konner M (1987) *Becoming a Doctor.* Viking, New York.

72 Stevenson RL (1886) *The Strange Case of Dr Jekyll and Mr Hyde.* Heinemann, London, 1934.

73 Doyle AC (1892–1922) *The Complete Sherlock Holmes.* Doubleday, Garden City, NY, 1938.

74 Knox R (1980) Studies in the literature of Sherlock Holmes: In: Haining P (ed.) *A Sherlock Holmes Compendium.* WH Allen, London, pp. 47–65.

75 Forster EM (1924) *A Passage to India.* Edward Arnold, London.

76 Durrell L (1974) *Monsieur.* Faber and Faber, London.

77 Ibid., p. 126.

78 Stevenson RL (1878) Story of the physician and the Saratoga trunk. In: Ball I (ed.) (1993) *Stevenson RL, The Complete Short Stories.* Mainstream Publishing, Edinburgh, pp. 183–204.

79 Ibsen H (1879) A Doll's House. In: Ibsen H (1965) *A Doll's House and Other Plays.* Translated by Watts P. Penguin, London, pp. 191–2.

80 Ibsen H (1884) The Wild Duck. In: Ibsen H (1957) *Three Plays*. Translated by Ellis-Fermor U. Penguin, Harmondsworth, p. 207.

81 Ibid., pp. 243–58.

82 Molière JBP (1665) Love's The Best Doctor. Translated by Waller AR. In: *The Plays of Molière*, vol. 4. John Grant, Edinburgh, 1926, pp. 291–7.

83 Molière JBP (1673) The Hypochondriack. Translated by Baker H and Miller J. In: *Molière's Comedies*, vol. 2. Dent, London, 1961, pp. 469–71.

84 Behn A (1678) Sir Patient Fancy. In: Summers M (ed.) (1967) *The Works of Aphra Behn*, vol. 4. Phaeton Press, New York, pp. 98–107.

85 Petersen CE (1938) *The Doctor in French Drama, 1700–1775*. Columbia University Press, New York.

86 Sterne L (1759–67). *The Life and Opinions of Tristram Shandy, Gentleman* (Work JA ed.) Odyssey Press, New York, 1940, p. 168.

87 Dickens C (1837) *Pickwick Papers*. Signet Classics, New American Library, New York, 1964, p. 726.

88 Trollope A (1858) *Doctor Thorne*. Oxford University Press, London, 1963, p. 123.

89 Melville H (1850) *White Jacket*. LC Page, Boston, MA, 1892, pp. 232–49.

90 Walter G (1992) The psychiatrist in American cartoons, 1941–1990. *Acta Psychiatr Scand*. 85: 167–72.

91 Ellis AE (1958) *The Rack*. Penguin Books, London, 1988, pp. 57–60.

92 Fitzgerald FS (1935) One Interne. In: Fitzgerald FS. *Taps at Reveille*. Charles Scribner's Sons, New York, pp. 294–313.

93 Van Der Meersch M (1943) *Bodies and Souls*. Translated by Wilkins E. William Kimber, London, 1953, pp. 9–11.

94 Adams P and Mylander M (1993) *Gesundheit*. Healing Arts Press, Rochester, VT, pp. 70–74.

95 Chekhov AP (1900–1) Three Sisters. In: *The Oxford Chekhov*, vol. 3. Translated by Hingley R. Oxford University Press, London, 1964, pp. 71–139.

96 Ibid., p. 113.

97 Ibid., p. 130.

98 Barnes D (1936) *Nightwood*. Faber and Faber, London, 1985.

99 Ibid., p. 29.

100 Ibid., p. 164.

101 Ibid., pp. 54–8.

102 Ibid., pp. 117–21.

103 Ibid., p. 232.

104 Bellow S (1956) *Seize the Day*. Penguin, New York, 1996, pp. 66–9.

105 Thwaites FJ (1939) *The Mad Doctor in Harley Street*. FJ Thwaites, Sydney, 1942.

106 Malmsheimer R (1988) 'Doctors Only': the evolving image of the American physician. *Contributions in Medical Studies*, Number 25, Greenwood Press, New York.

107 Apuleius L (2nd century AD) *The Golden Ass*. Translated by Graves R. Penguin, Harmondsworth, 1950, pp. 246–7.

108 Aesop (approx. 570 BC) *The Complete Fables.* Translated by Temple O and Temple R. Penguin, London, 1998, p. 69.

109 Martial MV (1st century AD) Epigrams. Translated by Ker WCA in *Loeb's Classical Library*, vol. 2. Heinemann, London, 1960, p. 291.

110 Yearsley M (1933) *Doctors in Elizabethan Drama*, Bale, Sons and Danielsson, London.

111 Hawthorne N (1844) Rappaccini's daughter. In: Hawthorne N. *Mosses from an Old Manse.* Ohio State University Press, 1974, pp. 91–128.

112 Christie A (1926) *The Murder of Roger Ackroyd.* Garland Publishing, New York, 1976.

113 Sayers D (1923) *Whose Body.* Gollancz, London, 1971, pp. 265–87.

114 Greene G (1943) *Ministry of Fear.* Heinemann and Bodley Head, London, 1973, p. 213.

115 Ouellette P (1996) *The Third Pandemic.* Pocket Books, New York.

116 Bellaman H (1940) *Kings Row.* Dymocks, Sydney, 1945, pp. 254–5.

117 Ibid., pp. 395–415.

118 Bridie J (1947) *Dr Angelus.* Constable, London, 1955.

119 Wycherley W (1675) The Country Wife. In: Friedman A (ed.) (1979) *The Plays of William Wycherley.* Clarendon Press, Oxford, pp. 248–354.

120 Dickens C (1843–4) *The Life and Adventures of Martin Chuzzlewit.* Oxford University Press, London, 1959, p. 437.

121 Danby F (Julia Frankau) (1887) *Dr Phillips: a Maida Vale idyll.* Garland Publishing, New York, 1984.

122 Thomas DM (1993) *Pictures at an Exhibition.* Bloomsbury, London.

123 Ariyoshi S (1967) *The Doctor's Wife.* Translated by Hironaka W and Kostant AS. Kodansha, Tokyo, 1989.

124 Mukand J, op. cit., p. xii.

125 Kafka F (1919) A Country Doctor. In: Kafka F (1978) *Wedding Preparations (In the Country) and Other Stories.* Translated by Muir W and Muir E. Penguin, Harmondsworth, pp. 119–24.

126 Beckett S (1934) A Case in a Thousand. In: Gontarski SE (ed.) (1995) *Samuel Beckett: the complete short prose 1929–1989.* Grove Press, New York, pp. 18–24.

127 Strong LAG (1945) The White Cottage. In: Strong LAG. *Travellers: thirty-one selected short stories.* Methuen, London, pp. 124–43.

128 Sexton A (1960) Unknown girl in the maternity ward. In: Sexton A. *To Bedlam and Part Way Back.* Houghton Mifflin, Boston, MA, p. 34.

129 Winick C (1963) The psychiatrist in fiction. *J Nerv Ment Dis.* **136**: 43–57.

130 Walter G (1989) The stereotype of the mad psychiatrist. *Aust NZ J Psychiatry.* **23**: 547–54.

131 Abe K (1991) *Kangaroo Notebook.* Translated by Mori MT. Knopf, New York, 1996, pp. 14–15.

132 Strindberg A (1898–1901) *The Road to Damascus.* Translated by Rawson G. Jonathan Cape, London, 1958, pp. 47–9.

133 Baum V (1929) *Grand Hotel.* Translated by Creighton B. Geoffrey Bles, London, 1930.

134 Herrick R (1900) *The Web of Life*. Macmillan, London.

135 Bashford HH (1911) *The Corner of Harley Street: being some familiar correspondence of Peter Harding MD*. Constable, London, 1913.

136 Proust M, op. cit., vol. 2, pp. 323–8.

137 Martin du Gard R (1922–9) *The Thibaults*. Translated by Gilbert S. John Lane, Bodley Head, London, 1939.

138 Simenon G (1950) The Heart of a Man. In: *The Second Simenon Omnibus*. Translated by Varèse L. Hamish Hamilton, London, 1974, pp. 151–62.

139 Mauriac F, op. cit., p. 58.

140 Stoeckle JD (1987) *Encounters Between Patients and Doctors*. MIT Press, Cambridge, MA, pp. 1–129.

141 Osler W (1906) Unity Peace and Concord. In: Osler W (1920) *Aequanimitas*. HK Lewis, London, pp. 447–65.

142 Plato (4th century BC) Protagoras. Translated by Jowett B. In: Buchanan S (ed.) (1979) *The Portable Plato*. Penguin, Harmondsworth, p. 103.

143 Corris P (1999) *The Other Side of Sorrow*. Bantam Books, Sydney, pp. 105–11.

144 Beaumont F and Fletcher J (1621) The Tragedy of Thierry and Theodoret (1621) Act II, Scene I. In: *The Dramatic Works in the Beaumont and Fletcher Canon*, vol. III. Cambridge University Press, Cambridge, 1976, p. 397.

145 Lewis S, op. cit., pp. 23–30.

146 Segal E (1988) *Doctors*. Bantam Books, New York, 1989.

147 Scott W (1831) *The Surgeon's Daughter*. Adam and Charles Black, London, 1892, pp. 56–9.

148 Gaskell E, op. cit., pp. 31–54.

149 Mauriac F, op. cit., p. 51.

150 Gaskell E, op. cit., p. 45.

151 Toner R (1994) The family doctor is rarely in. *New York Times*. 6 February, Weekend Review, p. 1.

152 Mauriac F, op. cit., p. 31.

153 Fearing K (1939) *The Hospital*. Ballantine Books, New York, p. 16.

154 Kornbluth CM (1950) The Little Black Bag. In: Conklin G and Fabricant ND (eds) (1963) *Great Science Fiction About Doctors*. Collier Books, New York, pp. 165–95.

155 Paton A (1994) Doctors in literature. In: Walton JN, Barondess JA and Lock S (eds) *Oxford Medical Companion*. Oxford University Press, Oxford, pp. 214–17.

156 Hamman L (1938) As others see us. *Transact Assoc Amer Physicians*. **53**: 22–45.

157 Poynter FNL (1968) Doctors in the human comedy. *JAMA*. **204**: 105–8.

158 Kail AC (1983) The bard and the body: 1. Shakespeare's physicians. *Med J Aust*. **2**: 338–44.

159 McLennan MF (1996) Images of physicians in literature: from quacks to heroes. *Lancet*. **348**: 458–60.

160 Jones AH (1997) Literature and medicine: Garcia Marquez' Love in the Time of Cholera. *Lancet* **350**: 1169–72.

161 McLay RN, Lutz B, Baden MM, Bray R and Griffies S (2000) Kind strangers? Physicians through the eyes of Tennessee Williams. *J Louisiana State Med Soc.* **152**: 405–9.

162 Snow CP (1973) Human care. *JAMA* **225**: 617–21.

163 Auden WH (1972) The Art of Healing, In Memoriam David Protetch MD. In: Auden WH. *Epistle to a Godson and Other Poems*, Faber and Faber, London, pp. 13–15.

164 Cleary PD, Edgman-Levitan S (1997) Health care quality: incorporating consumer perspectives. *JAMA.* **278**: 1608–12.

165 Lee Y and Kasper JD (1998) Assessment of medical care by elderly people: general satisfaction and physician quality. *Health Serv Res.* **32**: 741–58.

166 Plato (4th century BC) The Republic. Translated by Jowett B. In: Buchanan S (ed.) (1979) *The Portable Plato*, Penguin, Harmondsworth, pp. 396–7.

167 Mauriac F, op. cit., p. 60.

168 Cheever S (1987) *Doctors and Women*. Methuen, London, 1988, p. 21.

169 Hamman L (1938) As others see us. *Transact Assoc Amer Physicians.* **53**: 22–45.

170 Morris DB (1998) *Illness and Culture in the Postmodern Age*. University of California Press, Berkeley, CA.

171 Le Fanu J (1999) *The Rise and Fall of Modern Medicine*. Little Brown, London.

172 Cozzens JG, op. cit., pp. 36–40.

173 Davies R (1994) *The Cunning Man*. Viking, London, pp. 26–7.

174 Ellis AE. op. cit., pp. 99–100.

175 Sanders L (1973) *The First Deadly Sin*. Berkley Books, New York, 1974, pp. 61–2.

176 Neuberger J (1999) Do we need a new word for patients? Let's do away with 'patients'. *Br Med J.* **318**: 1756–7.

177 Tallis R (1999) Leave well alone. *Br Med J.* **318**: 1757–8.

178 Le Sage AR (1715) *The Adventures of Gil Blas de Santillana*, vol. 1. Translated by Smollett T. Oxford University Press, London, 1907, pp. 116–17.

179 Reade C (1863) *Hard Cash*. Chatto and Windus, London, 1894, p. 180.

180 Sanders L, op. cit., p. 83.

181 Winawer SJ, Stewart ET, Zauber AG, Bond JH, Ansel H, Waye JO, Hall D, Hamlin JA, Schapiro M, O'Brien MJ, Sternberg SS and Gottlieb LS for the National Polyp Study Work Group (2000) A comparison of colonoscopy and double-contrast barium enema for surveillance after polypectomy. *N Engl J Med.* **342**: 1766–72.

182 Moseley JB, O'Malley K, Petersen NJ, Menke TJ, Brody BA, Kuykendall DH, Hollingsworth JC, Ashton CM and Wray NP (2002) A controlled trial of arthroscopic surgery for osteoarthritis of the knee. *N Engl J Med.* **347**: 81–8.

183 Writing Group for the Women's Health Initiative Investigators (2002) Risks and benefits of estrogen plus progestin in healthy postmenopausal women: principal results from the Women's Health Initiative randomized controlled trial. *JAMA.* **288**: 321–33.

184 Ellis AE, op. cit.

185 James H (1881) *Washington Square*. Bantam Books, New York, 1959, p. 125.

186 McCullers C (1953) *Clock Without Hands*. Houghton Mifflin, Boston, MA, 1963, pp. 61–3.

CHAPTER 1

The physician's fee

Historical

As soon as medical characters make their appearance in literature, they attract attention on account of their remuneration. In general, the doctor is perceived to be obsessed with his payment, which is also seen as a poisonous element in his relationship with his patients. The earliest recorded decrees concerning doctors[1] are not devoted to codes of behavior or physicians' training, but almost in their entirety, to a regulation of medical fees. Asclepios, the mythical father figure of Greek medicine and the first doctor in 'Western' literature, is destroyed by his greed. This talented, semi-divine physician comes across as a recognizable type of general practitioner.[2] He treats patients suffering from 'sores of nature' as well as those presenting with traumatic injuries, 'their limbs wounded'. He is able to distinguish between patients who need reassurance ('tending some with kindly incantations'), those who require medications ('giving to others a soothing potion') and those who can be cured only by surgery ('restoring others by the knife'). Unfortunately, he is lured by 'a splendid fee of gold'[2] to attempt an illegal procedure and is punished accordingly.

The theme of the money-hungry doctor is repeated many times during the subsequent millennia. Amundsen[3] lists some of the references to greedy and corrupt physicians in classical literature. 'Is there a doctor now in all the town?' asks one of Aristophanes' characters rhetorically, and proceeds to answer his own question. 'There are no fees and therefore there is no skill.'[4] Pliny[5] fulminates against rapacious doctors, who introduce novel and dangerous treatments and 'enrich themselves even with the hazard of our lives'. Luckily, comments Pliny, medical services, like other commodities, are subject to the laws of supply and demand, so that with the large number of practicing doctors, 'the market is well fallen'.

Geoffrey Chaucer's physician,[6] who has 'a particular love for gold', makes a fortune during the plague years and is engaged in profit-sharing arrangements with an apothecary.[6] In the various versions of the Dance Macabre[7] the doctor is satirized for gazing at other men's urines in pursuit of money. But death comes and neither 'the gold that ye thereby have won' nor 'herb[s] and root[s]' will save the leech from having to report at the last judgement.

The Doctor of Physic in Shakespeare's *Macbeth*,[8] although portrayed with a great deal of sympathy, is made to discuss his remuneration at a most inappropriate moment. As a physician, this man displays considerable clinical skills. He attempts to take a medical history ('How came she by that light?'[8]); he comments on important physical signs ('You see her eyes are open'[8]); and, while he has some experience with sleepwalkers, he displays sufficient humility and tact to declare: 'This disease is beyond my practice'.[8] He gives appropriate therapeutic instructions

('Remove from her the means of all annoyance'[8]). Yet, trapped in the 'bunker' of Dunsinane Castle[9] and unlikely to escape alive, he still ruminates over his payment.

> Were I from Dunsinane away and clear,
> Profit again should hardly draw me here.[9]

Webster's *Duchess of Malfi*, whose followers have left on account of her 'decayed fortune', compares these fair-weather friends to doctors at a deathbed.

> This puts me in mind of death: physicians thus,
> With their hands full of money, use to give o'er
> Their patients.[10]

Humorous and not so humorous

The doctor's cash register continues to exercise the imagination of fiction writers down to the present age. The topic may be treated sarcastically, light-heartedly or resentfully, but it is never far from the surface, while the public's preoccupation with the subject transcends time, place and cultural backgrounds. Even in institutional settings, where one might expect money to play a very minor role, hostilities between former collaborators may ultimately be traceable to conflicts over money.[11]

One popular scenario consists of a dying patient attended by a physician whose main concern relates to the size of his bill.

> 'Is there no hope?' The sick man said.
> The silent doctor shook his head.
> And took his leave with signs of sorrow
> Despairing of his fee tomorrow.[12]

A more modern version of this setting occurs in Warren's *All the King's Men*,[13] when Governor Stanton

> died in a mahogany tester bed with a couple of high-priced doctors
> leaning over him and adding up the bill in their heads.[14]

Hilaire Belloc's cautionary verse[15] conveys much the same message: the doctors are not very good at treating the patient, but they are great at collecting their pay.

> Physicians of the utmost fame
> Were called at once but when they came
> They answered as they took their fees
> 'There is no cure for this disease.'[15]

Joseph Heller's Dr Daneeka,[16] like Chaucer's physician, has a kickback fee arrangement with drug stores. Unlike the other characters in *Catch 22*, who worry about staying alive or engage in personal squabbles with fellow members of the military establishment, Doc Daneeka spends his time brooding about what the war is doing to his income. 'I don't want to make sacrifices, I want to make dough.'[16]

The doctor's fee has even found its way into nursery rhymes:

> Miss Polly had a dolly who was sick, sick, sick.
> So they sent for the doctor to come quick, quick, quick . . .
> The doctor looked at dolly and he* shook his head
> And he said to Miss Polly 'put her straight to bed'.
> He wrote on a paper for a pill, pill, pill.
> 'I'll be back in the morning with my bill, bill, bill.'[17]

Other humorous references to the doctor's fee include Céline's account of Dr Baryton in *Journey to the End of the Night*.[19] Baryton, a cheerful rogue, runs a highly profitable asylum for mentally disturbed patients.

> In our nuthouse we had patients at all prices, the most opulent living in heavily padded Louis XV rooms. Baryton paid these a daily, highly priced visit. . . . Now and then he'd be welcomed with a . . . truly magnificent and long-premeditated sock on the jaw, which he'd enter on the bill under 'special treatment'

before sending the family an inflated account.[19] When Maurois' Dr O'Grady,[20] a psychiatrist in a private mental hospital, informs his chief, who is also the proprietor, that a particular patient has nothing wrong with him and should be discharged, the chief remarks:

> Your patient is suffering from congestion of the purse and I think we shall be able to give him some relief.[20]

The whining, dishonest, drunken migrant woman in William Carlos Williams' *The Girl with a Pimply Face*[21] has no intention of paying any sort of account. However, she evidently believes that if she promises to pay the doctor a large sum of money, he will intensify his efforts to cure her child.

> Doctor, you good doctor . . . I give you anything . . . I pay you twenty dollar. Doctor you fix my baby. You good doctor. You fix.[21]

The doctor's remuneration appears less humorous in *The Brothers Karamazov*,[22] where a famous specialist who has come from Moscow 'for a large fee'[22] visits a desperately poor and terminally ill school student (Ilyusha Snegiryov) in his hovel. Contemptuous of the Snegiryovs and their poverty, the doctor bellows in 'a loud peremptory voice' and gives totally inappropriate advice.[22] (*See also* p. 193.)

Leo Tolstoy, deeply suspicious of medical science, dislikes doctors and resents their fees. The chief character in *The Kreutzer Sonata*,[23] who regales a chance acquaintance on a train with the story of how he murdered his wife, complains bitterly about 'doctors who cynically undressed her and felt her all over (*see* pp 104–

---

* In some versions the doctor is (uncharacteristically) a female[18] (*see* Book IV).

5) – for which I had to thank them and pay them money'. He adds, 'I understand they want to earn money like lawyers and others',[23] but somehow this character (and Tolstoy) seem to find physicians' fees less appropriate than those of other professionals.

The fee-for-service system

The principle that medical care is a purchasable commodity, with qualities of service and price ranges that vary according to the patient's ability to pay, has divided the medical and lay communities for at least a century. Bernard Shaw, who favored a salaried medical service, argued at length that the doctor's fee constitutes a major conflict of interest.[24]

> That any sane nation . . . should . . . give a surgeon a pecuniary interest in cutting . . . [out your appendix] . . . is enough to make one despair of political humanity . . . What other men dare pretend to be impartial where they have a strong pecuniary interest on one side? . . . Nobody supposes that doctors are less virtuous than judges. But a judge whose salary . . . depended on whether the verdict was for plaintiff or defendant, prosecutor or prisoner, would be as little trusted as a general in the pay of the enemy.[24]

Remarkably, while the quality of medical care provided to the poor continues to be inferior to that enjoyed by the affluent even in developed countries,[25] suggestions that clinical decisions are made on the basis of mercenary considerations are relatively rare in fictional literature. Slaughter[26] writes about large numbers of hysterectomies on the private surgical floor of 'New Salem Memorial Hospital', but the clinical details are too sparse to indicate, even to a medical reader, whether these operations are performed for 'Shavian' indications.

Ravin's Dr Thomas McIlheny[27] fulminates against the size of the fee rather than the principle. McIlheny, a seriously flawed academic surgeon (*see* Book II, Chapter 7) expresses his views after imbibing a good deal of alcohol, but his misgivings regarding medicine as a trade rather than a profession seem genuine and the author appears to share them.

> [If] you want to be a millionaire . . . you go to Harvard Business School. Go into stocks and bonds. That's not what medicine is about. . . . Whatever happened to the old country doc who made house calls and charged a dollar for an office visit? Now all the offices have twenty women working computers, and doing the billing. You couldn't buy coffee for the office staff for what the old country doc charged for bringing a new life into this world.[27]

Current predictions that wealthy individuals will attempt to circumvent transplantation and cloning regulations were foreshadowed in Manzoni's *The Betrothed*.[28] The climax of that story takes place during a seventeenth-century plague epidemic. The rich, who develop suggestive symptoms and signs, but have no intention of complying with the isolation laws, pay their doctors handsomely for providing them with alternative diagnoses. Don Rodrigo, the villain of Manzoni's novel, has caught the disease and is casting around for a discreet physician who will keep him out of the lazaretto. His choice falls on Dr Chiodo, 'a good fellow who keeps quiet about his patients' illnesses if they pay him well'.[28] (Unfortunately for Don Rodrigo, his own servant, who has been dispatched to call the good doctor, summons the city functionaries instead. They drag the Don off to the public facility and divide his money with the treacherous servant.)

A system that allows successful physicians to extract large fees from poor patients was vigorously attacked by Robert Herrick in 1900. In *The Web of Life*[29] he describes Dr Lindsay's waiting room, where all patients wishing to see the doctor or his associates are first screened by a female clerk.

> 'What is your name please?' Her tones were finely adjusted to the caste of the patient. Judging from the icy sharpness on this occasion, the patient was not high in the scale . . . 'Have you been here before?' 'No mum.' 'You will have to pay the fee in advance.' 'What's that please?' 'Ten dollars.' 'Ten'? The clerk tapped irritably on her desk with a pencil. 'Yes. Ten dollars for the first visit; five after that; operations from fifty to five hundred.' The woman clutched tightly a small reticule. 'I hain't the money!' she exclaimed at last. 'I thought it would be two dollars.' 'You'll have to go to the hospital then.' The clerk turned to a pile of letters. 'Don't he see nobody here without he pays ten?' the woman asked. 'No.'[29]

The patient finally finds her way to Dr Sommers, Dr Lindsay's idealistic assistant, who agrees to treat her without charge, and is duly reprimanded for his non-businesslike attitude.

Money is not the only cause for Virginia Woolf's dislike of Sir William Bradshaw[30] (*see* p. 109) but it is certainly a contributory factor. Sir William, a poorly educated social climber, has managed to convince the medical and lay fraternities that he is now a leading London psychiatrist. His treatment methods may not be very effective but he is superb at extracting money from the affluent patients who have been referred to him. He

> would travel sixty miles or more down into the country to visit the rich, the afflicted who could afford the very large fee which Sir William very properly charged for his advice.[30]

The story ends in disaster, with one of Sir William's patients jumping out of a window rather than continue under the doctor's 'care'.

Thomas Mann's *Doctor Faustus*[31] contains yet another harrowing deathbed scene, together with an attack on the doctor's fee. The local physician, who cannot cope with the agony of a child dying of tuberculous meningitis, has asked for a consultation with a physician from the capital.

> The next afternoon the consulting authority arrived from Munich. He was a tall man . . . with a social presence . . . much sought after and high priced.[31]

The Doctor from Dunmore[32] is humorous rather than distressing, but its message is the usual one: doctors are so rapacious that they only care about one element in the Periodic Table. The chief character in the play, a greedy 'pagan' doctor, attempts to charge an exorbitant fee, but is outwitted by a group of Irish villagers who refer to him as a 'black-hearted old scoundrel . . . round shouldered with the weight of the gold he . . . is carrying in his pockets'. The doctor has been rowed over to an island off the West Coast of Ireland so as to examine and treat a woman with multiple fractures, for a stipulated fee of 'ten pounds'. When, at the end of the consultation he catches sight of a pile of money on the table, he makes a little speech to the assembled relatives and neighbors:

> You know we doctors have to live too . . . Unfortunately we have to charge what may sometimes seem like an exorbitant fee but . . . the trip here entails a long and dangerous crossing and . . . my time is valuable.

Condescension turns into sarcasm when the islanders inform the doctor that they have been able to collect only half the agreed fee. 'Now that you know the patient is out of danger . . . you don't intend to live up to your obligations.' Maureen O'Flaherty, a village girl about to be married, shocks everyone by adding her entire dowry (five pounds) to the sum on the table. The doctor counts his money and remarks, as he deposits it in his fat wallet, 'it's the principle of the thing'. The boatmen punish this medical Shylock for his greed by refusing to take him back to the mainland. 'You made a hard bargain Doctor. We kept our end of it. We took you here . . . you got your money. Now get back the best way you can.' After much teasing and some unseemly haggling, the doctor reluctantly agrees to return Maureen's dowry.[32]

Several stories describe physicians who have become so greedy, that they resort to fraudulent or unethical practices so as to augment their incomes. Lathen's *The Attending Physician*[33] is a superficial diatribe against the greed, the wealth and the mindless ostentatiousness of doctors. However, its catalog of medical misdeeds evidently reflects incidents that have occurred in the real world. Doctors in a group practice engage in Medicare and Medicaid fraud on an epic scale. They abandon all precautions, they submit impossible claims, and they bill the government several times for procedures that have not been performed at all. A Dr Yarborough claims for a vasectomy he has allegedly performed on a female,[34] while one of his colleagues demands a fee for an abortion on a Medicaid patient who has previously been billed for a hysterectomy.[35] Dr Costello, a previous member of the practice, who has been granted immunity and who is giving evidence against his former colleagues to a Congressional Committee, is asked why his group had 'billed Medicaid for non-existent services. "I really don't know why we bothered with that,"' admits Dr Costello. There are perfectly legitimate ways of milking the system. He explains the serial referral system ('Ping-ponging').

> 'We all have offices in the same building. So when someone on Medicaid comes to see me I look him over and say he ought to see the internist across the hall. Then the internist sends him to see the cardiologist, the cardiologist routes him to the neurologist and so on. By the time he gets to the end of the corridor we've got eight or nine racked up.'[36]

Dr 'Dump MacDonald', who is considered by the resident staff 'the dumbest human being ever to have been awarded the MD degree', is nevertheless a great financial success. He drives a Rolls Royce with MD plates and his grateful patients donate vast sums of money to the building fund at 'Manhattan Hospital'.[37] MacDonald has not become 'filthy rich' by entirely honest means. He comes in once a week to

> squeeze his notes into the charts so it would look as if he'd actually come into the hospital each day to see his own patients so he could bill the insurance companies for all the high-quality care he was not rendering.[38]

Arthur Miller's Dr Walter Franz, an entrepreneur as well as a surgeon, has made so much money out of his nursing homes[39] that he can now afford to spend time in public hospitals and to write newspaper articles with 'a genuine human quality'.[40] Despite his newly discovered altruism, the doctor has not lost his flair for making a fast buck and, during the discussion about the sale of his late father's furniture, he comes up with an ingenious income tax scam. The furniture, which is worth around two thousand dollars, is to be fraudulently valued at 25 thousand dollars, 'then I donate it to the Salvation Army. I pay around fifty per cent tax so if I make a twenty-five thousand dollar contribution I'd be saving around twelve thousand in taxes'.[41] Income tax evasion is not confined to the medical profession. However, this particularly crude scheme is obviously quite inappropriate for a prominent professional man.

Doctors feel guilty

While the fee constitutes an irritant to the patients, it may also engender a feeling of guilt in the doctor. This manifests itself in the form of certain types of jokes, in conjuring tricks, which remove the money ('the badge of shame') as soon as it is tendered, and in inappropriate acts of generosity, including a reluctance to collect outstanding debts. Occasional doctors complain bitterly about having to take money at all.

> I blushed scarlet when a patient put his twenty-five franc piece on my table and when he put it in my hand I felt as if I wanted to hit him . . . I said our profession was a holy office on the same level as that of the priest if not higher . . . Surplus money making should be forbidden by law . . . What was the proper fee for taking the fear of death out of a pair of terror stricken eyes by a comforting word or a mere stroke of your hand? How many francs were you to charge for every second of the death struggle your morphia syringe had snatched from the executioner?[42]

The doctor's coyness about accepting money can be circumvented, as in Julia Dodd's case,[43] by acrobatics that camouflage the shameful act. Julia, an essentially healthy teenager with non-specific symptoms, consults Dr Short, accompanied by her mother. The doctor diagnoses 'torpidity of the liver', he writes 'two elegant prescriptions', and he announces in extravagant terms that the prognosis is good. Mrs Dodd is most impressed.

'Oh thank you Dr Short . . . you inspire me with confidence and gratitude.' As if under the influence of these feelings only, she took Dr Short's palm and pressed it. . . . Both [hands] were . . . so equally adroit that a double fee passed without the possibility of a bystander suspecting it.[43]

In the same way, Turgenev's *District Doctor*[44] manages to make his payment disappear in minimum time. He 'deftly slid a five rouble note up his sleeve coughing dryly and looking away as he did so'.[44] In a somewhat blacker humor, Proust[45] describes a similar disappearance trick, performed during the theatrical scene enacted around a deathbed. Dr Dieulafoy, a prominent Paris physician, has been summoned. His main function consists of confirming that Marcel's grandmother is in extremis.

> In the majesty of his frock coat the Professor would enter the room, melancholy without affectation, uttering not a word of condolence that could have been construed as insincere . . . Having examined my grandmother . . . he murmured a few words to my father . . . bowed respectfully to my mother and made a perfect exit, simply accepting the sealed envelope that was slipped into his hand . . . He did not appear to have seen it . . . with such a conjurer's dexterity had he made it vanish.[45]

Young Dr Edward Lisse in *The Healers*[46] does not engage in sleights of hand, but he feels uncomfortable about repeatedly accepting payment for seeing 'Sir James Graye', a mentally handicapped British aristocrat,[47] and 'ventured to tell his chief that . . . he was doing nothing for the patient. "When you are as old as I am," replied this illustrious doctor, smiling, "you will wait till the patient discovers that."' Maartens leaves it to the reader to decide whether the 'illustrious doctor' is being cynical, ethical or a mixture of the two. Clearly, the doctor's visits may provide some comfort to the patient and his family, even when the situation is apparently 'hopeless'. In the end, Dr Lisse is able to improve the patient by performing a heroic and rather fanciful neurosurgical operation.[46]

The doctors' ambivalence towards accepting money for medical services may be transmitted to the patients, who worry about embarrassing their medical attendants. 'It's extraordinary how nervous people are about giving a doctor money,' observes Somerset Maugham's Dr Richard O'Farrell to one of his patients.[48] 'If you only knew how jolly glad he is to get it.' However, Dr O'Farrell strongly objects to the patient placing the fee on the mantelpiece, as he might in a whorehouse. 'There are limits.'[48]

Some fictional doctors who may be 'jolly glad' to receive money nevertheless back away from actually demanding payment. Dr Richard Mahony[49]

> might have pocketed his fee on the spot had he cared to ask for it. But the presenting of his palm professionally was a gesture that was denied him.[49]

In Mahony, this disinclination to ask for his fee is so strong that it persists even when his practice is falling apart.

> The older he grew, the more it went against the grain to badger patients for his fees. If they were too mean or too dishonest to pay for his services, he was too proud to dun them.[50]

Céline[51] expresses this sense of shame and guilt even more strongly.

> Medicine is a thankless profession. When you get paid by the rich, you
> feel like a flunkey, by the poor, like a thief. How can you take a fee from
> people who can't afford to eat or go to the movies? . . . When I was being
> escorted to the door after giving the family plenty of advice and handing
> them my prescription, I'd start talking about everything under the sun
> just to postpone the moment of payment a little longer. I was no good at
> playing the prostitute. Most of my patients were so wretchedly poor . . .
> that I always wondered where they would ever find the twenty francs
> owing to me . . . And yet I needed those twenty francs badly. Shameful! I
> still blush to think of it.[51]

Conan Doyle's Dr Horace Wilkinson,[52] whose practice is anything but flourishing,
asks a gypsy patient for 'half a crown' after bandaging her black eye and giving her a
bottle of 'cooling medicine' for her feverish child. The doctor alleviates his guilt
feelings about imposing a charge, by allowing this coarse woman to express her
anger and to introduce the 'class struggle' into the doctor's office:

> Where am I to get 'arf-a-crown? It is well for gentle-folk like you, who sit
> in your grand houses, an' can eat an' drink what you like, an' charge 'arf-
> a-crown for just saying as much as 'Ow d'ye do.' We can't pick up 'arf-
> crowns like that. What we gets we earns 'ard.[52]

Dr Jonathan Dakers' reluctance to accept his fee[53] leads to a tragedy. Jonathan has
been treating Lily Rudge, a seamstress, for a pulp space infection of her forefinger.

> Jonathan had incised the finger . . . and sent the girl home with the iron
> tonic that her bleached blood stream needed and the usual vain counsel
> of perfection; rest, fresh air, good food – all three unknown and
> unobtainable

in Lily's slum dwelling. Much to Jonathan's surprise and embarrassment, Lily
returns some days later to pay her account, and blushingly hands Jonathan

> a pathetic grubby florin . . . He patted the child's shoulder; refused it,
> telling her that she had much better spend it on the food that she
> obviously needed; that he himself would be convenienced if she would
> wait till the Christmas bills were sent out.

Lily cannot bear the thought of being in debt.

> 'You take the money now doctor, please do. I might be tempted to spend
> it and then I should be afraid to call you in if . . . I'm took bad again.' . . .
> Jonathan continued, good-humoredly to refuse; and that, perhaps, was
> the reason why some weeks later, the sister with whom Lily Rudge lived,
> sent for him so late.

That girl, who needs an appendectomy, develops peritonitis and dies.[53]

One of the most brilliant stories relating to a doctor who refuses payment is Richard Selzer's *The Consultation*.[54] An unnamed surgeon is attending an out-of-town conference, where he becomes bored with 'the lectures, the instruments, the whole gadgetry of surgery, the rooms full of well-dressed men', and decides to spend the night with 'Gloria', a woman from an escort agency. In the morning he discovers a suspicious lump in the sleeping woman's right breast. 'He showered deliberately' and as he is getting dressed,

> with his back to her, he said, 'I've got to talk to you.' 'It's a hundred dollars.' . . . He reached for his wallet counted out a fifty and five tens and held it out. She raised up on one elbow, watched this very carefully and said, 'put it on the table'. Then she sank back and watched him dress . . . 'There's something I've got to tell you,' he began again. 'You're not sick, are you?' She was paying attention now. 'No I'm not' . . . A pause. 'But you are.' 'What do you mean?' 'Listen, I'm a doctor, as you know.' His voice took on a deeper more professional tone . . . 'You've got a lump in your breast.'

Gloria promises to seek medical advice and the surgeon rises to leave.

> His fingers scuttled to the doorknob . . . which was a hard lump in his hand, . . . 'Wait.' She walked to the table and picked up one of the ten-dollar bills. 'Here. Thanks for the consultation.'

The doctor refuses on the grounds that he does not make 'house calls'.[54] He feels guilty about having 'exploited' a sick woman who may die of her cancer and he senses that under the circumstances any sort of payment is inappropriate. In addition, the doctor cannot bring himself to accept 'the hire of the harlot'[55] as his remuneration, even though he would no doubt have charged Gloria his usual fee had she consulted him in his office.

Even James Tate, not an admirer of the medical profession or its activities, acknowledges the doctors' suppressed sense of shame at being compared to armed robbers:

> What kind of human being
> Would grab all your money
> Just when you're down?
> I'm not saying they enjoy this:
> 'Sorry Mr Rodriguez, that's it
> No hope! You might as well
> Hand over your wallet.' Hell no.
> They'd rather be playing golf
> And swapping jokes about our feet.[56]

The convention that a doctor avoids this kind of embarrassment by collecting his fee through an intermediary is deeply rooted and widespread. ' "What do I owe you doctor?" ' asks the famous author after discussing his erectile dysfunction with a young psychiatrist.[57] He receives the appropriate response: ' "I'll send you a bill by and by." ' At an earlier age, when fees were lower and doctor's secretaries virtually non-existent, Trollope's *Doctor Thorne*[58] nonetheless provokes the disapproval of his 'Barchester' colleagues by not only charging less than the common fee but also by actually fishing around in his trouser pocket for the necessary change.

> A physician should take his fee without letting his left hand know what his right hand was doing. It should be taken without a thought, without a look, without a move of the facial muscles. The true physician should hardly be aware that the last friendly grasp of the hand had been made more precious by the touch of gold.[58]

In real life, the medical profession is very conscious of these sentiments and employs tens of thousands of receptionists whose principal function is to separate the 'handshake' from the 'gold'.

The fee as a positive aspect

Several writers portray the fee as a positive or amusing aspect of therapy rather than a cause for resentment or guilt. When Sigmund Freud proclaims that patients do not appreciate medical advice unless they pay a heavy price for it,[59] he is reiterating the sentiments of Samuel Richardson's *Clarissa Harlowe*,[60] who declines her physician's generous offer to waive his fee on the grounds that payment forms an essential part of the doctor–patient relationship. Clarissa insists, almost two centuries before Freud, that if her doctor were to see her without charging a fee, she might 'forget that he was her physician [and] she might be apt to abate of the confidence in his skill'.[60] The aphorism 'A physician who heals for nothing is worth nothing'[61]* goes back to the fifth century AD.

In a similar frame of mind, but in an early twentieth-century setting, Ellen Glasgow treats a meticulous medical accounts system as a sign of reliability. In *Barren Ground*[62] she contrasts a dependable, hard-working doctor with an idle, ineffectual medical drunkard (*see* Book II, Chapter 7). The 'good' doctor 'insisted on having his fees paid. . . . It was natural . . . to value advice more highly when it was not given away'. The 'bad' doctor, even before he became a total inebriate, could only whine about his inability to collect his fees. 'Since I've been here' complains Dr Jason Greylocks, 'I've made nothing. Down here the doctor gets paid after the undertaker or not at all'.[63]

Gide's amateur physiologist, Anthime Amand Dubois, a fanatical and somewhat unstable atheist, who does not want to be beholden to God or man for any improvement in his health, makes a fetish out of the doctor's fee.[64] ' "If I am to be cured, I want to owe it to no one but myself. So there!" "Then what about the doctor?" . . . "I pay him for his visits. We are quits." '[64]

---

* This statement, which is often quoted out of context, comes from a passage in the Babylonian Talmud[61] describing how a successful plaintiff in an assault case may foil the defendant's attempts to minimize his medical costs. If the defendant (presumably a physician who injured the plaintiff in the first instance) offers to treat him himself, the plaintiff is entitled to reject this 'generosity'. If the defendant tries to introduce the injured individual to a physician who will treat him free of charge, the plaintiff may counter by saying 'a physician who charges no fee is worth none'. If the defendant proposes to bring a physician from out of town, the plaintiff has the right to refuse this offer also.[61]

Conan Doyle's wealthy patients are quite happy to pay heavy medical fees in order to impress their impecunious physicians.[52] Jonathan Dakers' patients from the wealthier suburbs boast about their doctors' large fees so as to make an impression on their friends.

> [In the] high class residential neighborhood of Wednesford big fees were not only not resented but actually welcomed and referred to in public with a superior satisfaction.[65]

The patients' perception that the higher the fee, the better the service, is so deeply ingrained that when the senior partners in Nourse's *The Practice*[66] proposes that he and the junior man (Dr Robinson Tanner) charge different fees for confinements, his suggestion provokes outrage and is rejected out of hand. The older, more experienced doctor, who is overwhelmed with demands for obstetric services, wants to charge an extra hundred dollars with the stated intention of encouraging the poorer people in the town to consult the younger man who will continue to charge the present rate. Tanner is incensed by this allegedly harmless plan, which will send a message to the local population that two kinds of obstetric services are available: the good and the cheap. He refuses to be cast in the role of 'the slob in the corner office' who provides economy-class services while his more expensive partner offers quality treatment.[66]

Conversely, while a lack of money may constitute a barrier between the patients and medical treatment, it also acts as a deterrent against meddlesome and dangerous procedures. 'Isn't it fortunate for a lot of people', declares one of the 'progressive' young doctors in Caldwell's *Testimony of Two Men*,[67] 'that they can't afford some operations. Poverty has done more to save . . . lives than wealth.'[67]

Many instances of distinguished physicians submitting large medical bills are reported factually and without animosity. Henry James' Sir Luke Strett,[68] who has travelled from London to Venice to treat an American heiress 'for a huge fee', is admired rather than resented and certainly does not give the impression that he is anyone's lackey. Similarly, Sobel's Dr Jim Morelle[69] expresses no sense of guilt at sending an outrageous account to a wealthy patient who, in turn, evinces no sign of resentment. The action takes place around 1947.

> Even long afterwards when such a fee was not unusual he never forgot his amazement the first time [his secretary] asked his approval before sending out a bill for twenty-five hundred dollars for removal of a cancer of the colon; nor his even greater amazement when the check and a note of thanks were placed on his desk three days later.[69]

Another of Sobel's surgeons, Doctor Herman Augustus Emmerich, charges his rich patients enormous fees while treating the 'deserving' poor virtually free of charge. This 'Robin Hood' technique arouses neither resentment nor guilt feelings. Emmerich, the famous Chief of Surgery at 'McKinley Hospital'[70]

> did not favor a noisy waiting room filled with restless patients who had all been scheduled for the same time so that they would be impressed by the size of the doctor's practice. His fees, usually from five hundred to five thousand dollars for an operation were so large that he could afford

the luxury of a quiet office. In less than five minutes [after the arrival of a poor patient who is being charged a nominal fee] his . . . nurse . . . walked in briskly and whispered. 'Will you follow me please. He is ready for you now.' Her tone implied that 'He' was spelled with a capital H.[70]

Likewise, Dr Peter Harding,[71] a conservative and somewhat smug character in Edwardian England, whose clientele and fees are more modest, harbors no feelings of remorse over asking for money. On the contrary, in his scheme, the fixed fee and the absence of opportunities for haggling constitute an essential part of professionalism.[71] 'As a profession,' he writes to a younger colleague, '[we] have but lately differentiated ourselves from the ranks of retail commerce – so lately . . . that the barber tradition is far from being entirely defunct.' Harding goes on to tell a story, dating back to the 1870s, of a patient who wanted a young general practitioner to remove a tooth for half the regular price, which was 'one shilling'. When the doctor declines to bargain, the patient cheerfully consents to pay the scheduled fee; 'the shilling went into the till while the tooth, neatly wrapped in paper, was borne homewards for domestic inspection'. Many years later, when Harding is well established as an internist, and the tooth-extraction business is left to the junior staff in the Emergency Department,[72] his scheduled fee for an office consultation is 'two guineas', more than twice the weekly wage of one of his clinic patients. This discrepancy does not bother Dr Harding unduly. The patient, 'a stalwart gentleman who . . . does not stint himself in beer',[73] enjoys life in a swinish way and if he needs medical attention he is seen free of charge in a Charity Hospital.

The relatively large fee paid at the successful conclusion of a difficult confinement[74] generates only gratitude without a hint of resentment. Dr Miles, a general practitioner, who is having problems with a primipara going through a home delivery, needs an experienced obstetrician to provide 'a second opinion' and to help him with this 'nasty case'. The expectant father (Robert Johnson) is dispatched to summon Dr John Pritchard, 'a man who had been . . . driven, as so many others have been, by the needs of his increasing family to set the commercial before the philanthropic side of his profession'. Pritchard, who is awakened by Johnson's vigorous pulls at the night bell, wastes no time on clinical questions and immediately discusses the financial aspects. After being told the address, he informs Johnson that his consultation fee is 'three guineas, payable at the time' (one to two weeks' wages) and Johnson, who has been warned by Dr Miles that Pritchard is expensive, agrees at once. After the birth of the child, when Johnson feels for the first time in his life a 'turmoil of joy in his heart . . . his impulse was to fall upon his knees but he was shy before the doctors . . . "I'm very – I'm very" – he grew inarticulate. "There are your three guineas, Doctor Pritchard. I wish they were three hundred." "So do I," said the senior man and they laughed as they shook hands.'[74] The outcome is successful – the fee is a one-off event and the doctor-author, who tells the story, is aware of the financial problems of his colleagues.[72]

Poverty among doctors

In the days before Medicare and other managed care systems, patients had to pay for every visit to the doctor. While fees were low (one or two dollars in the USA in the first three decades of the twentieth century), many could not afford even these amounts, so that demands for doctors' services were made almost entirely during emergencies. Meanwhile, the doctors, especially those who had just gone into practice, sat in their offices, waiting for patients who did not show up. Dr Richard Mahony's 'plate had been on the door for two months . . . [but] all the new instruments . . . lay unused in their casings'.[75] One of Conan Doyle's doctors, recently established in practice and engaged in the 'terrible occupation of waiting' for patients, is visited by an officer of the gas company demanding money.[52] Dr Noel (Chris) Arden waits in his office for two weeks before the arrival of his first 'patient' – a dog with a bone in its throat.[76] Dr David Shelton[77] who is trying to re-establish a surgical practice after a prolonged illness, experiences 'the fickle economic realities of a medical specialty that was dependent on referrals from other physicians'. His financial situation is particularly precarious 'in a city like Boston with its surfeit of doctors'.[77]

Financial crises may occur late in doctors' careers. Dr Edward Hope, the hero of Martineau's *Deerbrook*,[78] who has fallen on hard times, is obliged to remind some of his patients that they owe him money.

> Money was due to him from some of his patients. To these he sent in his bills again and even made personal application. From several he obtained promises, from two or three, the amount of whose debt was very small, he got his money, disgraced by smiles of wonder and contempt.[78]

Zola's Dr Pascal Rougon[79] has much the same humiliating experience.

For some doctors this grinding poverty lasts all their lives. Dr Blenkinsop, one of Bernard Shaw's characters in *The Doctor's Dilemma*, is so poor that he is unable to afford winter clothes and has to stuff sheets of brown paper inside his shirt to keep himself warm.[80] Kingsley's Dr Levine,[81] who practices among 'fifty cent patients' in the tenements of New York's East Side, decides to leave the area because of his wife's pulmonary tuberculosis. The two of them move to Colorado where even the fifty-cent patients do not materialize. Doctor Levine's financial situation becomes so precarious that he has to humiliate himself and ask a successful surgical colleague to lend him twenty dollars.[82]

Dr Samuel Abelman, Gerald Green's *Last Angry Man*,[83] another impoverished New York general practitioner, remains at his post in the slums of Brooklyn, but his former patients abandon him. Those with any funds now see 'specialists and professors'. The poorer ones attend the 'dispensaries and free clinics'. Many of his 'old timers' have gone over to a rival practice. The year is 1955 and the doctor sits in his office waiting for patients. ''Most of the time they don't come' and when they do appear, there are sordid arguments about payment.[83]

> The door buzzer sounded and a dumpy woman of middle age, in a faded blue cotton dress entered. At her side was a small, terrified boy, clutching his injured right hand against his breast with the protective grasp of his left hand. . . . 'He broke his hand,' the woman said shakily. 'I told him not to play baseball with the big boys.' The doctor is examining the boy's hand when he suddenly remembers something. 'Aren't you Kalotkin?' 'Yes, doctor. You treated my husband two weeks ago.' 'That's what I mean. He never paid me. Two dollars for an office visit and three for a

house call. He said he'd send it over. I never saw it'. . . . 'I'm sorry, doctor, I don't have it with me.'[83]

Doctor Abelman treats the child's dislocated thumb despite the unpaid account, but Mrs Kalotkin does not even give him a chance to ask for payment. She 'yanked the boy from the examination table' as soon as the doctor had finished and 'with remarkable speed, she flew from the office, dragging the screaming boy, through waiting room and foyer and . . . into the street'. Abelman cannot understand why his rival, Dr Seymour Baumgart, who charges one hundred dollars for a consultation, has no problems with non-paying patients. 'He just charges and gets it.'[84]

Updike's *Doctor's Wife*[85] is set in a different environment but the culture of the impoverished doctor is very similar to that found in New York City. Updike's doctor, 'a slight, rapid-voiced man with a witty air of failure', is marooned in a Caribbean island because he is unable to find a position elsewhere. His wife is very bitter about the 'natives'.

> If you could see one-tenth of the antics and then the selfishness the doctor puts up with. At two in the morning, 'Doctor, Doctor, come save my child,' and then a week later when he tries to collect his poor little dollar or two, they don't remember . . . And if he insists – 'The white people are stealing our money.'[85]

In another short story also titled *The Doctor's Wife*,[86] Dr Pincus Silver practices in a decayed neighborhood among patients who come to see him for non-organic complaints. Most of them remain loyal to Silver 'because if they said they had no money to pay, he charged them only fifty cents for the visit and promised he would collect it next time. But next time he always forgot'. The doctor's patients are not ill in the accepted sense of the word, they receive no worthwhile treatment or advice and he evidently feels that he does not deserve to get paid.

In some doctors the preoccupation with money persists long after any threat of poverty has subsided. Dr Milton Haggett, the chief character in Sydney Howard's *The Late Christopher Bean*,[87] a general practitioner in a Massachusetts town during the depression years of the early 1930s, is not poor. The Haggetts can afford a maid and they have recently had their house painted. However, a family trip to Florida constitutes an expense that has to be discussed in great detail and in the end the doctor informs his daughters that he cannot afford to take them to Miami 'as long as I can't collect the bills my patients owe me'. This relative shortage of money is partially responsible for the doctor's loss of innocence. After he succumbs to a major financial temptation, Haggett can no longer state publicly 'No man has ever called me greedy for money'.[87]

Hank, a small town general practitioner in upstate New York,[88] also lives in moderate comfort but talks like a poor man. Although Hank is semi-retired, his bitterness on the subject of fees remains as active as ever. When his son, an internist visiting from Manhattan, asks whether the patients are paying their bills, the old man launches into a well-rehearsed tirade:

> The one about cheats and blackguards and villains, and how he worked late and early and in-between even with his cut-back schedule, and still they felt that they could call him at dawn for a sore throat or a boil they

should have seen to days ago, while they never, *never* felt they should pay within a month or two, the way Hank paid *his* goddamned bills.[88]

Atypical physicians. Indifference to money

Despite Freud's dire warnings against 'unsustainable' altruism,[59] some uncharacteristic fictional physicians display bursts of generosity on an apparently capricious basis. In a few, a lack of interest in money is a lifelong characteristic.

Dr H, the physician in Richardson's *Clarissa Harlowe*,[60] displays generosity as well as diagnostic acumen and clinical common sense. He recognizes, almost as soon as he enters the sick-room, that Clarissa's problems are not 'organic' in origin and tells the patient: 'You can do more for yourself than all the faculty can do for you.' [The doctor] would fain have declined his fee as her malady was rather to be relieved by the soothings of a friend than by the prescriptions of a physician . . . ,[60] but as Clarissa insists on paying (*see* p. 33), he decides not to call on a daily basis. 'He knew her case could not so suddenly vary as to demand his daily visits.'[89]

Mrs Esther Woodcourt, wife of Dr Allan Woodcourt in Dickens' *Bleak House*,[90] who considers her husband a perfect physician, emphasizes his altruism and his lack of interest in money.

> We are not rich in the bank but we have always prospered and we have quite enough. I never walk out with my husband but I hear the people bless him. I never go into a house of any degree but I hear his praises or see them in grateful eyes. I never lie down at night but I know that in the course of that day he has alleviated pain and soothed some fellow creature in the time of need. I know that from the beds of those who were past recovery thanks have often gone up in the last hour for his patient ministration. Is not this to be rich?[90]

Dr Cukrowicz in Tennessee Williams' *Suddenly Last Summer*[91] is tempted, like Asclepios, by a 'splendid fee of gold'[2] to carry out a forbidden procedure, but is able to resist. Initially Cukrowicz makes a very unfavorable impression. His remark 'Call me Doctor Sugar'[92] is fit for a buffoon rather than a physician, while the account of his financial difficulties, 'I'd like to marry a girl I can't afford to marry',[93] is totally inappropriate. Mrs Venable wants the doctor to perform a pre-frontal lobotomy on Catherine, the fiancée of her late son ('Sebastian'), so as to stop the girl 'babbling' and destroying Sebastian's reputation for chastity. (Sebastian had in fact been a promiscuous homosexual and pederast.) Doctor Cukrowicz is to be handsomely rewarded if he 'cuts this hideous story out of her brain'.[94] The doctor does not reject the offer out of hand as he should have done, and as Mrs Venable half expected him to. However, as the details gradually emerge, he decides that Catherine's sordid tale may well be true and that the girl does not require a lobotomy. He regains his dignity when he decides to remain poor rather than accept financial support from the 'Sebastian Venable Memorial Foundation'.

Dreiser's Dr Gridley[95] is the epitome of the 'priestly' physician, discussed in meticulous detail in Norris' dissertation.[96] He had

> a head like Plato's or that of Diogenes, the mild, kindly, brown-gray eyes peering, all too kindly into the faces of dishonest men.

Despite his isolation, Dr Gridley is extremely knowledgeable.

> Other physicians from . . . so far away as Chicago were repeatedly calling him into consultation.

Gridley is, of course, totally indifferent to money. On one occasion, he is hailed simultaneously by two potential patients.

> One was a prosperous farmer who had always paid his doctor's bills and the other was a miller, a ne'er-do-well with a delicate wife and a family of sickly children . . . who only occasionally and at great intervals handed the doctor a dollar in payment for his many services.

The good doctor, naturally, goes off with the poor man arguing that the prosperous farmer can afford to go to another physician while the miller 'can't get anyone but me'.[95] He is

> fascinated . . . by . . . something in the very poor [which] made him a little more prone to linger at their bedsides.

Sinclair Lewis' Dr Will Kennicott, a general practitioner in a small town in Minnesota,[97] who is very conscious of money, is asked by an immigrant farmer's wife 'Vell, how much ve going to owe you doctor?' The bill (for a nocturnal house call) came to eleven dollars. 'I dunno ve can pay you, yoost a little w'ile, doctor.' Kennicott declares loudly that they can pay him in the fall after they have harvested their crop.[97]

Similarly, Arnold Bennett's Dr Raste is normally very careful with money.[98] He has been taught by experience 'never to disburse money for patients', and when Violet Earlforward needs to go to hospital by taxi, he makes sure that she has sufficient funds[98] so that the account does not ultimately get sent to him. This tightfisted character suddenly becomes generous towards Violet's live-in maid who confesses that she is hiding and nursing her sick lover in her garret.[99] Elsie's conviction that doctors take no trouble with poor people turns out, on this occasion, to be uncharitable. Dr Raste examines 'Joe', he makes a diagnosis of malaria and arranges a very prompt supply of quinine, despite the couple's poverty.

Dr Coutras, the French physician in Somerset Maugham's *The Moon and Sixpence*,[100] with his French middle-class prejudices, his 'enormous paunch' and his 'comfortable home in Papeete' freely admits that he did not appreciate the painter Charles Strickland, his art and his Bohemian way of life.

He was an idle, useless scoundrel who preferred to live with a native woman rather than work for his living like the rest of us. Mon Dieu, how was I to know that one day the world would come to the conclusion that he had genius?[100]

Despite his lack of sympathy for Strickland and his way of life, Dr Coutras behaves in an exemplary fashion during the painter's final illness when he displays considerable generosity and compassion. He walks seven kilometres to Strickland's hut, he refuses payment, and his 'bedside manner' in breaking the dreadful news to Strickland is perfect[100] (*see* pp 127–8). On leaving Strickland's hut

I told [the boy] I would send some medicine that might be of service; but my hope was small that Strickland would consent to take it and even smaller that if he did, it would do him good. I gave the boy a message for Ata that I would come whenever she sent for me. Life is hard and Nature sometimes takes a terrible delight in tormenting her children.[100]

After Strickland's death, Dr Coutras helps to bury the body because the locals are terrified of catching leprosy.[100]

Sinuhe, Mika Waltari's Egyptian physician,[101] exceptionally conscious of money, status and power, abandons his ambitions and his somewhat precarious lifestyle for a few months in order to provide medical care to the disadvantaged population in a poor neighborhood. 'Thus began my life in the poor quarter of Thebes . . . I had many patients and lost more money than I earned. The gifts I received were of small value though they gave me joy, and even greater joy was it to learn that the poor had begun to bless my name.' Sinuhe soon finds that the poor are as suspicious of their physicians as the rich, and abandons his benevolent medical practice.[101]

Balzac's Dr Benassis, who leaves his Parisian environment for a miserable Alpine village as a penance, keeps his 'vow of poverty' for the rest of his life.[102] He refuses to name a fee to Commandant Genestas, who wants his advice and help.[103] 'If you are wealthy, you will repay me amply . . . and if you are not, I will take nothing whatever.' Benassis adds:

'Rich people shall not have my time by paying for it; it belongs exclusively to the folk here in the valley. I do not care for fame or fortune and I look for neither praise nor gratitude from my patients. Any money which you may pay me will go to the druggists in Grenoble to pay for the medicine required by the poor of the neighborhood.'[103]

Similarly, Dostoyevsky's saintly Dr Herzenstube[104] is a 'kind-hearted, humane man who treated his poor patients . . . for nothing, went into their hovels . . . [and] left money for medicine'.[104] Dr Dubois, one of the physicians in Ellis' *The Rack*,[105] initially seems somewhat aloof, presumably as the result of a letter from one of Paul Davenant's previous medical attendants, implying that Paul is a 'difficult' patient.[106] Despite this inauspicious beginning, Dubois turns out the most helpful, the most professional and the most generous of Paul's doctors. He pays the hospital bills of several inmates, using money obtained from his wealthier patients. After the doctor's sudden death, it is found that his house did not belong to him. He possessed neither stocks nor shares. He left a widow, the love and gratitude of a multitude of patients and nothing else.[105]

More recent idealistic physicians include Max Loeb in Lapierre's *City of Joy*.[107] Dr Loeb gives up a life of luxury in Miami to minister to the lepers in Calcutta under the most primitive conditions. In his new environment he witnesses large rats running over the belly of a woman in labor. 'One wizened old man . . . obligingly coughed up a great clot of blood into his hand and showed it to me with supreme satisfaction.'

Unlike these 'Mother Theresa-type' physicians, Dr Benjamin Phillips, *The Maida Vale Idyll*,[108] can hardly be described as an honest and moral individual. He deceives his good-natured wife, insults her[109] and, in the end, murders her.[110] He keeps a mistress, but deceives her also.[111] His patients are objects of dangerous experiments performed for the sake of excitement rather than in pursuit of knowledge.[111] One might have thought that this thoroughly evil man who gambles heavily[112] would be quite ruthless in his pursuit of money. Surprisingly, generosity in financial affairs, especially where his patients are concerned, is one of Phillips' redeeming virtues. After he obtains his additional qualification he is entitled to charge higher fees 'but he had not taken this degree until he had been established in practice and those patients he had attended for . . . "ten shillings", he continued to charge ten shillings. . . . He never asked for his money and in cases of real illness he came just as readily whether he had been paid or not'.[112]

Generosity or rather an indifference to money, may also be found among 'earthy' physicians. 'Did you ever hear of me worrying a fellow before he was ready to pay?' Faulkner's Dr Peabody[113] reprimands Anse Bundren, who is too mean to call for medical help until it is too late, and whose wife dies during the doctor's visit.[114] Peabody feels nothing but contempt for Anse, a selfish, canting, mean tyrant who ruins the health of his wife and children through a series of inappropriate omissions[114] and commissions.[115,116] Yet, when one of Anse's sons is brought to the doctor's office with a broken leg that had been set in cement, and Peabody is almost beside himself with rage at Anse's mistreatment of his family, he gives the young man enough money to pay the family's hotel bill.[117]

Another earthy physician, Cozzens' Dr George Bull,[118] is lazy, slovenly and aggressively incompetent. He is also careless about money – his appetites are more primitive. When at the age of sixty-seven Bull is called before a town meeting that will determine whether he should be dismissed from his post as Local Officer of Health, his sloppy accounts are represented as signs of generosity and offered in his defense. 'Some paid him and some didn't but he never worried over that.' Although Dr Bull loses his temper at the meeting, the motion of dismissal is not put, and he is allowed to remain in his position.[118]

Dr Sevier 'laid his left hand on the rich and his right hand on the poor and he was not left-handed'.[119] ' "Yes I have money", Doctor Sevier declared, "but I don't go after it. It comes to me because I . . . render service for the service's sake." '[119] William Wharton's Dr Delibro[120] ridicules the 'Freudian idea [that] you need to make it expensive so the treatment will be appreciated',[59] which he considers a 'bit of Viennese sadomasochistic nonsense',[120] and is quite happy to accept Medicare payments for his elderly patients.

Occasionally, doctors may refuse a fee not from a sense of generosity but in order to show that they are not the flunkeys of wealthy patients. Dr Kate Hunter in *Nothing Lasts Forever*[121] refuses a gangster's 'C-note' so as to assert her independence. 'The cashier's office is outside', she remarks as the money is flashed in front of her, and then walks off with a curt 'no, thanks', when he tries to make her keep it as a mark of his appreciation.

Dr Kirilov's refusal of money in Chekhov's *The Enemies*[122] is more complicated. The doctor has been dragged away from the deathbed of his only child to attend to a rich man's wife. This woman has simulated an attack of unconsciousness in order to abscond with her lover while her husband is summoning medical help. Kirilov feels that the entire exercise is an 'insult' to himself and that he is being used as a 'prop' for the rich man's melodrama.

> Hurriedly Aboghin thrust his hand into his side-pocket, pulled out a wallet and taking out two bank notes, flung them on to the table. 'That's for your visit,' he said, his nostrils quivering. 'Now you've been paid.' 'Don't you dare offer me money!' the doctor shouted and swept the bank notes off the table. 'You don't pay a man for insulting him.'[122]

Medical missionaries like Dr Owen Jones in Somerset Maugham's *The Vessel of Wrath*[123] and Ira Hinckley in *Arrowsmith*[124] are obviously not motivated by monetary considerations. Similarly, non-religious but 'priestly'[96] physicians like Dr Adam Stanton in *All The King's Men*[125] and Dr Colin in *A Burnt-Out Case*[126] think very little about their earnings. Sawako Ariyoshi's throw-away line: 'Of course it was expected that the family of a doctor live frugally'[127] implies that in late eighteenth-century Japan, the doctor's priestly role was considered incompatible with a vulgar display of wealth. A few other altruistic physicians exist, especially in Balzac's writings, but they are in the minority, even in the nineteenth century.

'The doctor who has no money cannot be any good'

In general, non-medical authors appear so obsessed with the doctor's payment, his wealth and his greed, that the physician who is poor, whether by choice or by misfortune, is automatically assumed to be eccentric or incompetent or both. Dr Owen Jones[123] comes across as a pious ass. Dr Adam Stanton[13] is a great surgeon but an impractical do-gooder who, in the end, becomes violent. Kindly and generous Dr Herzenstube[104] is regarded as a useless old pedant whose visits 'were of little avail'.[22] Céline's Dr Ferdinand Bardamu[128] who has recently put up his plate in a poor suburb of Paris feels guilty about accepting fees (*see* p. 31) and gives gratuitous medical advice. He recognizes that there is something incongruous about a doctor who fails to charge, and he is despised by his patients.

> People avenge themselves for the favors done them. Bébert's aunt, took advantage of my lofty disinterestedness. In fact, she imposed on me outrageously. . . . 'Bébert, Doctor, I have to tell you because you're a doctor – he's a little pig! . . . He touches himself! I noticed it two months

ago and I wonder who could have taught him such a filthy habit . . . I've always brought him up right! . . . I tell him to stop . . . but he keeps right on . . . .' I gave her the classic advice: 'Tell him he'll go crazy.' Bébert, who'd been listening, wasn't pleased. 'I don't touch myself, it's not true. It's the Gagat kid who suggested . . .' 'See?' said the aunt. 'I suspected as much. The Gagats, you know, the people on the fifth floor . . . They're all perverts.'[128]

Dr Bardamu follows up by prescribing an 'anti-vice syrup' for the boy but the aunt is unimpressed.

> Her favorite doctor is Frolichon. She always recommends him when she can and runs me down at every opportunity. . . . Except that this Frolichon she admires makes her pay cash, so she consults me on the run.[128]

Dr Bardamu's altruism gains him no admirers. On the contrary, the neighbors smile contemptuously when they meet him in the street coming home from the shops, carrying his own purchases. He is obviously too poor to afford a maid.[51]

Poverty in doctors becomes self-perpetuating. Balzac's Dr Poulain,[129] who looks after poor patients in the Marais district of Paris, lives frugally with his mother who launders his clothes at home.

> For a long time their neighbors had been accustomed to seeing the doctor's and his mother's linen hanging out in the garden . . . This domestic economy did considerable harm to the doctor for people could not credit him with talent when they saw he was so poor.[129]

Poulain's wealthier clients pay him

> only a couple of francs for his visits which he made on foot. For a doctor a cab is even more necessary than a knowledge of medicine.[129]

Lawrence Sanders[130] tells of an encounter between Captain Edward X Delaney, a senior New York police officer, and a Dr Spencer, who informs him that his wife will have to have an operation for kidney stones.

> 'Do you anticipate any trouble, doctor?' he asked. The surgeon . . . looked at him coldly. 'No' he said. 'I trust him,' Delaney said (to his wife, before the operation) . . . 'He's a professional. I asked Ferguson to check him out and he said Spencer is a fine surgeon and a wealthy man.' 'Good,' Barbara smiled faintly, 'I wouldn't want a *poor* surgeon.'[130]

Dr Spencer subsequently performs a nephrectomy and Mrs Delaney dies as a result of a Proteus infection.

Why the resentment and the guilt?

Why is the physician's fee resented and commented upon more disparagingly than that of the builder or the dressmaker? Why should an appropriate remuneration be considered incongruous in a doctor? Is it reprehensible that a physician should try to compensate himself for lean times, when 'money stops coming in, the moment [the doctor] stops going out'?[24] Would not any prudent person make provision for such a contingency? Here is Shaw again: '[The doctor] dare not stop making hay while the sun shines, for it may set at any time'.[24] Why should the doctor have to pose as a philanthropist when he is obviously not capable of maintaining such a pretense indefinitely?[59] Henry Handel Richardson, a doctor's daughter, asks the same question the other way around: 'Who could blame a man for hesitating of a pitch dark night in the winter rains or on a blazing summer day whether or no he should set out on a twenty-mile ride for which he might never see a ghost of a remuneration?'[49]

Fiction writers do not specifically address these questions, which presumably reflect the ambivalence of patients in all ages towards their physicians, whom they need but mistrust. The layman, who is not in a position to differentiate between real dangers and minor ailments, suspects that the doctor might misrepresent trivial symptoms as major illnesses, in order to enhance his income. '[The doctor] looked grave and mentioned a string of grievances that the flesh is heir to – most ending in "itis". I immediately paid him fifteen dollars . . . .'.[131]

There is obvious resentment of a fee for treatment that fails to lead to any improvement in the patient's condition or actually makes matters worse. The biblical patient who 'had a flow of blood for twelve years and who had suffered much under many physicians and who . . . was no better but rather grew worse', is understandably resentful about having 'spent all that she had'.[132]* Little 'Echo' in Thomas Mann's *Doctor Faustus* dies of tuberculous meningitis notwithstanding the Munich consultant's 'high price'.[31] Septimus Warren Smith in Virginia Woolf's *Mrs Dalloway*[30] kills himself in spite of (or possibly because of) Sir William Bradshaw's fees and his fashionable institutions. Eugene O'Neill's Professor Henry Leeds,[134] whose daughter's bizarre sexual behavior has not responded to medical treatment, briefly toys with a scheme of refusing to pay the doctor's enormous fee, but goes on to reject the idea. Here is Professor Leeds brooding about his medical expenses.

> I'll have to call in a nerve specialist . . . but the last one did her no good . . .
> his outrageous fee . . . he can take it to court . . . I absolutely refuse . . .
> but if he should bring suit? . . . What a scandal . . . no, I'll have to pay . . .
> somehow . . . borrow . . . he has me in a corner, the robber.[134]

Fees that are inappropriately high for a particular service[135,136] also elicit adverse comments even if there is no apparent danger. Samuel Richardson's complaints concerning physicians' earnings[135] sound almost contemporary:

---

* 'Doctor' Luke's account of the same patient[133] is less emotive. It makes no mention of money or unpleasant treatment but states simply that she 'could not be healed by anyone'.[133]

Gentlemen of the faculty should be more moderate in their fees or take more pains to deserve them; for, generally, they only come into a room, feel the sick man's pulse, ask the nurse a few questions, inspect the patient's tongue, and perhaps his water; then sit down look . . . wise and write. The golden fee finds the ready hand, and they hurry away, . . . valuing themselves upon the number of visits they make in a morning and the little time they make them in.[135]

Flannery O'Connor, who had a good deal of personal contact with the medical profession, also complains about the combination of little visits and big bills.[136] One of her characters wonders 'why a doctor with as much money as they make, charging five dollars a day to just stick their head in the hospital door and look at you – couldn't afford a decent-sized waiting room'.[136] Similarly, Sylvia Plath[137] comments on the contrast between the size of the doctor's fee and the miniscule service provided:

> And there is a charge, a very large charge
> For a word or a touch
> Or a bit of blood.[137]

An extreme form of perceived extortion is described in Levenkron's *The Best Little Girl in the World*,[138] where Dr Alexander Smith, a Park Avenue psychiatrist, charges fifty dollars for fifty minutes' non-attendance (in 1978). Dr Smith is 'treating' Francesca Dietrich, a fifteen-year-old, for anorexia nervosa. He has warned her parents that he will not communicate with them, and he has told them that they will be billed if the child misses an appointment. Two months and eight hundred dollars later, Harold Dietrich, Francesca's father, telephones Dr Smith enquiring about his daughter's progress.

> 'She's been seeing you for two months. According to my wife, she's still losing weight and according to her school, she has serious problems. I was wondering how things looked to you?'

Harold Dietrich is incensed when the doctor informs him that Francesca has missed several appointments.

> 'How many is several?' There was a silence and Harold could picture Dr Smith leafing through an expensive leather-bound calendar book. 'The last time I saw her was April twenty-third.' 'That was more than a month ago! More than six goddamn weeks ago!' 'I understand your anger but I don't think it's me you're angry at.' 'You don't, do you. Well I'll tell you something you goddamn thief. It is you I'm angry at. Angry as hell at someone who forgets to mention that my daughter isn't showing up for appointments, but doesn't forget to send the bills.'

Dietrich threatens a malpractice suit but the doctor hangs up on him, obviously unimpressed with this threat.[138]

A great deal of the resentment against the doctor's fee stems from the perception (by both parties) that payment is an incongruous part of the doctor–patient relationship. Demanding a fee might be appropriate behavior for a barber surgeon (a one-off fixer), a dentist or an apothecary. It might even be appropriate for a nineteenth-century medical practitioner who supplies his patients with 'pink and brown mixtures'[139] and who provides 'something measurable' for which he can submit an itemized account. It is evidently considered inappropriate for the physician who is perceived to function as a hybrid between a Good Samaritan and a Faustian seeker of knowledge. Moreover, the priest-like figure with his ritual, his vestments and his specialized vocabulary, with his ability to examine body and soul, suddenly becomes a common tradesman when he demands a fee. The quotation 'We are angels when we come to cure, devils when we ask for payment' comes from Walter Scott,[140] but the same sentiment is expressed repeatedly over the centuries.[141] Cobb illustrates the incongruity of the doctor's roles as healer and recipient of fees in one very brief sentence

[The doctor] took my temperature and fifteen dollars.[142]

The paradox of the doctor's greed is summed up by Noah Gordon in biblical terms.[135] Gordon's Dr Silverstone 'wanted to be a healer and a capitalist, Jesus Christ and the money changers all rolled into one'.[143]

Summary

For more than two and a half millennia, the doctor's payment has been an integral aspect (and, for the most part, an annoying aspect) of the doctor–patient relationship. Both patient and doctor are aware of the incongruity of the fee, and various methods have been devised to minimize the direct passage of money from one hand to the other. The perception that financially poor doctors are also professionally poor is deeply entrenched and leads to the inevitable paradox that patients want their doctors to be financially successful, but resent this success and are reluctant to contribute to it.

References

1 Hammurabi (23rd century BC), Code of Laws. In: Johns CHW (1903) *The Oldest Code of Laws in the World*. T and T Clark, Edinburgh, pp. 45–7.

2 Pindar (approx. 474 BC) Pythian Odes. In: *The Odes of Pindar*. Translated by Sandys J. Loeb Classical Library. Heinemann, London, 1946, pp. 189–91.

3 Amundsen DW (1977) Images of physicians in classical times. *J Popular Culture*. 11: 643–55.

4 Aristophanes (388 BC) The Plutus. Translated by Rogers BB. *Loeb's Classical Library*, vol. III. Heinemann, London, 1963, p. 399.

5 Pliny the Elder (Gaius Plinius Secundus) (1st century AD) *Natural History*. Translated by Holland P. Southern Illinois University Press, 1962, Book 29, pp. 294–7.

6   Chaucer G (approx. 1390) Canterbury Tales. In: Fisher JH (ed.) (1977) *The Complete Poetry and Prose of Geoffrey Chaucer*. Holt, Rinehart and Winston, New York, pp. 17–18.

7   Anonymous (15th century) *The Dance of Death*, Warren, Florence (ed.), Early English Text Society, Kraus Reprint Co, New York, 1971, vol. 181, 118 pp.; pp. 53–55.

8   Shakespeare W (1606) In: Wright LB and LaMar VA (eds) (1969) *The Tragedy of Macbeth*, Act V, Scene I. Washington Square Press, New York, pp. 77–8.

9   Ibid., Act V, Scene III, p. 84.

10 Webster J (1623) The Duchess of Malfi, Act III, Scene V. In: Brown JR (ed.) (1976) *The Revels Plays*. Manchester University Press, Manchester, p. 98.

11 Segal E (1988) *Doctors*. Bantam Books, New York, 1989, pp. 579–81.

12 Gay J (1727) The Sick Man and the Angel (Fable 27). In: Gay J (1969) *Fables*. Scolar Press, Menston, England, p. 90.

13 Warren RP (1946) *All the King's Men*. Modern Library, New York, 1953.

14 Ibid., p. 113.

15 Belloc H (1940) *Selected Cautionary Verses*. Penguin, Harmondsworth, 1973, pp. 23–4.

16 Heller J (1962) *Catch 22*. Dell Publishing Co, New York, 1974, pp. 33–41.

17 Anonymous (1987) Miss Polly had a Dolly. In: Pooley S. *A Day of Rhymes*. Knopf, New York, p. 65.

18 Anonymous (1978) In: Turner I, Factor J and Lowenstein W. *Cinderella Dressed in Yella*. Heinemann Educational, Richmond, Victoria, Australia, p. 32.

19 Céline LF (1932) *Journey to the End of the Night*. Translated by Manheim R. New Directions, New York, 1983, p. 359.

20 Maurois A (1921) *Colonel Bramble*. Translated by Wake T. Jonathan Cape, London, 1937, p. 222.

21 Williams WC (1938) The Girl with a Pimply Face. In: Williams WC (1984) *The Doctor Stories*. New Directions, New York, pp. 49–53.

22 Dostoyevsky F (1880) *The Brothers Karamazov*, vol. 2. Translated by Magarshak D. Penguin, Harmondsworth, 1978, p. 633.

23 Tolstoy L (1891) The Kreutzer Sonata. Translated by Maude A. In: Simmons EJ (ed.) (1966) *Leo Tolstoy, Short Novels*, vol. 2. Modern Library, Random House, New York, 1966, vol. 2, pp. 148–149.

24 Shaw GB (1906) The Doctor's Dilemma. In: *The Bodley Head Bernard Shaw's Collected Plays With Their Prefaces*, vol. 3. Max Reinhardt, The Bodley Head, London, 1971, pp. 228–43.

25 Fiscella K, Franks P, Gold M and Clancy CM (2000) Inequality in quality: addressing socioeconomic, racial and ethnic disparities in health care. *JAMA*. **283**: 2579–84.

26 Slaughter FG (1964) *A Savage Place*. Arrow Books, London, 1966, p. 77.

27 Ravin N (1987) *Evidence*. Charles Scribner's Sons, New York, pp. 151–8.

28 Manzoni A (1827) *The Betrothed*. Translated by Penman B. Penguin, Harmondsworth, 1983, p. 609.

29 Herrick R (1900) *The Web of Life*. Macmillan, London, pp. 117–20.

30 Woolf V (1925) *Mrs Dalloway*. Zodiac Press, London, 1947, p. 105.

31   Mann T (1947) *Doctor Faustus*. Translated by Lowe-Porter HT. Secker and Warburg, London, 1949, pp. 475–6.

32   Dillon TP and Leary N (1940) The Doctor from Dunmore. In: Fowler HG (1957) *Curtain Up: ten short modern plays*. Melbourne University Press, Carlton, Victoria, pp. 117–43.

33   Lathen E (Dominic RB, pseudonym) (1980) *The Attending Physician*. Macmillan, London.

34   Ibid., p. 10.

'35   Ibid., p. 34.

36   Ibid., p. 123.

37   Ravin N (1989) *Mere Mortals*. MacDonald, London, 1990, p. 27.

38   Ibid., p. 48.

39   Miller A (1968) *The Price*. Secker & Warburg, London, pp. 81–2.

40   Ibid., p. 17.

41   Ibid., p. 72.

42   Munthe A (1929) *The Story of San Michele*. John Murray, London, 1950, pp. 188–9.

43   Reade C (1863) *Hard Cash*. Chatto and Windus, London, 1894, pp. 31–2.

44   Turgenev I (1852) The District Doctor. Translated by Garnett C. In: *The Novels of Ivan Turgenev*, vol. 1. Heinemann, London, 1920, p. 56.

45   Proust M (1913–22) *Remembrance of Things Past*, vol. 2. Translated by Scott-Moncrieff CK and Kilmartin T. Penguin, Harmondsworth, 1987, pp. 354–5.

46   Maartens M (1906) *The Healers*. Constable, London.

47   Ibid., pp. 82–3.

48   Maugham WS (1909) Penelope. In: Maugham WS (1960) *The Collected Plays*, vol. 1. Heinemann, London, p. 40.

49   Richardson HH (1917–29) *The Fortunes of Richard Mahony*. Penguin, London, 1990, pp. 188–9.

50   Ibid., p. 680.

51   Céline LF, op. cit., pp. 227–8.

52   Doyle AC (1894) A False Start. In: *Round The Red Lamp*. John Murray, London, 1934, pp. 65–88.

53   Young FB (1928) *My Brother Jonathan*. Heinemann, London, pp. 322–32.

54   Selzer R (1972) The Consultation. In: Selzer R (1974) *Rituals of Surgery*. Harpers Magazine Press, New York, pp. 18–23.

55   The Bible (approx. 7th century BC) Revised Standard Version. Oxford University Press, New York, 1977, Deuteronomy, 23: 18.

56   Tate J (1976) On the Subject of Doctors. In: *Viper Jazz*. Wesleyan University Press, Middletown CT, p. 36.

57   Lewisohn L (1928) *The Island Within*. Harper and Brothers, New York, pp. 215–17.

58   Trollope A (1858) *Doctor Thorne*. Oxford University Press, London, 1963, p. 302.

59   Freud S (1913) On Beginning the Treatment. Further Recommendations in the Technique of Psychoanalysis. In: Strachey J (ed.) (1958) *The Standard Edition*

of the Complete Psychological Works of Sigmund Freud, vol. 12. Hogarth Press, London, pp. 131–3.

60 Richardson S (1747–8) The History of Clarissa Harlowe. In: Stephen L (ed.) (1883) *The Works of Samuel Richardson*, vol. 7. Henry Sotheran, London, pp. 377–8.

61 Babylonian Talmud (approx. 450 AD) Epstein I (ed.) (1964) *Baba Kamma*. Translated by Kirzner EW. Soncino Press, London, p. 85a.

62 Glasgow E (1925) *Barren Ground*. Virago, London, 1986, p. 262.

63 Ibid., p. 89.

64 Gide A (1914) *The Vatican Caves*. Translated by Bussy D. Penguin, Harmondsworth (with 'Strait is the Gate'), 1965, p. 150.

65 Young FB, op. cit., pp. 227–8.

66 Nourse AE (1978) *The Practice*. Futura Publications, London, 1979, pp. 378–80.

67 Caldwell T (1968) *Testimony of Two Men*. Collins, London, 1990, p. 348.

68 James H (1902) *The Wings of the Dove*. Signet Classics, New York, 1964, pp. 400–37.

69 Sobel IP (1973) *The Hospital Makers*. Doubleday, Garden City, NY, p. 325.

70 Ibid., pp. 68–9.

71 Bashford HH (1911) *The Corner of Harley Street: being some familiar correspondence of Peter Harding MD*. Constable, London, 1913, p. 74.

72 Ibid., p. 260.

73 Ibid., p. 201.

74 Doyle AC (1894) The Curse of Eve. In: Doyle AC (1934) *Round the Red Lamp*. John Murray, London, pp. 89–108.

75 Richardson HH, op. cit., pp. 165–7.

76 Rinehart MR (1935) *The Doctor*. Farrar and Rinehart, New York, pp. 19–21.

77 Palmer M (1982) *The Sisterhood*. Bantam Books, New York, 1995, p. 14.

78 Martineau H (1839) *Deerbrook*. Virago Press, London, 1983, p. 426.

79 Zola E (1893) *Doctor Pascal*. Translated by Kean V. Elek Books, London, 1957, pp. 201–2.

80 Shaw GB, op. cit., p. 375.

81 Kingsley S (1933) Men in White. In: Kingsley S (1995) *Five Prize Winning Plays*. Ohio State University Press, Columbus, p. 37.

82 Ibid., p. 67.

83 Green G (1956) *The Last Angry Man*. Charles Scribner's Sons, New York, pp. 46–8.

84 Ibid., p. 424.

85 Updike J (1963) The Doctor's Wife. In: Updike J. *Pigeon Feathers and Other Stories*. Andre Deutsch, London, pp. 197–210.

86 Ozick C (1971) The Doctor's Wife. In: Ozick C (1983) *The Pagan Rabbi and Other Stories*. Penguin, New York, p. 181.

87 Howard S (1932) The Late Christopher Bean. In: Warnock R (1952) *Representative Modern Plays*. Scott Foresman and Company, Chicago, pp. 118–24.

88 Busch F (1984) A History of Small Ideas. In: Busch F. *Too Late American Boyhood Blues*. David R. Godine, Boston, pp. 150–70.

89 Richardson S, op. cit., vol. 7, p. 397.

90 Dickens C (1852–3) *Bleak House*. Collins, London, 1953, p. 796.

91 Williams T (1958) Suddenly Last Summer. In: *The Theatre of Tennessee Williams*, vol. 3. New Directions, New York, 1971, pp. 343–423.

92 Ibid., p. 351.

93 Ibid., p. 365.

94 Ibid., p. 423.

95 Dreiser T (1919) The Country Doctor. In: Dreiser T (1930) *Twelve Men*. Constable, London, pp. 102–22.

96 Norris CB (1969) The Image of the Physician in Modern American Literature, PhD dissertation, University of Maryland.

97 Lewis S (1920) *Main Street*. Harcourt Brace and Company, New York, 1948, pp. 176–9.

98 Bennett A (1923) *Riceyman Steps*. Cassell, London, 1947, p. 230.

99 Ibid., pp. 271–81.

100 Maugham WS (1919) *The Moon and Sixpence*. Penguin, Harmondsworth, 1953, pp. 198–212.

101 Waltari M (1945) *The Egyptian*. Translated by Walford N. Panther Books, London, 1960, p. 194.

102 Balzac H de (1833) *The Country Doctor*. Translated by Marriage E. Dent, London, 1923.

103 Ibid., p. 32.

104 Dostoyevsky F, op. cit., p. 790.

105 Ellis AE (1958) *The Rack*. Penguin, London, 1988, pp. 342–3.

106 Ibid., pp. 260–1.

107 Lapierre D (1985) *City of Joy*. Translated by Spink K. Arrow Books, London, 1991, pp. 335–45.

108 Danby F (Julia Frankau) (1887) *Dr Phillips: a Maida Vale idyll*. Garland Publishing, New York, 1984.

109 Ibid., pp. 27–30.

110 Ibid., pp. 276–86.

111 Ibid., pp. 95–7.

112 Ibid., pp. 186–7.

113 Faulkner W (1930) *As I Lay Dying*. Vintage Books, New York, 1985.

114 Ibid., p. 44.

115 Ibid., p. 204.

116 Ibid., p. 237.

117 Ibid., p. 260.

118 Cozzens JG (1933) *The Last Adam*. Harcourt Brace and Company, New York, pp. 284–9.

119 Cable GW (1883) *Dr Sevier*. James R Osgood and Company, Boston, pp. 6–8.

120 Wharton W (1981) *Dad*. Alfred A Knopf, New York, p. 346.

121 Sheldon S (1994) *Nothing Lasts Forever*. HarperCollins, London, p. 74.

122 Chekhov AP (1887) The Enemies, also titled Two Tragedies, also titled Antagonists. In: Chekhov AP (1994) *Short Stories*. Translated by Fen E. Folio Society, London, pp. 58–72.

123 Maugham WS (1933) The Vessel of Wrath. In: Maugham WS (1975) *Collected Short Stories*, vol. 2. Pan Books, London, pp. 9–46.

124 Lewis S (1924) *Arrowsmith*. Signet Books, New York, 1961, pp. 16–17.

125 Warren RP, op. cit., p. 257.

126 Greene G (1961) *A Burnt-Out Case*. Heinemann and The Bodley Head, London, 1974, p. 15.

127 Ariyoshi S (1967) *The Doctor's Wife*. Translated by Hironaka W and Kostant AS. Kodansha, Tokyo, 1989, p. 76.

128 Céline LF, op. cit., pp. 209–11.

129 Balzac H de (1847) *Cousin Pons*. Translated by Hunt HJ. Penguin, Harmondsworth, 1968, pp. 172–3.

130 Sanders L (1974) *The First Deadly Sin*. Berkley Books, New York, p. 92.

131 Henry O (Porter WS) (1910) Let Me Feel Your Pulse. In: Henry O (1974) *Roads of Destiny and Other Stories*. Hodder and Stoughton, London, pp. 174–86.

132 The Bible (1st century AD) Revised Standard Version. Oxford University Press, New York, 1977, Mark, 5: 25–6.

133 The Bible (1st century AD) Revised Standard Version. Oxford University Press, New York, 1977, Luke, 8: 43.

134 O'Neill E (1928) Strange Interlude. In: O'Neill E (1988) *Complete Plays*, vol. 2. Library of America, New York, p. 642.

135 Richardson S, op. cit., vol. 8, pp. 113–14.

136 O'Connor F (1964) Revelation. In: O'Connor F (1988) *Collected Works*. Library of America, New York, p. 634.

137 Plath S (1965) Lady Lazarus. In: Plath S (1976) *Ariel*. Faber and Faber, London, p. 18.

138 Levenkron S (1978) *The Best Little Girl in the World*. Penguin, London, 1988, pp. 65–89.

139 Eliot G (1871–2) *Middlemarch*. Penguin Books, London, 1988, pp. 484–5.

140 Scott W (1831) *The Abbot*. Adam and Charles Black, London, 1893, p. 280.

141 Strauss MB (1968) *Familiar Medical Quotations*. Little Brown and Company, Boston, pp. 175–8.

142 Cobb IS (1915) Speaking of Operations. In: Zevin ED (ed.) (1945) *Cobb's Cavalcade*. World Publishing Company, Cleveland, pp. 17–37.

143 Gordon N (1969) *The Death Committee*. The Book Society, London, undated, p. 35.

CHAPTER 2

Time

The busy doctor: genuine or sham?

Time constitutes a constant source of frustration and irritation. There are long waits for appointments to see the doctor and there may be further delays before the relevant tests are performed. The patients complain that they spend too much time in the waiting room or too little time in the office. They are made to stay in hospital to await the arrival of a consultant, who invariably has more urgent business than clearing someone for discharge. Physicians seem not to share their patients' sense of urgency and take an unconscionably long time to obtain a laboratory result, to come up with a diagnosis or to start treatment. They refuse to provide accurate time frames for the duration of a particular illness. Patients become particularly angry when the doctor's behavior (or his receptionist's remarks) suggest that every minute is precious to him while they have unlimited time at their disposal. Alison Lurie,[1] in a nostalgic mood, has one of her characters compare the Norman Rockwell-type doctors of her childhood days ('calm, slow, patient'), with their modern counterparts.

> Now, of course, they're all computers, ticking out a diagnosis as fast as possible and on to the next case.[1]

Patients may declare with varying degrees of sincerity 'I know you're a busy man', but Raymond Chandler[2] sees the doctor's lack of time as a total pretense.

> I had some trouble getting through to Dr Lagardie himself. When I did, his voice was impatient. He was very busy, in the middle of an examination, he said. I never knew a doctor who wasn't.[2]

Alice Westerley, the wealthy, self-confident, cosmopolitan widow in Weir Mitchell's *In War Time*,[3] is not herself a patient and can afford to declare herself amused by a young doctor's unpunctuality.

> I know you will have some delightful excuse . . . I envy you doctors your wealth of excuses.[3]

The office visit

Alison Lurie's historical comparison[1] notwithstanding, the crowded waiting room, the brusque physician and the abrupt termination of the interview were well described in the 1860s, though the patients of that period seem more accepting of these annoyances than their modern counterparts. In Reade's *Hard Cash*,[4] Mrs Dodd, who has consulted several 'Barkington' doctors about her nineteen-year-old daughter Julia (who is 'love-sick'), has now decided to see a nationally renowned specialist and the two of them are sitting

> patiently at the morning levee of an eminent and titled London surgeon. Full forty patients were before them so they had to wait and wait. At last they were ushered into the presence chamber, and Mrs Dodd entered on the beaten ground of her daughter's symptoms. The noble surgeon stopped her civilly but promptly. 'Auscultation will give us the clue,' said he and drew his stethoscope.[4]

He finds a 'very slight diastolic murmur', writes a prescription, asks Julia to come again in a month and 'Ting! He struck a bell' to indicate that the cash register was ready to receive another patient's fee.[4]

One hundred and forty years later, the waiting room scene in Lightman's *The Diagnosis*[5] epitomizes the time element that causes patients to become angry and frustrated. Bill Chalmers, the afflicted hero, has a ten thirty appointment with his physician, Dr Armand Petrov. He hurries from the subway station but when he reaches Petrov's office with two minutes to spare he finds half a dozen patients ahead of him.

> At 10.35 a man leaped out of his chair and advanced upon the receptionist. 'I can't wait any longer . . . my appointment was at ten . . . Does Petrov think he's the only one whose time is valuable?' The receptionist retreated a few paces and whispered something to an assistant behind her. 'I'm sorry,' she said, returning to the front desk. 'Dr Petrov is busy with another patient at the moment. Would you like me to reschedule your appointment?' 'Reschedule!' the man shrieked. 'So that I can waste another half-day waiting?'[5]

A young woman in the same waiting room, who also has a ten o'clock appointment, has been typing away on her laptop computer and now needs an important document. She asks the receptionist whether she might receive a fax so that she can continue working, but is informed that fax services are not available for patients.

> From somewhere behind her, the assistant whispered something and the receptionist stifled a laugh.

The woman with the laptop objects:

> 'It would not be at all unreasonable for you to offer fax service to your patients . . . especially when you keep us waiting so long . . . Hotels offer fax service.' 'Maybe you should walk over to the Holiday Inn across the street,' blurted the invisible assistant, and she released a loud guffaw.[5]

(The fax machine is turned off and the waiting continues.)

Once a patient has penetrated the inner sanctum, a 'double-standard' applies and the doctor becomes very parsimonious with his time.[4-6] A patient arriving behind schedule may even receive a lecture on the virtue of punctuality. Thomas Mann's Dr Behrens, who thinks nothing of confining his patients to bed for weeks, reprimands the two cousins, Hans and Joachim, for being a few minutes late for a consultation in his office. Ostentatiously looking at the wall-clock, he tells them to hurry. 'We are not here simply and solely for the honorable gentlemen's convenience.'[7] This newly discovered promptness also annoys Harold Dietrich, the aggressive father of an anorectic daughter in Levenkron's *The Best Little Girl in the World*.[8] Dr Smith, a psychiatrist, terminates his consultation with Francesca Dietrich and her parents after fifty minutes. When the family has been ushered out of the doctor's office, Harold 'looked at his watch. It was precisely ten minutes to two. "Prompt son of a bitch, isn't he"'.[8] (*See also* p. 201)

The hospital

In hospital settings, patients become resentful or openly hostile when they have to wait, for no obvious reason, to receive treatment or to undergo tests. Major John Morton, who has been transferred to a Philadelphia military hospital after sustaining a gunshot wound in the leg at Gettysburg,[9] and who is clearly in a great deal of pain, is made to wait for his opium. Instead of providing instant relief for the wounded soldier, Dr Ezra Wendell,[6] one of Weir Mitchell's 'inferior' physicians,[10] concentrates on preserving his own status.

> 'We'll see about it . . . when we make evening rounds.' 'Confound the fellow and his evening round!' growled the major under his mustache. 'I wish he had my leg.'[9]

By contrast, Pavel Nikolayevich Rusanov, a Communist Party Functionary in Alexander Solzhenitsyn's *Cancer Ward*,[11] does not suffer in silence. Rusanov, who has been admitted to a provincial hospital because of lymphoma, believes he is not being treated expeditiously and vents his impatience on Dr Ludmila Afanasyevna Dontsova, a docile female oncologist.

> Pavel Nikolayevich . . . waited until Ludmila Afanasyevna was quite close to his bed then he adjusted his glasses and declared . . . 'I shall inform the Ministry of Health of the way things are conducted in this clinic . . . I have been here for eighteen hours and nobody is giving me treatment.' Dontsova . . . said in a quiet conciliatory tone, 'That's why I'm here, to give you treatment.' 'No, it's too late. I've seen quite enough of the way things are done here and I'm leaving. No one shows the slightest interest, nobody bothers to make a diagnosis.'[11]

This scene, which is witnessed by several other patients, ends in reconciliation. The patient, who has nowhere else to go, accepts medical advice to have chemotherapy, although there is a further outburst when he is told that, for some bureaucratic reason, he can not commence treatment on a Saturday.[11] This confrontational scene occurs in Communist Russia but the conflict over time could equally well have taken place in a Western country.

In the days of long rest cures in mountain sanatoria, the patients had to put up with apparently arbitrary decisions involving weeks or months of restricted activities leading to much resentment and an occasional confrontation. Hans Castorp, the principal character of Thomas Mann's *Magic Mountain*,[12] who has been confined to bed for three weeks

> reminded the head physician ['Hofrat' Behrens] on his morning round that the three weeks were out and asked leave to get up. 'What the deuce – you don't say!' said Behrens. 'Time's up is it? Let's see: Yes, you're right – good Lord how fast we grow old! . . . Well Castorp, I won't grudge you human society any longer. Up with you man and get on with your walks.' . . . [Hans] raised the question . . . [with his cousin] how long the Hofrat might have let him lie had he not been reminded.[12]

On another occasion, when Hans' cousin, Joachim, asks how much longer he has to stay in the sanatorium, the Hofrat becomes irritated. 'So are going to pester me again? . . . Have a little ordinary politeness.'[13]

A somewhat similar scene (also in a sanatorium setting) is described by AE Ellis in *The Rack*.[14] Paul Davenant, an intelligent, sensitive university student who has just been admitted, asks for information about his future.

> 'Excuse me, but how long do you think I shall have to stay here?' Dr Bruneau glanced over his shoulder: 'You should know, monsieur, that this is not the sort of place to which you come for three weeks.' 'Yes, yes, of course. All I ask is the very least idea.' 'Monsieur, we are doctors, not prophets.'[14]

When, after months of inaction, Paul is suddenly summoned (at half past twelve on a Saturday afternoon) for the induction of a pneumothorax,[15] the nurse 'chided him for his slowness as he tried to pull on a pair of heavy socks, bustled him into his ancient and shabby dressing gown and preceded him from the room'.[15] There is a delay at the elevator so that Paul has to walk down several flights of stairs. In the treatment room, three obviously impatient physicians are awaiting him. When he is a little slow at getting undressed, one of them remarks: 'We are waiting, monsieur'.[15] Davenant bears his tribulations without protest.*

On a subsequent occasion Paul Davenant has to put up with yet another time-related frustration – the interruption of a diagnostic procedure with prolongation of his discomfort.[17] Dr Vernet, who is performing an old-fashioned bronchogram, has just injected contrast medium into an endobronchial tube, when he has to take an urgent long-distance call. During his absence his assistant and one of the nurses discuss the performance of an American actor in a recent movie. The nurse is 'bent double with laughter' while Paul is waiting anxiously for the 'next item on the program'.[17]

---

* Through judicious selection of patients and various Machiavellian tactics, the physician in charge of Somerset Maugham's *Sanatorium*[16] avoids impatience for discharge as a cause of resentment in his establishment.

Time is not the only issue in Lars Magnussen's resentment of the medical profession but it is a major factor. Magnussen, the principal character in Ravin's *Informed Consent*,[18] is the archetype of the 'difficult' patient – difficult to handle because he hates doctors and hospitals, and difficult to diagnose because he suffers from a rare disease – Multiple Endocrine Neoplasia Type II. During a herniorrhaphy, his blood pressure fluctuates wildly, so, at 11 am on the day after the operation, the surgeon asks him to stay until Dr McCullough, the internist, has checked him out.

> McCullough didn't get . . . [the surgeon's] message until three thirty and he had two patients to see in his office. At four o'clock Lars walked out of his room, suitcase in hand, trailed by . . . the head nurse who wanted him to wait for McCullough or sign the Against Medical Advice form. Lars had no intention of doing either.

When reproached by his wife for not waiting, he is quite unrepentant. He argues that if he had waited, Dr McCullough would no doubt have behaved as he had during the preoperative visit, when he presented his card, asked Lars to see him at his office and

> stepped into the hall where he noted Lars' name and Blue Cross number so he could bill him for taking his blood pressure and giving him his card.[18]

Occasionally patients complain, mostly inappropriately, that they require two surgical operations and that the doctors, through indifference or lack of organizational skills, fail to have the two procedures performed simultaneously. Alfred Groves, Dr Rushton's truculent patient, who requires an emergency aortic embolectomy,[19,20] feels aggrieved because his bunions are not fixed while he is anesthetized. Groves cannot understand that quite apart from the dangers inherent in orthopedic procedures on ischemic feet, it would be most disruptive for the orthopedic surgeons and their other patients if Groves' bunionectomy were to be scheduled as an emergency procedure.

The confrontational scene in the surgeons' waiting room in Lawrence Sanders' *The First Deadly Sin*[21] is also related, at least in part, to a perceived lack of urgency in a doctor's attitude. Police Captain Delaney has been waiting for many hours to interview Dr Spencer, the surgeon who operated on his wife earlier in the day but who has subsequently been caught up in some other surgical disaster. In the small hours of the morning Delaney finds his way to the surgeons' lounge.

> He saw a small room, one couch, two armchairs, a TV set, a card table and four folding chairs. There were five men in the room wearing surgical gowns, skull caps and masks pulled down over their chests . . . One man was standing, staring out a window, one was fiddling with the knobs on the TV set . . . one was trimming his fingernails with a small pocket knife. One was seated at the card table, carefully building an improbable house of leaned cards. One was stretched out on the floor raising and lowering his legs doing some kind of exercise. 'Dr Spencer?' Delaney said sharply. The man at the window turned slowly, glanced at the uniform, turned back to the window. The Captain said 'My name is Delaney. You operated on my wife earlier this evening. Kidney stones. I want to

know how she is.' Spencer turned again to look at him. The other men did not pause in their activities. 'Delaney,' Spencer repeated. 'Kidney stones. Well, I had to remove the kidney.' 'What?' 'I had to take out one of your wife's kidneys.' 'Why?' 'It was infected, diseased, rotted.' 'Infected with what?' 'It's down in the lab. We'll know tomorrow.' The man building a house of cards looked up, 'You can live with one kidney,' he said mildly to Delaney. 'Listen,' Delaney said choking, 'listen, you said there'd be no trouble.' 'So?' Spencer asked. 'What do you want from me? I'm not God.'[21]

Sanders' description is significant, not so much because of the 'I'm not God' remark, which is not unusual among doctors who have run out of therapeutic options,[22] but because of the clash of two different timescales. The surgeons and anesthetists are presumably waiting for another patient and engage in time-wasting pursuits, while the patient's husband is infuriated by this inaction.[21] Delaney is also incensed at the surgeon's apparent mañana attitude towards the bacteriological results.

Childbirth

The doctor's late appearance or non-appearance at a confinement is rarely commented upon even in the days of home deliveries, though there are some notable exceptions. Robert Johnson, the expectant father in Conan Doyle's *The Curse of Eve*,[23] is outraged by his doctor's relaxed attitude. Johnson's wife has gone into labor and he has finally tracked down Doctor Miles after searching for him all over town.

> 'If you please doctor, I've come for you,' he cried; 'the wife was taken bad at six o'clock.' He hardly knew what he expected the doctor to do. Something very energetic, certainly – to seize some drugs, perhaps and rush excitedly with him through the gas-lit streets.

Instead, the doctor declares that he is going to have some dinner first.

> A sort of horror filled Robert Johnson as he gazed at this man who could think about his dinner at such a moment . . . To Johnson he seemed little better than a monster. His thoughts were bitter as he sped back.[23]

(The story ends happily.)

The Jessup baby in *Home is the Sailor*[24] has been born in the absence of the family's regular doctor.

> Although a young doctor from Monson successfully delivered a fine boy weighing eight pounds . . . the Jessups as a family remained unsatisfied. They felt they had been slighted and their injured feelings over-rode all the usual relief and joy, which goes along with young parenthood . . . what other professional call, they reasoned loudly in a chorus, could possibly be more important than the arrival of this child![24]

Doctor Gray and the local nurse have been busy in his laboratory, operating on cats. Within days the Jessups' righteous indignation turns into open slander.

The doctor's recreational activities

Doctors, like all other persons, are allowed some leisure time. On Sundays, one finds

> doctors at country clubs, doctors at the seaside, doctors with mistresses, doctors with wives . . . doctors everywhere resolutely being people, not doctors.[25]

However, many of the doctors' spare-time pursuits are resented or at least perceived as incongruous. How dare this man enjoy himself with his mistress or his wife (in that order[25]) while his patients are suffering and dying? Esther Greenwood[25] who is bleeding from a post-coital vaginal tear on a Sunday cannot believe that the doctors' trivial spare-time activities would take precedence over her medical emergency.

Fancy dress parties seem particularly inappropriate. Van der Meersch's *Bodies and Souls*[26] begins with the annual medical dinner where, once a year, the students stage a revue lampooning the faculty members who also attend on these occasions. One talented performer has dressed up in a waitress' apron and is about to launch into a satirical song concerning the activities of one of the professors, when he is summoned to a suburban house where a young girl is bleeding to death. As he leaves the party he finds that he is still wearing the symbolic and ridiculous apron.[26]

In Ellis' *The Rack*,[27] Doctors Vernet and Bruneau hurriedly leave the hospital fancy dress ball because a delirious woman with tuberculous meningitis has climbed over a number of balconies, landing in another patient's room. 'The door was thrown open and in ran the doctors . . . unbuttoned white coats flying, flapping over carnival costumes.' During her forcible removal the woman hits her face against the door handle and screams that the staff are trying to assassinate her. Presently, Dr Vernet returns 'now carrying his white coat over his arm; he was dressed as a rather stocky harlequin'. Dr Bruneau, who has been deputed to give the woman a sedative, joins his colleague a little later.

> In one hand he was carrying a hypodermic syringe with a long needle attached, in the other, a false nose. He went straight over to a mirror, slipped off his white coat and rearranged his costume, that of a Renaissance jester.[27]

The sedative proves ineffective and the agitated woman kills herself by jumping out of a fourth-floor window before the doctors have a chance to return to their festivities. When Dr Bruneau emerges from the entrance to examine the body, he is still carrying his false nose.[27]

Jean Stafford's Dr Nicholas, who is singled out for special scrutiny and a great deal of distaste,[28] participates in a great many extracurricular activities. He is

> young, brilliant and handsome . . . an aristocrat, a husband, a father, a clubman, a Christian, a kind counsellor and a trustee of his preparatory school.

We do not observe Nicholas functioning in his various non-medical roles, but whatever his achievements in these endeavors, as a doctor he is a disaster[28] (*see* Chapter 3).

Visits to the theatre are suspect,[29] departures during a performance to attend to an emergency even more so.[30] Robertson Davies' Dr Bliss

> had tiptoed out with that stealth peculiar to doctors which is so much more noticeable than a frank exit.[30]

Patients take exception to Wednesday afternoon golf on the grounds that the morning patients are given short shrift so that the doctor can tee off on time.[31] The unnamed Palm Springs 'desert' physician, who is unable to distinguish between exercise-induced hematuria and glomerulonephritis, spends insufficient time considering his patient's condition, he looks at the clock while delivering his death sentence because of a Wednesday afternoon golf date,[31] and he provides a totally incorrect survival time, 'two years maybe'.

Even the doctor's home comforts are considered incongruous. Maugin, Simenon's famous actor, whose lifestyle is chaotic and who is consulting Dr Biguet out of hours and in his home[32] (*see* pp 87–8 and p. 108) is resentful of the doctor's domesticity. Admittedly, he has other reasons to feel aggrieved. The doctor, who presumably smells cheap wine on Maugin's breath, does not bother to ask questions about his alcohol intake.

> Did he resent Biguet's discretion in not mentioning wine or alcohol? Or was it only the specialist's silence that irritated him, his calm, his apparent serenity or, even more, his luck in being on the other side of the [fluoroscopic] screen?[32]

Maugin is particularly annoyed by the coziness of the Doctor's apartment, 'the drawing room with the log fire and the grand piano, even the doctor's velvet smoking jacket'.

When Dr Zajac in *The Fourth Hand*[33] makes a special appointment to see his patient, Patrick Wallingford, on a Saturday morning

> it was deeply disconcerting to Patrick that Dr Zajac, specifically his face, smelled of sex. The evidence of a private life was not what Wallingford wanted to know about his hand surgeon.[33]

Chess and jogging generate less resentment than other recreational activities, presumably because chess is perceived to provide training in problem solving,[34] while jogging, an intrinsically unpleasant activity, is practiced by eccentric, obsessive individuals and provides physical training.[35]

The doctor's assistant

The presence of an assistant, however inexperienced, *as well as* the nominated doctor, provides the chief with additional status and is rarely resented.[36] By contrast, the arrival of an assistant *instead of* the doctor sends a message to the patient that the senior person does not have the time to come himself, because he is engaged in more important medical or non-medical activities. The resulting resentment is vividly described in the Bible.[37] In more contemporary literature, 'Doctor Harding'[38] explains this 'syndrome' in some detail. Trying to reassure a young 'locum tenens' who has been dismissed in favour of an older man, Harding tells his young colleague of his own experience.

> When I was about twenty-four, [I was] called up . . . to attend a confinement. It was three o'clock in the morning and . . . walking down the empty streets in a pallid drizzle of rain, a certain sense of heroism came to my rescue. After all, it was a noble thing to be doing; and no doubt my patient would be proportionately grateful. As a matter of solemn fact, on setting eyes upon me she lifted up her voice and wept incontinently . . . She had expected to see the genial, middle-aged physician who had often attended her; and behold, in his stead, a pale-faced boy who might very nearly have been her son! It was no wonder that she burst into tears.[38]

(The lady delivers a normal baby and becomes reconciled to the boy-doctor.)

John O'Hara's *The Doctor's Son*[39] is set in a small colliery town during the 1918 influenza epidemic. 'Doctor' Myers, a final-year medical student from the University of Pennsylvania, is taking Dr Michael Malloy's calls while James, the doctor's son, is driving the car and telling the story. The head of the Loughran family who belongs to the 'lower classes' (*see* Chapter 10) is furious when, instead of Dr Malloy, a young relieving doctor comes to examine a sick family member. Loughran does not accept this state of affairs with quiet resignation.

> Doctor Myers went in. He came out in less than two minutes, followed by Mr Loughran. Loughran walked over to me. 'You,' he said. 'Ain't we good enough for your Dad no more? What kind of a thing is this he be sending us?' 'My father is sick in bed like everybody else, Mr Loughran. This is the doctor that is taking all his calls till he gets better.' 'It is, is it? So that's what we get and doctoring with Mike Malloy since he come from college and always paid the day after payday. Well young man, take this back to Mike Malloy. You tell him for me if my woman pulls through it'll be no thanks to him. And if she don't pull through and dies, I'll come right down to your old man's office and kill him with a rock. Now you and this one get the hell outa here before I lose me patience.'[39]

Nourse's Herman Barney, a patient with morbid obesity and pulmonary edema,[40] expresses himself in very similar terms when faced by a new doctor. Having squeezed himself into the passenger seat of his car, Barney is now unable to walk the few steps from the parking lot to the doctors' office, and insists on being examined and treated where he is. Furthermore, despite his precarious state of health, he is seething with hostility, because Dr Martin Isaacs, his regular physician, is unavailable. Dr Rob Tanner, Isaacs' new assistant, and Agnes, the clinic nurse, are standing by the open car window, barely able to avoid the jets of Barney's pink frothy sputum.

> He sat back to catch his breath . . . then looked malevolently up at Rob.
> 'Where's Isaacs?' he said in a wheezy rasp. Agnes stepped forward. 'Mr
> Barney, Dr Isaacs had to go up to the hospital.' 'Hospital my ass. I saw
> the goddam bastard drive out of here when we drove in.' He pointed a
> thumb at Rob. 'Who's this?' 'This is Dr Tanner, our new doctor.' . . .
> 'Goddam bastard said he'd be here this afternoon. I don't want to see no
> new doctor.' 'Well he's gone and he won't be back,' Agnes said. 'I think
> he's delivering a baby.' 'Baby my ass,' the fat man snorted. 'Goddam
> bastard's hiding.' . . . Agnes started to say something but Rob shushed
> her. 'Look Mr Barney, maybe I can help. What's the trouble?' 'What the
> hell does it look like?' the fat man roared. 'I can't breathe, that's what's
> the trouble.'[40]

Surprisingly, Rob's emergency treatment is successful despite the unusual circumstances and Barney's hostility. The two establish a reasonable relationship, much to
Dr Isaacs' disgust, and Barney actually loses some weight.

Robert Berquam, a medical technologist whose anger against doctors forms the
central theme of *Ward 402*, is furious at having to deal with the house staff rather
than the head of the unit.[41] Determined to transmit his hostility to the parents of
other children on the ward, he is lecturing Herbert Handleman, the father of a boy
with renal failure, whose second renal allograft has to be removed because of acute
rejection. The chief resident (Dr Cane) performs the operation because the head of
the Transplant Unit (Dr Kadden) is out of town.

> 'Believe me, Herb,' . . . [Robert] was saying, 'I've been round hospitals
> long enough to know they could have got Kadden if they'd wanted to.
> How hard do you think Cane tried? If you were a bank president or the
> head of a big company, you can bet they would have let Kadden know.'
> . . . 'He was out of town,' Handleman said. 'It's been eighteen hours
> since. Have you heard from him yet? There is absolutely no reason why
> you should have to deal with anybody but the boss, especially with . . .
> residents you've never seen before. He's your child, not theirs.'[41]

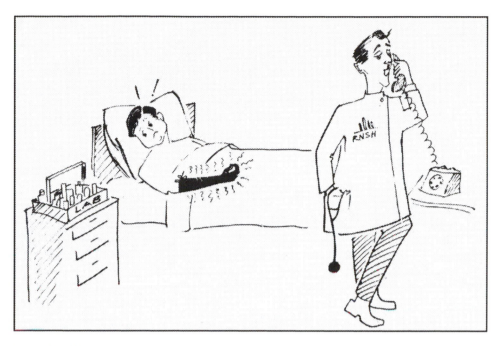

Figure 2.1 The perception of time is a constant source of friction between doctors and patients. Reproduced by permission of Royal North Shore Hospital, Sydney, Australia.

Time constraints as perceived by the doctor

From the doctor's perspective, the problem of time looks quite different. There are patients to see, procedures to perform, telephone messages to answer, not to mention domestic commitments; now comes a 'demanding' patient wanting urgent attention. Ever since doctors first appear as fictional heroes in the early nineteenth century, their capacity for hard, unpleasant and dangerous work, while a major source of strength, has also been a source of annoyance to individual patients who want attention now. Harriet Martineau's Dr Edward Hope, who leaves 'a warm room to go out into the cold night',[42] will not be available if some other caller arrives during his absence. When he is summoned to see a patient in a geriatric establishment, he comes back late because other inmates develop the 'While-You're-Here-Doctor' syndrome.

> They could not expect to see Edward for some hours as he had been sent for to the almshouses . . . When he was sent for by one of the inmates, nearly all the rest were wont to discover that they ailed more or less; so that their medical guardian found it no easy matter to get away and his horse had learned, by practice, to stand longer there than anywhere else without fidgeting.[42]

During cholera and plague epidemics physicians continue working, oblivious of any danger to themselves. Naturally, during these crises, anyone with what the doctor considers 'trivial' complaints will receive short shrift. In Charles Kingsley's *Two Years Ago*,[43] Dr Tom Thurnell

> thought nothing about death and danger at all. Always smiling, always cheerful, always busy yet never in a hurry, he went up and down, seemingly ubiquitous. Sleep he got when he could and food as often as he could. [He was] the only person in the town who seemed to grow healthier and actually happier as the work went on.[43]

Doctor Rieux, the main character and chronicler in Camus' *The Plague*,[44] is not as cheerful as Thurnell, but just as dedicated. Rieux has set up a hospital in

> a requisitioned school house. [It] now contained five hundred beds, almost all of which were occupied. After the reception of the patients which he personally supervised Rieux injected serum, lanced buboes, checked the statistics again and returned for his afternoon consultations. Only when night was setting in, did he start on his round of visits and he never got home till a very late hour . . . His visits were beginning to put a great strain on his endurance. Once the [disease] was diagnosed, the patient had to be evacuated forthwith. Then . . . began . . . a tussle with the family . . . When he came home at two in the morning . . . his mother was shocked at the blank look he gave her.[44]

Even during normal times physicians have to endure punishing work schedules both within and outside hospitals. Hospital interns are on duty for thirty-six hour shifts,[45–48] and have to work either Christmas Day or New Year's Eve.[49] Physicians in practice have 'to face all weathers at all hours of the night and day, often not enjoying a complete night's rest for a week'.[50] They get out of bed in the small hours of the morning to attend to their patients though they may express some resentment at not having been called sooner.[51,52] Here is Sinclair Lewis' 2 am encounter between a migrant farmer and Dr Will Kennicott, who practices in a small Minnesota town.[51] The two speak in a mixture of Pidgin-German and English.

> 'Morgen, doctor. Die Frau ist ja awful sick. All night she been having an awful pain in the belly.' 'How long she been this way? Wie lang, eh?' 'I dunno, maybe two days.' 'Why didn't you come for me yesterday instead of waking me up out of a sound sleep?' . . . 'She got soch a lot vorse last evening. I t'ought maybe all de time it go away but it got a lot vorse.'[51]

A few minutes later Kennicott is on his way to a homestead 'hungry, chilly and unprotesting', while his wife, Carol (who stays in bed), fantasizes about 'the drama of his riding by night to the frightened household on the distant farm; pictured children standing at a window waiting for him'.[51] He was back four hours later and by 7.15 he was grumbling 'Aren't you ever going to get up for breakfast?'[51]

Mauriac's unnamed doctor who is summoned after one of Thérèse's midnight 'crises'[53] has obviously been pulled out of bed but does not impose a similar ordeal on the patient's relatives. The doctor arrives still half asleep with puffy eyes and his hair tousled. He had put on a topcoat over his nightshirt. After listening to Thérèse's heart, he followed Marie into the passage. Their whispering was interspersed with bursts of louder talk. 'But of course you must get them . . . Tomorrow morning . . . first thing . . . not later.'[53]

The constant demand on the doctor's time forms a common denominator between the most diverse members of the profession. Dr Ludovic Vallorge,[54] a scheming French medical academic, who spends a good deal of time and effort in furthering the advancement of his career, has little in common with Dr Benedict Mady Copeland,[55] a black American general practitioner, except that both are capable of honest hard work which they do not resent.

> Vallorge, without . . . neglecting the backstairs intrigues . . . that went on at the Faculty, prepared, revised and produced his lectures immaculately. He did the rounds . . . at the hospital every morning. He never disconnected the night bell . . . He could be summoned at midnight or in the course of . . . a party . . . to go to a [poor] patient with colic; Vallorge would slip into his overcoat, go and get his car out in the snow and drive off; and then for three francs sixty which the municipality might or might not pay him, he would spend the rest of the night at his patient's bedside, without ill-humor or the slightest trace of being put out.[54]

Dr Copeland,[55] one of the few black medical practitioners in fictional literature, fails in his attempt to instill a Marxist philosophy into the black community in his home town. Indeed, his unrealistic ideology has alienated his own wife and children (*see* Book II, Chapter 1). However, he is able to sublimate his frustrated political ambitions by engaging in a constant grind of hard medical work.

> He went from one house to another and the work was unending. Very early in the morning he drove off in his automobile and then at eleven o'clock the patients came to the office . . . The benches in the hall were always full of sick and patient Negroes who waited for him and some-times even the front porch and his bedroom would be crowded. All the day and frequently half the night there was work.[55]

Even office practice may create inevitable disruptions to the doctor's schedule. William Carlos Williams' doctor[56] has been seeing patients in his office since 1 pm; it is now half past three

> and a number of calls still to be made about the town . . . 'Anybody left out there?' I asked the last woman, as I thought, who had been waiting for me. 'Oh yes, there's a couple with a baby.'

The doctor conceals his impatience, he suppresses his desire to walk out and he complies with the migrant parents' request that the child be fully examined. A long discussion about feeding problems ensues. When that is over, and the doctor makes a second attempt to leave his office, 'the man stopped me. Doc, he said, I want you to examine my wife'.[56] Resistance is considered useless. 'I simply gave up and returned to my desk chair. Go ahead. What's the matter with her?' The doctor is rewarded for his forbearance by the discovery of a diagnostic problem. It turns out that the woman who is severely bow-legged suffers from nocturnal pains in the legs. There is also a large ecchymosis near the left knee 'where in all probability a varicose vein had ruptured . . . "Is that what makes her have the pain?"' When the doctor has finished answering questions and giving advice concerning lifestyle, he finally relents and gives the woman what she has come for – a prescription.

> 'Can you swallow a pill?' . . . 'Let see,' said the woman. I showed a few of the pills to her on the palm of my hand. 'For pain in leg?' 'Yes,' I told her.

At that point the doctor receives a second reward.

> For the first time since I had known her a broad smile spread all over her face. 'Yeah,' she said, 'I swallow him.'[56]

Dr Macklin Riley, an oncologist at the 'Parkinson Cancer Center', is exhausted as he returns to his office around 7 pm.[57] He has spent the afternoon seeing multiple patients at the clinic, he then discussed a management problem with two colleagues, he has been to visit a ten-year-old boy with leukemia and he is longing to go home even though home is 'a little room piled with packing crates'.[57] (His wife recently decamped; *see* Book II, Chapter 1.)

> He shuffled through the pink message slips as if there might be something there to lighten his spirits. Mr Donaldson had abdominal pains. Mrs Ingall's leg was worse. Janet Owsley had trouble breathing. Would he write another prednisone prescription for Annie Golden? Barbara Morse was having a bad reaction to the adriamycin – her doctor had called. Dorothy Clay wanted to know if she should come in next week.[57]

Dr Riley is hungry and tired but it will be a long time before he gets 'home'. Instead of a game of tennis followed by a proper meal, he has to make do with a substitute for both, a symbolic chocolate tennis racket, which provides no physical or culinary pleasure but staves off his hunger pangs for a while.

> He reached over . . . to an open box of fancy chocolates in the shape of sports equipment, the latest of the gift boxes from patients. He . . . bit into the chocolate tennis racket . . . it tasted like sawdust. Still chewing, he began to dial the first of his calls.[57]

Riley is not a medical hero. His ex-wife accuses him of having become a social climber[58] and he proves her right by marrying a divorcee from one of the wealthiest New York families.[59] His research activities are 'inadequate and badly prepared'.[60] Artistically he is totally illiterate; even the paintings at the Frick Gallery 'give him the creeps'[61] (*see* Book II, Chapter 5). He lets himself be seduced by the married daughter of one of his patients and then complains about his guilt complexes.[59] He has become 'depressed about his medical skills',[59] he feels insecure and he needs something doctors are not supposed to need – reassurance.[62] Despite all his flaws and despite the wealth and power of his new wife, he keeps up a grueling work schedule and may well continue to do so.

Jim Wyatt, the idealistic young doctor in *Bright Scalpel*,[63] on a visit to an elderly woman in a nursing home, obviously underestimates the time required to listen to her complaints, and is duly reprimanded.

> He sat down at Mrs Bathgate's bedside and let the old shrew tell him how terribly Annie neglected her, how awful the food was and how ungrateful her children were to put her in such a place.[63]

When Dr Wyatt decides he has listened long enough and leaves the room, he can hear 'Mrs Bathgate's announcement that she was going to change doctors'.[63]

Frederick Busch provides timescales for the activities taking place on both sides of the partitioning wall. In the office is Dr Eli Silver, a pediatrician conducting an office practice in Upstate New York,[64] who feels frustrated by the repetitive nature of the work and the pressure of multiple patients in the waiting room, though he experiences brief bursts of professional satisfaction.

> There is croup. There is diarrhea, there are mouth lesions from Coxsackie A virus, . . . a baby vomiting, an infant's arm that is covered with flea bites . . . an older hyperactive boy who crawls in circles, jumps from the table, pushes at chairs. He talks with . . . parents of pregnant girls, with women whose children are swallowing their mother's lives. He tells the mother of a six-months infant that her baby gains weight and is perfect. 'You're doing a perfect job.' He . . . caution[s] the mother of an eight year old boy not to worry about bed-wetting. 'How many fifty year olds do you know who wet their beds?' The boy, his face set and crimson, doesn't smile.[65]

Working away at his challenging tasks inside the office, the doctor may give a brief thought to his waiting area where bored patients have nothing to do but appraise the hairstyle of the receptionists, criticize the size, shape and decor of the room, and become annoyed by the 'limp-looking magazines'.[66]

> In the waiting room he can hear the ringing of the telephone, the high tin music of the TV . . . the crying of the children, [and the] low disgruntled tones of impatient parents.[65]

But Dr Silver does not have the time to worry about these issues. He has to concentrate on his patients.

> He sees a mongoloid child cared for by his grandmother. She does it, she says, 'because it's a little too much for Jeff's mother. But Jeffie's kind of special to me.' . . . When the grandmother dresses him while he sits on the examination table Jeff's arm goes along her shoulder in total confidence.[65]

There are literally hundreds of references to long hours, to night calls, to disrupted schedules and to doctors' 'workaholic' attitudes. A few physicians who have come to dislike their trade (*see* Book II, Chapter 4) and some impaired individuals (*see* Book II, Chapter 7) do not fit the pattern of the hard-working doctor but, as a general rule, unlike arrogance, acquisitiveness and alcoholism, laziness is not a medical vice.

Summary

Unless patients have a doctor, a hospital and a laboratory all to themselves, there will be occasions when they will have to wait, for administrative reasons. Until the complexity of physiological processes is totally explicable in terms of physics and chemistry, some imprecision concerning life expectancy and the time course of diseases will remain inevitable, for scientific reasons. In a non-Utopian world, frustrations associated with such problems of time can be mitigated if the patients can be made to understand that delays are not entirely due to bureaucratic bungling and that the doctor's lack of time is not due, as a rule, to a capricious or callous attitude.

References

1   Lurie A (1974) *The War Between the Tates*. Heinemann, London, pp. 57–70.
2   Chandler R (1949) *The Little Sister*. Houghton Mifflin, Boston, MA, p. 31.
3   Mitchell SW (1885) *In War Time*. The Century Company, New York, 1913, p. 81.
4   Reade C (1863) *Hard Cash*. Chatto and Windus, London, 1894, pp. 32–3.
5   Lightman A (2000) *The Diagnosis*. Pantheon Books, New York, pp. 107–14.
6   Cobb IS (1915) Speaking of Operations. In: Zevin ED (ed.) (1945) *Cobb's Cavalcade*. World Publishing Company, Cleveland, OH, pp. 17–37.
7   Mann T (1924) *The Magic Mountain*. Translated by Lowe-Porter HT. Penguin, Harmondsworth, 1960, pp. 176–8.
8   Levenkron S (1978) *The Best Little Girl in the World*. Penguin, London, 1988, pp. 65–77.
9   Mitchell SW, op. cit., p. 14.
10   Malmsheimer R (1988) 'Doctors only': the evolving image of the American physician. *Contributions in Medical Studies*, Number 25, Greenwood Press, New York.
11   Solzhenitsyn A (1968) *Cancer Ward*. Translated by Bethell N and Burg D. Bodley Head, London, 1971, pp. 57–8.
12   Mann T, op. cit., p. 203.
13   Ibid., p. 179.
14   Ellis AE (1958) *The Rack*. Penguin Books, London, 1988, p. 33.
15   Ibid., pp. 71–2.
16   Maugham WS (1947) Sanatorium. In: Maugham WS (1976) *Sixty-Five Short Stories*. Heinemann/Octopus, London, pp. 541–56.
17   Ellis AE, op. cit., pp. 64–7.
18   Ravin N (1983) *Informed Consent*. GP Putnam's Sons, New York, pp. 79–84.

19 Russell R (1985) *While You're Here, Doctor*. Souvenir Press, London.

20 Ibid., pp. 8–11.

21 Sanders L (1973) *The First Deadly Sin*. Berkley Books, New York, 1974, p. 102.

22 Dostoyevsky F (1880) *The Brothers Karamazov*, vol. 2. Translated by Magarshack D. Penguin, Harmondsworth, 1978, pp. 655–9.

23 Doyle AC (1894) The Curse of Eve. In: Doyle AC (1934) *Round the Red Lamp*. John Murray, London, pp. 89–108.

24 Blodgett R (1932) *Home is the Sailor*. Harcourt Brace, New York, p. 289.

25 Plath S (1963) *The Bell Jar*. Bantam Books, New York, 1972, pp. 189–90.

26 Van Der Meersch M (1943) *Bodies and Souls*. Translated by Wilkins E. William Kimber, London, 1953, pp. 9–11.

27 Ellis AE, op. cit., pp. 57–60.

28 Stafford J (1953) *The Interior Castle*. Harcourt Brace and Company, New York, p. 206.

29 McCarthy M (1942) *The Company She Keeps*. Penguin, Harmondsworth, 1975, pp. 185–6.

30 Davies R (1951) Tempest-Tost. In: Davies R (1986) *The Salterton Trilogy*. Penguin, London, p. 240.

31 Wambaugh J (1985) *The Secrets of Harry Bright*. Sphere Books, London, 1987, p. 93.

32 Simenon G (1950) The Heart of a Man. Translated by Varèse L. In: *The Second Simenon Omnibus*. Hamish Hamilton, London, 1974, pp. 151–62.

33 Irving J (2001) *The Fourth Hand*. Bloomsbury, London, p. 169.

34 Remarque EM (1945) *Arch of Triumph*. Translated by Sorell W and Lindley D. Appleton Century, New York, p. 48.

35 Irving J, op. cit., p. 31.

36 Thompson M (1949) *The Cry and the Covenant*. Pan Books, London, 1969, p. 123.

37 The Bible (6th century BC) Revised Standard Version. Oxford University Press, New York, 1977, 2 Kings, 5: 11.

38 Bashford HH (1911) *The Corner of Harley Street: being some familiar correspondence of Peter Harding MD*. Constable, London, 1913, pp. 76–7.

39 O'Hara J (1935) The Doctor's Son. In: O'Hara J (1984) *Collected Stories*, MacShane F (ed.). Random House, New York, pp. 8–9.

40 Nourse AE (1978) *The Practice*. Futura Publications, London, 1979, pp. 219–20.

41 Glasser RJ (1973) *Ward 402*. Garnstone Press, London, 1974, pp. 135–44.

42 Martineau H (1839) *Deerbrook*. Virago Press, London, 1983, pp. 173–8.

43 Kingsley C (1857) *Two Years Ago*. Macmillan and Co., London, 1884, pp. 303–4.

44 Camus A (1947) *The Plague*. Translated by Gilbert S. Penguin, Harmondsworth, 1960, pp. 75–6.

45 Doctor X (Alan E Nourse) (1965) *Intern*. Harper and Row, New York, p. 87.

46 Ravin N (1981) *MD*. Delacorte Press/Seymour Lawrence, New York, 1981, pp. 28–31.

47 Sheldon S (1994) *Nothing Lasts Forever*. HarperCollins, London, pp. 43–5.

48   Ibid., p. 97.

49   Frede R (1960) *The Interns*. Corgi, London, 1965, pp. 19–37.

50   Shaw GB (1906) The Doctor's Dilemma. In: *The Bodley Head Bernard Shaw Collected Plays with their Prefaces*, vol. 3. Max Reinhardt, The Bodley Head, London, 1971, p. 243.

51   Lewis S (1920) *Main Street*. Harcourt Brace and Company, New York, 1948, pp. 176–9.

52   Faulkner W (1930) *As I Lay Dying*. Vintage Books, New York, 1985, p. 44.

53   Mauriac F (1927–35) *Thérèse*. Translated by Hopkins G. Penguin, Harmondsworth, 1959, p. 312.

54   Van der Meersch M (1943) *Bodies and Souls*. Translated by Wilkins E. William Kimber, London, 1950, p. 152.

55   McCullers C (1943) *The Heart is a Lonely Hunter*. Cresset Press, London, 1953, p. 138.

56   Williams WC (1938) A Face of Stone. In: Williams WC (1984) *The Doctor Stories*. New Directions, New York, pp. 78–87.

57   Cheever S (1987) *Doctors and Women*. Methuen, London, 1988, p. 21.

58   Ibid., p. 18.

59   Ibid., pp. 236–8.

60   Ibid., p. 229.

61   Ibid., p. 197.

62   Ibid., p. 219.

63   Seifert E (1941) *Bright Scalpel*. Aeonian Press Inc., New York, 1973, pp. 7–8.

64   Busch F (1979) *Rounds*. Farrar, Straus and Giroux, New York, p. 38.

65   Ibid., pp. 80–1.

66   O'Connor F (1964) Revelation. In: O'Connor F (1988) *Collected Works*. Library of America, New York, p. 634.

CHAPTER 3

The bedside manner

Lady Visitor: 'Oh that's your doctor, is it? What sort of a doctor is he?'
Lady Resident: 'I don't know much about his ability but he's got a very
good bedside manner.'[1]

The professional manner that he ridiculed so often . . . covered up
incompetence and hypocrisy . . . but . . . was . . . useful in . . . such cases
as this . . . One could not be straightforward with women and fools.[2]

Helpful or harmful?

Long before Ivan Illych's attack on what he saw as the 'redundancy' of the doctor–
patient relationship,[3] there was a good deal of discussion, particularly within the
medical profession, concerning the non-scientific component of medical care. Is the
bedside manner necessary? Is it helpful or harmful? The subject is reviewed in detail
by Stoeckle.[4]

The dictionary definition of the term bedside manner ('the deportment of a
medical man towards his patient'[5]) is neutral and carries no pejorative overtones.
After all, the ability to convey information and advice has been a recognized part of
the art of medicine since classical times. Plato even describes medical doctors with
substandard communication skills, who went on their rounds, accompanied by a
'spin-doctor', so as to enhance their credibility. Gorgias the rhetorician[6] successfully
served in that capacity on multiple occasions:

Many and many a time have I gone with my brother or other doctors
to visit one of their patients and found him unwilling either to take
medicine or to submit to the surgeon's knife . . . and when the doctor
failed to persuade him, I succeeded.[6]

Formal courses in communication training are being offered in a number of medical
schools,[7] though there is at present no evidence that such courses enhance patient
satisfaction.

Despite the obvious need for the effective transmission of messages, there is a
widespread perception that the doctor's conduct towards his patients serves as a
substitute for clinical competence[3] and that

the worse the . . . [physician], the better the bedside manner.[8]

Bogus doctors such as Molière's Sganarelle[9] and his English counterpart, Lacy's 'Doctor' Drench,[10] use their superficial acquaintance with bedside patter to convince potential clients and victims that they are genuine members of the profession. Drench is a particularly fast learner:

> 'Let me see how to behave myself like a doctor now. I will first take your mistress by the pulse and look up gravely at the ceiling all the while; then ask what she took last, and when she's had a stool and there's half a doctor's work.'[10]

In this context, the term 'bedside manner' carries intensely negative connotations, implying that doctors are insincere in their dealings with sick people, and that meaningless rituals replace the history and the physical examination. 'Professional' behavior patterns, facial expressions and catch phrases are utilized to impress gullible patients (particularly the rich patients) who, at the end of the consultation, are told what they want to hear or what the doctor thinks they want to hear. One of the young doctors in *The Cry and the Covenant*[11] finds this aspect of medicine particularly repulsive.

> I went with the eminent Dr Brauner the other day to a rich patient. The moment we entered, he set the servants to work. This one to fetch water, the other to bring wool, a third for milk. 'Make your presence felt,' he whispered to me. 'Set everybody running.' One of the family entered and instantly he pulled a grave and portentous face. Now that rigmarole isn't science and it isn't art. It's acting.[11]

Morton Thompson and his characters[11] may not like the play-acting part of medicine, but some pretense is often required for an effective relationship between doctor and patient, whether during a trivial office consultation or at a deathbed. The pretense is resented only when it is recognized as such.

Dress; voice; facial expressions; gestures

The white coat, which has been invested with a good deal of symbolic significance,[12] is, in real life, considered appropriate medical attire by most patients.[13,14] In literature it is resented as an unwarranted badge of authority. Dr Vernet, the authoritarian head of Paul Davenant's tuberculosis sanatorium, who is about to torture Paul with a bronchogram (*see* p. 56), wears, for the occasion, 'a white jacket which was so starched that it crackled when he moved'.[15] Bernhard, one of the most hostile anti-doctor writers of the twentieth century (*see* p. 196), fulminates against 'the white-coated impotence of the medical profession'.[16] The young doctor who inserts a nasogastric tube into Francoise de Beauvoir[17] is characterized by a 'white coat . . . [and an] unresponsive face' as if the two somehow go together. Dr Samuel Abelman, in *The Last Angry Man*,[18] envies his colleague Dr Vogel, who distances himself from his patients by wearing a 'forbidding'[19] white coat. Abelman evidently does not wear any sort of white coat, forbidding or otherwise. Unlike Vogel, he allows his patients to call him by his first name,[19] a practice considered inappropriate by most patients even at the end of the twentieth century.[20,21]

The bedside manner may incorporate a distinctive 'bedside voice' (*see also* p. 180). Dr Amos Varley in Raymond Chandler's *The Long Good-Bye*[22] is, like several of Chandler's physicians, a somewhat dishonest character, but his assumed bedside manner is impeccable.

> 'What can I do for you, Mr Marlowe?' He had a rich soft voice to soothe the pain and comfort the anxious heart. Doctor is here, there is nothing to worry about; everything will be fine. He had that bedside manner, thick honeyed layers of it.[22]

Dr Varley's mask comes off abruptly when Philip Marlowe (a private detective posing as a patient) asks a few awkward questions. 'The sun had set in Dr Varley's manner. It was getting to be a chilly evening.'[22]

Osler has no doubts concerning the doctor's need for a bedside manner, with the most important ingredient comprising an apparent imperturbability. His mantra

> The physician who . . . shows in his face the slightest alteration expressive of anxiety or fear . . . is liable to disaster at any moment[23]

is widely quoted, though the nature of the 'disaster' is not made clear. Arnold Bennett's Dr Raste[24] has learnt this Oslerian precept well.

> He was impenetrable . . . He might be tired or he might not be tired. He might have been roused from his bed at 2.00 am; he might have slept excellently in perfect tranquility . . . The secrets of the night were locked up in that trimly dressed bosom.[24]

Elsie (the housemaid) considers him 'stand-offish, stony', but William Osler would have given him full marks. Michael Crichton's Dr John Berry has also been trained in the school of 'equanimity'.[25] When a policeman provides him with a startling piece of information, he keeps his face absolutely blank.

> Fortunately you have a lot of practice at that in medicine; you are trained to show no surprise if . . . patient[s] tell you they make love ten times a night or have dreams of stabbing their children or drink a gallon of vodka daily. It is part of the mystique of the doctor that nothing surprises him.[25]

Harmless and possibly beneficial[26] gestures like holding a patient's hand during a bedside visit may be perceived as out of place and hypocritical. Roy Basch in *The House of God*,[8] who dislikes most forms of medical practice, is particularly resentful of Dr Putzel, an attending physician who has built up a large and lucrative private practice. Putzel, 'a hand-holding doctor from the suburbs', sits on the side of his patients' beds, holding their hands, with (to Basch) obviously dishonest motives.[8] Jason Posner MD, the biochemistry major in *Wit*[27] who looks forward to returning to the laboratory, but is currently working as a fellow in oncology, finds the hand-holding process ridiculous for different reasons. Bedside behavior does not come naturally to Jason.

> There's a whole course on it in med school . . . colossal waste of time for researchers . . . we have to hold hands to discuss a creatinine clearance.[27]

Pasternak's Yury Zhivago[28] worries over his own bedside manner after visiting Anna Ivanovna, his future mother-in-law. Anna, who knows she is dangerously ill, is terrified. The two of them discuss Life after Death and similar topics and, towards the end of the visit, Zhivago, in a symbolic gesture, touches Anna on the forehead.

> 'What's come over me?' he thought [after leaving Anna's room]. 'I'm becoming a regular quack – muttering incantations, laying on the hands' . . . Next day Anna was better.[28]

Inappropriate phrases; stale jokes

Many doctors develop a bedside jargon, which they use exclusively in their conversations with patients. Most of the time this form of speech goes unnoticed, but it may lead to resentment and preventable tensions. One of the commonest features of the bedside patter is the use of the pronoun 'we' instead of 'you',[29–31] as in 'How are we today?'[32,33]* When Dr Allison Baydee examines Katie Rostova, a self-mutilating teenage athlete with multiple injuries, and remarks: 'I'd say we got off lightly', Katie reflects 'What do you mean "we"?'[31] Judge Clane in Carson McCullers' *Clock Without Hands*, who has plenty of other grievances, also complains volubly about the doctors' use of the first person plural instead of the second person singular.[30] The judge finds it particularly annoying when his doctor, who prescribes a diet, tries to soften the blow by observing: 'We won't find the diet too hard, Judge'. He grumbles to his friend after his return from Johns Hopkins Hospital:

> 'Don't you loathe it when doctors use the word "we" when it applies only and solely to yourself? He could go home and gobble fifty biscuits and ten baked Alaskas . . . while me, I'm starving on a diet.'[30]

Jean Stafford's Pansy Venneman in *The Interior Castle*[29] also expresses considerable irritation against her nose doctor who speaks of 'our nose' when he means 'your nose' and says ' "we" would be a new person when we could breathe again'.[29] She is also annoyed by the doctors' tired clichés, and their pathetic attempts at reassurance. Pansy, in her sixth week in hospital after a vehicular accident, writes these messages to her friends:

> Dr Nash says my reflexes are shipshape (*sic*) . . . Dr Nicholas, the nose doctor, promises to operate as soon as Dr Rivers gives him the go-ahead sign (*sic*). . . .[34]

---

* The term 'we' only occurs in the English translation.[33] Mauriac's original reads 'Et cette santé?'

On the day of the operation, when Dr Nicholas arrives with his entourage of 'white-frocked acolytes'[35] and his surgical toys, which his hands are 'aching' to use,[29] Pansy feels exceptionally threatened. She is afraid of the instruments on the surgical trolley, the 'knives and scissors and pincers, cans of swabs and gauze'. Even the iodine-containing mixture, 'a bowl of liquid whose rich purple color made it seem . . . like the brew of an alchemist',[35] makes her apprehensive.

Dr Nicholas turns out just the sort of person one would have anticipated from his little phrases. He is not deliberately cruel. In fact, he and his team make several dismal attempts to put Pansy at ease while operating on her nose.[36] However, the chit-chat between Nicholas and his associates produces quite the opposite effect so that, at the end of her 'treatment', Pansy feels that she has been subjected to an outrage. Dr Nicholas begins by remarking to no one in particular 'I couldn't start my car this morning. Came in a cab'.[37] For the sake of conducting some sort of conversation with his patient he asks Pansy whether she likes chicory in her coffee.[36] During the procedure, Dr Nicholas whispers to her

> in the voice of a lover, 'If you can stand it five minutes more I can perform the second operation now and you wont have to go through this again. What do you say?' The intern said 'You don't want your nose packed again, do you?' The surgical nurse said 'She's a good patient, isn't she, sir?' 'Never had a better,' replied Dr Nicholas.

When the painful process is over

> the surgeon, squeezing her arm with avuncular pride, said 'Good girl' as if she were a bright dog that had retrieved a bone.[36]

In *Not as a Stranger*[32] the pronoun 'we' is partially to blame for an open confrontation in the surgical ward of a Community Hospital. The participants are two interns, Drs Avery and Marsh, who are making rounds, and an uninsured, thirty-nine-year-old mechanic whose appendix has been removed three days earlier and who now has some abdominal distension.

> 'Well,' said Avery going forward, 'how are we today?' 'I don't know how you are but I'm in pain!' 'Gas troubling you?' 'You're goddamned right it's troubling me!' . . . 'Let's take a look!' . . . 'Son-of-a-bitch!' the man yelled suddenly. 'It's not necessary to yell.' Avery straightened. 'It isn't hurting you.' 'Nor use profanity.' 'You just take it easy!' 'It's all over now –' 'God damn it!' 'I'm not going to ask you again, Mr Jones – ' 'If I was rich you wouldn't be yanking me like that!' 'Now that's hardly the attitude for a sick man we've just done our best to help – ' 'I got gas pain enough without you monkeying where I was cut' . . . The ward listened, watched, waited.[32]

The situation was probably out of control before Dr Avery even appeared in the ward. Mr Jones has not been sufficiently well informed about the various complications he might encounter and he feels he is being treated differently from an insured patient. His resentment surfaces when he senses that he is being patronized by Dr Avery who uses the term 'we' instead of 'you'.

Other expressions that come up repeatedly in bedside parlance include 'What seems to be the problem?'[38] The term 'little' is used to indicate the relative mildness of a disease in a particular case (a few 'little' tuberculous spots[39]), the harmlessness of a 'little' prescription[40] and the simplicity of the procedure required for dealing with 'this little problem' (an unwanted pregnancy).[41] Dr Philip Denny who, despite his alcoholism, is the most likable medical character in *The Citadel*,[42] detests all aspects of the bedside jargon but reserves a particular derision for the word 'little' when used in this context. 'Don't use your bedside manner on me. I've used it plenty in my time,' he growls at a colleague who is trying to put him to bed during one of his drinking bouts. Denny, in his inebriated state then goes on to mimic a fashionable physician trying to impress a rich hypochondriacal woman.

> 'And how are you today, my dear lady? A leetle better I fancy. A leetle more strength in the pulse. Sleep well? Ha! Hum! Then we must prescribe a leetle sedative.'[42]

Malègue, who devotes almost the entire second volume of *Augustin, ou, Le maître est là*[43] to the fatal illnesses of three members of the Méridier family, resents the physicians' impotence rather than their incompetence or conduct (*see* pp 199–201). However, at times, irritating forms of speech obtrude, particularly the use of the word 'little'. When Christine's infant son is dying of tuberculous meningitis the doctor, in order to relieve the tension, prattles to him in baby language.[44] 'What's that? You don't want to? . . . You'll go straight back to beddie byes.' (Non? Tiens? Vous ne voulez pas? . . . On vous remettra tout de suite dans le dodo.) None of the adult family members pays the slightest attention to this 'smokescreen of idle chatter' (rideau de mots vains). When the doctor orders a sedative for the child's convulsions he uses the term 'little', to reassure the mother.

> 'Just a little injection – it's not dangerous' . . . the small size no doubt representing a guarantee for its harmlessness.[44] (Une petite piqûre sans aucun danger . . . la petitesse étant sans doubt garante de l'innocuité.)

Some physicians make up their own annoying special idioms. Hellerstein's insensitive gynecologist welcomes each of his patients with the greeting 'Scoot down to the edge of the table, hon'.[45] Susan Cheever's cancer surgeon,[46] who distributes his compassion in small quantities (*see* pp 182–3)

> had verbal formulas to deal with the awkwardness of the physical exam. 'Let's get you elegant,' he would say as he wrapped the flimsy gown around the patient's body.[47]

The use of the expression 'dear' when addressing female patients evidently troubles *Clarissa Harlowe*'s physician,[48] who finds himself looking after a young girl who has run away from her family and her lover, and now finds herself isolated in a strange city. The doctor calls the patient 'Dear Madam' but immediately goes on to reassure her that this appellation is not meant to indicate any unseemly familiarity.

'A father of children, some of them older than yourself, may be excused for his familiar address.'

Clarissa clearly does not regard the doctor's remarks as unprofessional and 'looked upon him . . . with a regard next to filial'.[49]

Even Margaret Drabble, who is usually kind to her fictional doctors, has her Rosamund Stacey express considerable bitterness against the expressions used by Dr Protheroe, a cardiac surgeon. Rosamund, the unmarried mother of Baby Octavia, has been informed that the child requires surgery for a congenital cardiac defect (? patent ductus).[50] The doctor has apparently contradicted himself – he previously mentioned five or six years as the usual age for this type of surgery and he now proposes to operate on the infant at the age of six months. He tries to explain this change of plans but the message is not being received.

> 'I was trying to explain to you,' he said, 'that we really have no choice. The severity of the condition varies, so . . . ' 'But there has been no sign of anything . . . She's always been so well.' 'As I was saying,' he said 'certain symptoms are not . . . likely to become manifest until the child becomes more active.'[50]

Then there is the question of prognosis. Again the doctor's language is inappropriate as well as imprecise and the statistics are obscure.

> 'Five years ago, in an infant of this age, I should have said the chance of survival was about five to one. Now we could put it at four to one.' I almost think he expected me to congratulate him, but instead I burst into tears. It was the first time anyone had used the word survival to me, so bluntly.'[50]

What particularly offends Rosamund is the use of the word 'luck'. The baby's cardiac murmur was discovered during a routine physical examination.

> 'It was really a stroke of extraordinary luck, that we discovered it at this stage' . . . 'Luck you call it, luck,' I said, unable to speak. 'Luck, is it?' It has never ceased to amaze me that they showed, at this stage, so little professional sympathy. I see now and I suspected then that his only emotion was professional curiosity. She was an odd case, my baby was a freak.'[50]

Peace is restored when Rosamund discovers Dr Protheroe and her father had been at university together and that the doctor is of the 'correct' political persuasion.[50] (The operation is a success.)

Inappropriate touching, backslapping and laughter may prove unsettling to the patient and ruin what might otherwise have been a smooth doctor–patient relationship. Selzer's introverted twenty-five-year-old man who worries about his falling hair and his seborrheic hyperkeratoses finds himself in the hands of a laugher.[51]

> 'Don't be silly,' says your doctor the next day, and he laughs. A doctor who laughs is bad news. 'You're in your prime,' he says. You whisper

your secret to him. About your hair. 'You're shedding more than your hair my friend,' he says. 'A hundred thousand brain cells per day.' . . . It occurs to you that he is the most repellent man you know – short, fat, bald and with dangerously bulging eyes. The only prime I am in is the prime of my senility. And he gives that terrible laugh. Caligula you decide would be more simpatico than this doctor.[51]

Dr Lewis Worship in Frede's *The Interns*[52] expresses considerable misgivings about his own bedside manner, which consists largely of stereotyped answers and stale jokes. A young primipara whose membranes have just been ruptured is asking the usual questions in the obstetric ward:

'Will it be soon?' 'Before Christmas, I guarantee.' Christ, he thought, if you have to talk to her on that level, don't talk to her at all. She deserves more than clichés. She had giggled. But now she said with more concern than she was able to hide . . . 'Does it take very long? Usually? The whole thing?' 'Long enough to be interesting . . . and short enough to just cover the subject.' Christ! He thought, furious at himself. She giggled again and then, still smiling, said, 'I bet that's the same question all the time. And the same answer too.'[52]

The brutal style

During the nineteenth and early twentieth centuries, several prominent physicians are portrayed as having developed or cultivated a deliberately intimidating bedside manner in order to prove to the patients and to themselves that they are in absolute control. A typical story is that of Dix[53] and his two female relatives whom he escorts to see a popular London doctor. When, after a seemingly interminable wait, the three are at last admitted into the consulting room, they find the doctor standing in front of the fireplace, warming his posterior.

'Now then, which of you wants me?' were his first words, which he uttered without removing from his elegant position before the fire. The elder lady, by a sign, indicated that her daughter was the patient and was about detailing the symptoms when he interrupted her with – 'There, hold your tongue madam!' then sitting by the young lady, he felt her pulse, asked her a few questions, gave a peculiar shrug with his shoulders

and after advising the patient and her mother to read his book, unceremoniously ushered the trio out of his room.[53] The same physician, when consulted by a Boston clergyman who repeatedly mentions his 'little flock', becomes impatient and rudely calls out:

'Damn your little flock, sir, stick out your tongue.'[53]

It seems almost inconceivable that private patients would travel long distances and pay exorbitant fees for a ten-minute office consultation during which they were abused and insulted. And yet, if authors of fictional works are to be believed, one hundred years ago, some physicians' reputations were built on exorbitant charges and dictatorial posturing. The patients are shown as anticipating this sort of approach, accepting it without protest and returning for more of the same. Indeed, Dr Richard Mahony's patients,[54] who consider him supercilious because he refuses to threaten them, take themselves off to other physicians for hectoring and harassment. Mahony who

> had not one manner for the bedside and another for daily life . . . never sought to ingratiate himself with people or to wheedle them; still less would he stop to bully and intimidate. He was always by preference the adviser rather than the dictator. And men did not greatly care for this arms length attitude; they wrote him down haughty and indifferent and pinned their faith to a blunter, homelier manner.[54]

The veterinary method seems to have been particularly well developed in France. Dr Finet in Zola's *The Earth*[55] despises the local peasants (who are indeed a vicious and brutalized lot) and treats them like animals.

> Monsieur Finet . . . spent a long time examining . . . [Lise's sick father, while she] and her husband watched anxiously. The doctor's silence confirmed their anxiety. When he sat down in the kitchen to write a prescription they decided to question him. 'So, it's serious is it? Might last a week eh? Heavens, what a long prescription. What's all that you're writing?' Monsieur Finet made no reply. He was used to this sort of interrogation by peasants bewildered and upset by the sight of illness, and he had taken the wise decision of treating them like horses, refusing to enter into conversation with them . . . Since he blamed his patients for having ruined his career he treated them roughly, thereby making them all the more deferential.[55]

Lise and her husband decide not to have the prescription filled and employ a different 'treatment' for the 'useless' old man. They suffocate him and then set fire to his bed, watched by their horrified children.[56] When Dr Finet is summoned again, his 'bedside manner' is one of cynical indifference.

> The doctor's only worry was to expedite the signing of the death certificate to save himself unnecessary journeys . . . If he did harbor any suspicions he took good care to keep them to himself. Good God! Suppose they had crisped their old father a bit since he was in no hurry to die! He'd seen it all; and such things hardly mattered. In his indifference born of contempt and resentment, he was content merely to shrug his shoulders: a dirty, rotten lot, these peasants.[56]

Daudet's *Les Morticoles*[57] is a satire against medicine in general and the leaders of the profession in particular. The patients, who are totally dominated by the physicians, are addressed in terms that would have been considered outrageous by the most menial servant, even at that time. Wabanheim, the Jewish doctor, is as savage as his gentile colleagues.

> He was particularly rough with women . . . He would growl at them: 'Get undressed.' Then he became impatient. 'Do I have to help you? You don't know how to undo your corset? Your underwear too . . . yes your underwear . . . Are you deaf? . . . You are looking for your stockings? I haven't stolen them! I'm not a collector of stockings! What's happening now? Tears! Why doesn't someone get me a bucket.'

Wabanheim is equally brutal with children, who are terrified of him.

> 'Come here, you idiot. Get your fingers out of your nose. His father died of dementia? That's where the boy gets it from. (Il tient de lui.) Put your hand on your forehead. On – your – forehead. You see, he doesn't hear a thing. Do you have any other children? No? Pity. You're not going to raise this one.'[57]

Simenon's Dr Mandalin, 'a formidable authoritarian',[58] uses a similarly boorish, 'take it or leave it' style. Mandalin has set up as a 'specialist' in a French provincial town and is now 'caring' for Marthe Cosson, who is expecting her first child and who has been admitted in labor. In the early hours of the morning, Mandalin the obstetrician and Bergelon the family doctor arrive together, from a party, at Mandalin's private establishment. Here they find

> Cosson standing at his wife's bedside, holding her hand, his lips trembling and a look of despair in his eyes. 'Tell me doctor . . . ' 'Now listen to me, I want you out of here, and the sooner the better. Go and wait in the grounds. I'll send for you when it's all over.' A broad wink at Bergelon, as if to say, 'that's the stuff to give the troops!' (Marthe Cosson and the baby both die.)[58]

By the 1930s this brutal method has become attenuated, especially in English-speaking countries, though the underlying contempt for the patient is still in evidence especially among older, earthy doctors. Francis Brett Young's Dr Jacob Medhurst,[59] a 'gross . . . cynical, crude old man', considers the physical examination, the diagnosis and the treatment as parts of a massive fraud, designed to deceive the patients and their families. His 'Ten Commandments' included such precepts as

> Never leave a case, however trivial it may be, without putting a name to it. If your patient's wife or aunt can't pronounce the name, so much the better; it'll do him a world of good.[59]

Medhurst also has strong views concerning treatment, which he considers useless unless it produces immediate and spectacularly unpleasant results[59] (*see* pp 163–4).

Cozzens' Dr George Bull,[60] lazy, ignorant, and boorish,[61] is too indifferent to the opinion of his patients to cultivate any sort of bedside manner or to hide his deficiencies with a camouflage of explanations, outlandish diagnoses or dramatically unpleasant medications. Bull, a graduate of the University of Michigan (Class of 1889) but not a particular ornament to that institution,[62] has been 'practicing' for over forty years[62] in 'New Winton, Connecticut' where, at the age of sixty-seven,[63] he narrowly escapes a motion of no confidence at a 'town meeting'.[64] Towards his patients, Bull tends to be argumentative rather than dictatorial. When a patient phones to tell the doctor her husband is feverish, he is skeptical. '[Did you] take his temperature? Well, how do you know he's feverish? Oh, he says so, does he? Give him a dose of castor oil and make him stay at home.'[65] When Dr Bull is summoned to see Sally Peters, who is dying of eclampsia, he is his usual argumentative self. Pa Peters, Sally's father in law, begins the telephone conversation:

> 'Doc, you'd better come down. Sal's awful sick. She . . .' 'What the hell do you mean, awful sick?' he answered. 'She's only eight months gone.' Someone took the telephone away, protesting. 'Aw, you old fool, let me . . .' The stronger voice was Jeff Peters and he said, 'Hello! Doc! Listen, come down right away, can you! She's pretty near unconscious. She can't see anything.' 'If she's unconscious, how do you know she can't see anything?'[66]

Bull's behavior contrasts strongly with that of his younger colleague, Dr Verney, whose bedside manner is superbly developed. When Virginia Banning, the daughter of New Winton's richest man, develops typhoid fever, Verney organizes two nurses 'to see that complications don't get a chance to start . . . What he meant was that complications when they started would not be overlooked'.[67] Of course complications do start[68] and while Virginia does not receive Dr Bull's favorite treatment (a dose of castor oil), she nevertheless dies from intestinal perforation. The dead girl's father is most appreciative of Dr Verney's attention, and thanks him in a little formal speech: 'I only want to say that I know you've done everything humanly possible. I want you to know what a comfort it's been . . .'[69] We do not hear Dr Bull's comments on this sad scene, which he would have found distasteful and hypocritical. When one of his own patients dies he turns up the next day to sign the death certificate, because he can see no point in the public relations exercise of attending a deathbed scene.[70]

Insensitive behavior; purposeless remarks; fun at the patient's expense

Many physicians, while not deliberately cruel to their patients, nonetheless behave inconsiderately and in a way that is bound to give rise to physical or mental anguish. Louisa Alcott's military surgeon is obviously insensitive to the pain he is inflicting on his patients who are totally in his power (*see also* Chapter 10). The doctor

> could not grasp the fact that there was some connection between the patient and his wound. The more complex the wound, the better he liked it and on at least one occasion he made a patient hold his injured arm with his good arm while he poked around in the wound examining various anatomic structures.[71]

Wambaugh's 'Desert Physician',[72] who is in a hurry (*see* Chapter 2) and has come up with the wrong diagnosis, treats Barney Wilson, a Palm Springs policeman, with unbelievable thoughtlessness. He called the twenty-nine year old cop into his office and gave him the good news first. No, he didn't have the clap as he'd feared. He could keep the same girlfriend and he wouldn't have to make any confessions to his wife. The bad news was that he'd only have the girlfriend for two years. Ditto for the wife. The doctor looked mildly cranky . . . 'You've got red blood cells in your urine. Acute glomerulonephritis. Two years maybe.'[72]

George Sava's *No Man is Perfect*[73] is a fanciful account of the career of Dr Anthony Sommers, who functions as a neurologist as well as a miracle-working neuro-surgeon. When Jonathan Davies, a wealthy financier, has recovered from a massive stroke and the situation has stabilized, Davies' wife, who has designs on Dr Sommers as a future son-in-law, asks him to continue to make house calls. 'What should we do if he had another of those terrible strokes?' At this point Sommers, who has to decline a patient's unreasonable request, becomes somewhat abrupt (possibly in a vain attempt to ward off Mrs Davies' advances) though his response is factually correct: 'My calling twice a week won't hold it off'.[73]

Proving a point to a belligerent patient is generally regarded as futile, so that most doctors avoid remarks or questions that may lead to arguments.

> It's the same between doctor and patient as it is between man and woman. Do you want to prove things to her or do you want to keep her?[74]

Similarly, reproaches for past actions or inactions are not generally considered part of a doctor's function. When rare physicians comment on such topics, their remarks are at best useless and at worst, mischievous. What is 'Doctor Thomas' trying to establish when he asks *Miss Gee*[75] why she has been neglecting the symptoms of her endometrial carcinoma?

> Doctor Thomas looked her over.
> And then he looked some more
> Walked over to his wash basin
> Said, Why didn't you come before?[75]

Robertson Davies' Dr James Cobbett[76] makes a similarly futile comment. One of his patients, appropriately named Mrs Gall, who suffers from empyema of the gall bladder, requires urgent surgical intervention. Unfortunately, the old lady, who belongs to some obscure religious sect, rejects Dr Cobbett's advice, she refuses to go to hospital and she dies at home of peritonitis. While filling out the death certificate, the doctor feels constrained to remark to the late Mrs Gall's daughter, 'I think it is my duty to emphasize once again that this need not have happened'. He is suitably rebuked: 'My mother was always used to having her own way . . . and there is no point in discussing that now.'[76]

Mario Puzo in *The Godfather*[77] has a gangster give a lesson in bedside behavior to an unsympathetic and culturally unattuned young resident who attempts to use the authoritarian approach. The scene takes place outside the hospital room of one of the godfather's henchmen who is dying of some unidentified malignancy. Corleone, his family and hangers-on have come to pay a final visit, but the nurses and residents consider such tribal rites unseemly.

> Dr Kennedy looked over the large group with exasperation. Didn't these people realize that the man inside was dying? 'I think just the immediate family,' he said in his exquisitely polite voice . . . 'My dear doctor,' said Don Corleone, 'is it true he is dying?' 'Yes,' said Dr Kennedy. 'Then there is nothing more for you to do . . . We will comfort him . . . we will close his eyes . . . we will bury him and weep at his funeral.' Dr Kennedy shrugged. It was impossible to explain to these peasants.

The 'peasants', who understand the dying man's needs, proceed into the room while Dr Kennedy disappears 'down the corridor his white coat flapping'.[77]

Some physicians find their patients' questions and complaints amusing and provide 'smart' or funny bits of advice, especially in the presence of an audience. Hierocles and Philagrius[78] tell the story of a patient with a chronic pain syndrome who complains that he is unable to lie down, to stand up or even to sit. His doctor suggests that he might try hanging himself. A nineteenth-century doctor, who dislikes requests for dietary advice, tells a patient, in response to such a request: 'You must not eat the poker, shovel or tongs for they are hard of digestion; nor the bellows because they are windy; but [you can eat] anything else you please'.[79] This type of inappropriate conduct is uncharacteristic even in collections of medical jokes, but 'wisecrack' answers to patients' questions continue to turn up in contemporary fiction.

AE Ellis[80] describes the protracted illness of Paul Davenant, an English university student who suffers from tuberculosis and who spends several years in Alpine sanatoria. In spite of (or possibly as the result of) multiple therapeutic procedures, Paul develops one complication after another. He has seen a number of doctors and he is now being advised by yet another physician. Professor Klauss, the famous Swiss expert, asks Paul how he feels about a thoracoplasty.

> Paul made no reply. 'I said what would you think of such an idea?' 'It depends . . . I don't know.' Paul looked about him. What was he meant to say? 'How many ribs would have to be removed?' he murmured. Professor Klauss led the chorus of laughter . . . 'How many ribs indeed? My goodness what a question.' He blew his nose loudly. 'You mean,' he continued turning to Paul, 'that if I said six ribs you would accept but if I said nine you would refuse!' . . . He started to laugh again

ably assisted by a retinue of sycophants. The professor's witty observations are technically correct and would have been entirely suitable for scoring points off a colleague at Grand Rounds. In the presence of a sick and depressive patient, Klauss' remarks and his underlying attitude are obviously unacceptable and it is no wonder that this semi-autobiographical book, which is full of such incidents, is named *The Rack*.[80]

Luke Rhinehart's *Dice Man*[81] is essentially a caricature of psychiatry and psychiatrists and the 'smart' answers to Pastor Cannon, whose son is being committed to a state institution, are meant to be tragic rather than funny. Eric Cannon, a child of the manse, has been, since the age of five 'both remarkably precocious and a little simple-minded'. After multiple deviant acts (including an attempt at suicide), Eric is being admitted to a mental hospital. As the adolescent is being led away, the Pastor asks whether it might be possible for his son to be given a single room. The psychiatrist replies:

> 'This is a Christian institution . . . We firmly believe in the brotherhood of all men. Your son will share a bedroom with fifteen other healthy normal American mental patients. Gives them a feeling of belonging and togetherness. If your son feels the need for a single, have him slug an attendant or two and they'll give him his own room; the state even provides a jacket for the occasion.'[81]

The black humor inherent in these crude wisecracks suggests that no kind of bedside manner can overcome the parents' anguish at the moment when the gates of a psychiatric hospital close behind their sick child.

Favorable accounts of the bedside manner

Fortunately, some doctors know how to behave even under difficult circumstances, and succeed in alleviating or at least not augmenting the patient's anxieties. Dr John Finch, the uncle of Jean Louise Finch ('Scout') in Harper Lee's *To Kill a Mocking-bird*,[82] evidently strikes the right note with the little girl, though other doctors do not. Dr John

> never terrified me, probably because he never behaved like a doctor. Whenever he performed a minor service for Jem and me as removing a splinter from a foot, he would tell us exactly what he was going to do, give us an estimation of how much it would hurt and explain the use of any tongs he employed.[82]

Mary Rinehart's Dr Chris Arden,[83] who spends some years in general practice, knows better than to concentrate on 'diet and bowel movements' when the patients want to discuss more important matters.

> The patients waited for the ritual of pulse and temperature; but the real moment came for them when, having put away thermometer and watch, he sat back in his chair beside the bed. . . . This was their hour, the one time when as to a priest they poured out their anxieties and griefs and even their sins. 'I suppose that's the reason I can't sleep. I get to thinking I'll go crazy. To have done a thing like that.' . . . Often he failed them. . . . Now and then, however, he found the right answer. A face would brighten or relax.[83]

Chris entertains considerable doubts about this aspect of the doctor's role and complains to a colleague

> 'only half . . . [my work] is medicine.' 'What's the rest? Babies?' 'Psychology.'

The colleague reassures him that psychology is part of medicine.

'Tell 'em they're better and they get better.'[83]

However, Chris evidently finds 'real' medicine more congenial than playing the part of priest and confessor. He turns into a full-time surgeon, who can declare with fake modesty 'I'm just a carpenter'.[84]

Four British general practitioners and one French internist stand out for their faultless bedside behavior. One of the British doctors has to deal with the diagnosis and treatment of sciatic pain in an elderly woman,[85] the second with a chest infection in an impoverished young mother,[86] the third with the family of a well-to-do demented patient[87] and the fourth with the eccentric inhabitants of a refined but threadbare boarding house.[88–91] The French internist[92] is consulted by a nationally famous film actor with self-destructive habits (*see also* p. 109). All five behave impeccably.

Arnold Bennett's 'Doctor Stirling',[85] urbane and well-read, gives old Mrs Constance Povey his full and concentrated attention as she describes her symptoms.

> He seemed to regard . . . [Constance's sciatica] as the one case that had ever aroused his professional interest; but as it unfolded itself in all its difficulty and urgency, so he seemed, in his mind, to be discovering wondrous ways of dealing with it; these mysterious discoveries seemed to give him confidence and his confidence was communicated to the patient by faint sallies of humor. He was a very skilled doctor. This fact, however, had no share in his popularity, which was due solely to his rare gift of taking a case very seriously while remaining cheerful.[85]

Unfortunately, Stirling's treatment, while 'correct' in theory, is inappropriate in this particular case (*see* p. 149) but his combination of seriousness and optimism is perfect.

Dr John Bradley,[86] on the point of retirement, is shown reproaching an impoverished, sick woman for coming to his office rather than having him visit her in her home because she could not afford the cost of a home visit.

> Often enough, the difference was theoretical and the sum, small or large, unlikely to be paid.[86]

During the physical examination, Dr Bradley, outwardly gruff but essentially compassionate, displays a paternalistic attitude, which his poor patients not only do not resent, but actually seem to expect.

> Keep this thermometer under your tongue and don't bite it through or you'll have to pay for it. Let's feel your pulse . . . Now come over here and lie down. I must run over your chest (*see* Chapter 4). Put the baby on the floor: it won't hurt. . . . His face . . . had first been angry (though the violence was often assumed for their benefit) and then brusquely kind for fear that he had scared her too much.[86]

The consultation ends with the patient being presented with a bottle of medicine (free of charge).[86]

Muriel Spark's unnamed physician in *Memento Mori*[87] obviously deals with a more prosperous clientele. In this case, he has to cope with the family of a physically and mentally frail patient (Charmian Colston), who is still being cared for at home but is heading towards institutional care. The doctor remains polite but firm. He indicates to Charmian's husband (Godfrey Colston) and her scheming housekeeper (Mabel Pettigrew) that while Charmian is demented and may even have to go into a nursing-home, his main concern is for her and not for them.[87]

> Later in the morning when the doctor called, Godfrey [Colston] stopped him in the hall. 'She is damned difficult today, doctor.' 'Ah well,' said the doctor, 'it's a sign of life.' 'Have to see about a home if she goes on like this.' 'It might be a good idea if only she can be brought around to liking it,' said the doctor. 'The scope for regular attention is so much better in a nursing home . . . She has extraordinary powers of recovery, almost as if she had some secret source.' Godfrey thought: This is his smarm. Charmian has a secret source and I pay the bills. He said explosively 'Well sometimes I feel she deserves to be sent away.' 'Oh, deserves,' said the doctor, 'we don't recommend nursing-homes as a punishment.'[87]

A little later, Mrs Pettigrew tells the doctor her version of the story.

> 'We wouldn't,' said Mrs Pettigrew, 'take our pills this morning, doctor, I'm afraid.' 'Oh that doesn't matter,' he said. 'I did take them,' said Charmian, 'I took them with my early tea . . . and just suppose I'd taken a second dose.' 'It wouldn't really have mattered,' he said. 'But surely,' said Mrs Pettigrew, 'it is always dangerous to exceed a stated dose.'[87]

The doctor has no intention of engaging in an argument with Mrs Pettigrew, who is courteously sent out of the room.

> The doctor said as he took [Charmian's] pulse, 'Mrs Pettigrew, if you would excuse us for a moment.'[87]

Dr Mainwaring, Kingsley Amis' rural general practitioner, 'much despised' among his shabby-genteel patients,[88] is nonetheless 'much in demand'. Mainwaring, who is unable to 'treat' any 'real' disorders, functions as a provider of fatuous advice,[89] a prescriber of sedatives and an arranger of hospital admissions.[90] However, the behavior of this lowly doctor towards the bizarre inhabitants of the 'Tuppeny-Hapenny' boarding house is exemplary and one is not surprised at his popularity. Dr Mainwaring not only keeps his composure when Marigold Pyke, aged seventy-three, talks in terms of having a 'drinkle-pinkle' and her friend being a 'sweetle-peetle,'[89] but also manages to reassure her about her memory lapses. Derrick Shortell the alcoholic, homosexual clown of the establishment who suffers from one of the 'gay bowel' syndromes greets the doctor with prolonged and parodied ceremony.[89] . . . 'Do I take it that thou cravest audience with thy unworthy servant, O mighty bearer of the staff of Hippocrates?'[90]

The doctor, who is accustomed to this nonsense, replies: 'Just a very brief word, Mr Shortell'. When the two are alone, the doctor asks:

'How much do you drink a day?' 'About a bottle.' There were in existence, after all, bottles that would hold the true amount. 'Not a bottle of spirits?' 'No fear. Kind of wine.'

The doctor makes no attempt to turn Shortell into an abstemious citizen and after a cursory abdominal examination reassures him that things are no worse than on previous occasions.[91] Bernard Bastable, another homosexual, but of the aggressive variety, has inoperable rectal cancer. Instead of complaining, Bastable, an ex-Brigadier General, comforts himself during his last few weeks by playing nasty practical jokes on the other members of the household. Dr Mainwaring knows better than to make compassionate remarks.[90]

'Good morning, Mr Bastable . . . Any change?' 'Nothing dramatic; I seem to be passing more blood.' . . . 'What about the pain?' 'I can stand it at the moment.' 'You're sure you don't want surgery?'

Bastable has previously been told the chances of success are less than five per cent and again declines Dr Mainwaring's offer of a referral to a surgeon. The doctor is very practical.

'Mr Bastable, when . . . this phase seems like coming to an end, I'd be grateful if you'd warn me in good time. I may not be able to find you a [hospital] bed immediately.'

Bastable is not disturbed by this allusion to terminal care and the doctor's final visit (as it turns out) ends with a handshake.[90]

Dr Mainwaring is undoubtedly despised not only by his patients but also by the junior staff at the tertiary referral centre who regard him as practicing a 'primitive' sort of medicine. The demented old lady is not subjected to any cerebral imaging procedure, the alcoholic clown is let off without liver function tests and no heroic attempts are made to treat the irascible former brigadier with radiotherapy or chemotherapy. However, as the story evolves, it transpires that expensive investigations or unpleasant therapeutic measures would have made no difference whatever to the outcome in these three cases.

Simenon in *The Heart of a Man*[92] provides an excellent account of a physician confronted by a distinguished and widely admired performing artist who has to make a choice between either terminating his career or persisting in his self-destructive habits. The patient is Émile Maugin, the most famous film and stage actor in the country who suffers from alcoholism and cardiomyopathy and cannot or will not change his lifestyle. Maugin has fortified himself with two glasses of cheap wine before surreptitiously visiting Dr Biguet, a leading Paris consultant, after regular office hours. In response to Maugin's ostensible request for 'advice', Biguet performs credibly though, from a clinical point of view, nihilistically.

> 'You are fifty-nine, Maugin . . . Well, here in front of me I have a seventy-five-year-old-heart.' . . . 'I see.' 'You must remember that a man of seventy-five still has time ahead of him, it may be considerable time.' 'In other words I can go on living if I'm careful.' 'Yes.' 'If I don't indulge in any excesses.' 'If you don't live at too rapid a pace.' . . . 'That's the treatment you order? No women, no tobacco, no alcohol and, I suppose, not too much work either?' 'I prescribe no treatment. Here is the outline of your heart. This pouch here is your left ventricle and here, in red, you see it as it should be at your age . . .' 'No pills, no drugs?' 'You tell me that you have five films to make. And your stage part until the fifteenth of March. What can you change in your way of living?' 'Nothing.' 'And on my side, all that it is within my power to do for you is to spare you pain.'[92]

The doctor, who has a high regard for Maugin's talents, cannot bring himself to advise this great performing artist to cancel all his engagements, sign up with Alcoholics Anonymous and live out the remainder of his life in a suburban cottage, tending his garden, eating a healthy diet and drinking fruit juice. In the unlikely event of such advice being accepted, the rustic lifestyle would obliterate 'Maugin' as everyone knows him.[92]

> What more had they to say to each other now? Neither of them wanted to look at his watch. Maugin could not ask the specialist how much he owed him . . . He had better go. They were going to find themselves, both of them, obliged to resort to banalities. 'Thank you Biguet.' . . . A handshake without insistence, almost brusque, out of diffidence, out of decency. 'Don't hesitate to telephone me any time.' . . . While they were standing together in the doorway, all [the doctor] allowed himself was a tap on the shoulder as he said: 'You're a hell of a chap, Maugin.' . . . A few moments later, a moist hand was turning the door handle of the bar on the Rue de Courcelles and the proprietor at his counter, trying not to look surprised, said . . . quickly: 'A glass of red, Monsieur Maugin?'[92]

(Maugin goes on acting and drinking and dies suddenly a few months later.)

The expression 'you're an intelligent person' as a prelude or an accompaniment to bad medical news sounds patronizing, but unlike some other medical jargon, it does not seem to provoke resentment. Indeed, it evidently works in widely different settings. In the Chinese classic *The Dream of the Red Chamber*,[93] Dr Chang, a scholarly, self-deprecating physician has been summoned to see a young woman with an undiagnosed disorder (from which she subsequently dies). The medical aspects are handled in the traditional Chinese style. Dr Chang impresses the family by guessing the patient's symptoms (insomnia and menstrual irregularities) and by writing a prescription containing fourteen ingredients. However, his handling of the husband's question 'Is her life in danger?' is masterful and universal: 'You are an intelligent young man . . . When an illness has reached this stage, it is not going to be cured in an afternoon'.[93] Dr Vernet in *The Rack*[94] also uses this approach.

'Mon cher,' said Dr Vernet, taking a chair and sitting down, 'you are an extremely ill man – to tell you otherwise would be to insult your intelligence.'[94]

The dying patient

The physician's performance at a dying patient's bedside comes in for a good deal of discussion in fictional literature. In the presence of death (which doctors have to recognize and 'pronounce') they behave appropriately though there are a few exceptions. Cynical Dr Medhurst[59] wants nothing to do with dying patients and advises his young assistant to 'shove them into hospital and you won't get the blame'.[59] The disgusting surgical professors in *Bodies and Souls*[95] argue about a patient

> who presented an interesting case. Heubel claimed it was a benign tumor, Geoffroy a cancer, Géraudin an abscess. Standing around the dying man they hurled barbaric terms at each other, expressions that were incomprehensible to the patient. A mysterious phrase would close the argument: 'Oh well, we'll see at Morgagni's.' To go to Morgagni's . . . meant carrying out an autopsy.[95]

Thomas Mann's Dr Grabow looks after Elizabeth Buddenbrook during her final illness.[96] His interaction with the patient and her family is described in considerable detail and in very unfavorable terms. The doctor's initial oily optimism is inappropriate.

> 'There is positively no reason for serious disquiet at present . . . Our honored patient's powers of resistance [are] . . . simply astonishing for her years.'

When Mrs Buddenbrook's son, the senator, appears skeptical, Grabow covers himself by adding:

> 'I don't say that your dear mother will be walking out tomorrow . . . the lung is slightly affected.'[96]

Grabow's assistant, who will shortly be taking over the practice, is more direct and tells the senator that his mother has pneumonia, but Grabow continues to be breezy. He even enumerates the various symptoms (dyspnea, hemoptysis, confusion) and goes on reassuringly, like Aesop's physician[97] (*see* pp 129–30), that all these complications are 'to be expected, entirely regular and normal'. He advises the senator not to notify his brother who is out of town.[96] As the patient gets worse Dr Grabow changes his tactics.

> 'Yes my dear senator,' Dr Grabow said and took Thomas Buddenbrook by the hand, 'it is now both lungs – we have not been able to prevent it . . . I should not attempt to deceive you . . . the condition is serious.'

On this occasion Grabow advises the senator to telegraph his brother but then becomes effusive once again.

> 'For heaven's sake my dear senator, don't draw any exaggerated conclusions from what I say. There is no immediate danger – I am foolish to take the word in my mouth! . . . We are well satisfied with your mother as a patient.'

Frau Consul Buddenbrook continues to deteriorate and Dr Grabow continues to give inappropriate advice. When her son and daughter express their concern about the old lady's physical and mental anguish, Grabow declares 'in a tone of authority' that there is no suffering, '[her] consciousness is very clouded'. . . . However, 'a child could have seen from the Frau Consul's eyes that she was entirely conscious'.[96] Towards the end Mrs Buddenbrook gasps:

> 'Have mercy gentlemen, let me sleep!' . . . But the physicians knew their duty – [they had] to preserve life at any cost. So they strengthened the heart action by various devices and even improved the breathing by causing the patient to retch.[96]

Not one of the participants in this drama (except the dying patient) is shown in a favorable light, but Mann's harshest treatment is reserved for the doctor. The family members cry and squabble, the servant steals the patient's belongings, the nurse engages in superstitious practices but at least these 'lay' individuals show a realistic awareness of their impotence in the face of death.

> They were alive . . .they were able to breathe . . . but they could help her no more (except by) watching her die.[96]

Dr Grabow on the other hand, while behaving 'correctly' from the medical point of view, is lacking in diagnostic acumen, sincerity and compassion.

Most fictional doctors faced with potentially lethal diseases are more helpful and, occasionally, more useful. In a romantic passage,[98] Conan Doyle shows that, at times, the best bedside manner consists of being there and saying nothing. Dr James Winter, whose knowledge of medical theory and practice has been acquired fifty years earlier, is a positive menace when it comes to diagnosing and treating patients. He is so deaf that he can no longer distinguish between 'a mitral murmur and a bronchial rale' while his therapeutic armamentarium consists of 'senna and calomel'.[98] Yet,

> his mere presence leaves the patient with more hopefulness and vitality. . . . At a dying patient's bedside it is of more avail than all the drugs in his surgery. Dying folk cling to him as if the presence of his bulk and vigor gives them more courage to face the change and that kindly wind-beaten face has been the last earthly impression which many a sufferer has carried into the unknown.[98]

In a few masterly sentences, William Carlos Williams[99] indicates how a physician may reduce a dying patient's fears by treating imminent death as a matter of fact[100] (*see also* p. 126) and using only a minor degree of deception. Williams' physician, writing in the first person,[99] has been called out at three o'clock in the morning to examine a man with erysipelas of the face, a lethal condition in the pre-antibiotic days. The 'wildly excited' patient wants the doctor to witness his will. 'Will it be legal? Yes, of course. He signs. I sign after him.' Reassurances such as 'You don't need a will right now' are considered inappropriate while the inevitable flaws in a hastily drawn-up, unprofessional document seem irrelevant at this point in time. The doctor's main concern is to calm the patient. The wailing wife – 'Oh my God what will I do without him' – is reprimanded.

> Kindly be quiet, madam. What sort of a way is that to talk in a sickroom?
> Do you want to kill him? Give him a chance if you please.[99]

One might be tempted to criticize the physician's domineering approach, but the stern reprimand to the distraught wife may actually have a therapeutic benefit: it carries the implication that the situation is not entirely hopeless.

Louisa May Alcott[71] believes that at the bedside of a dying patient a poorly trained but sympathetic nurse may be more useful than an aggressive interventionist surgeon. Dr Thomas More, the flawed psychiatrist in Walker Percy's *The Thanatos Syndrome*,[101] takes this concept a stage further. When the priest in charge of a hospice for incurable patients calls for the doctor, 'when the depression and the terrors of his AIDS patients are more than he can handle', More abandons his role of adviser and intervener and presents himself to the patients as a fellow-sufferer.[101] He and the priest (who is also flawed)

> do little more than visit with them, these haggard young men, listen, speak openly, we to them, they to us and we to each other in front of them about them and about our own troubles, we being two old drunks and addled besides. They advise us about alcohol, diet and suchlike. It seems to help them and us. At least they laugh at us.[101]

When Louise Cooper in Leavitt's *Equal Affections*[102] makes an unscheduled visit to her oncologist because of a recrudescence of her lymphoma, his greeting is phrased in a way that expresses concern but not necessarily a fear of an impending disaster.

> 'Well, Louise,' he said, 'I can't exactly say I'm pleased to see you here.'[103]

Dr Thayer, who has to prepare the Cooper family for Louise's imminent death, lectures somewhat inappropriately and uses clichés like 'tough as an ox', 'I wouldn't have put money on her getting this far' and 'insult added to injury'.[104] However, he is able to convey bad news to her family clearly and without undue brutality. The key message is:

> 'I've had twelve cases like this and I've lost eleven of them.'[104]

Louise's academic husband (computer science) and her two somewhat unusual children (both homosexual) evidently understand the significance of this statement and believe that the information has been transmitted appropriately.[104]

Dreiser's idealized Dr Gridley[105] knows exactly what to say and do around a deathbed. When a little boy is dying from meningitis, Dr Gridley declares, 'He is passing as free from pain as ever I knew a case of this kind'. At the deathbed of a farmer, who is about to succumb to traumatic bile peritonitis, Dr Gridley indicates by non-verbal gestures that the situation is hopeless.

> He walked down the yard to a chair under a tree some distance from the house where he sat drooping and apparently grieved. There was no need for words. Every curve and droop of his figure . . . told all of us . . . that hope was gone.[105]

Body language is also used by Guterson's Dr Williams,[106] an old-fashioned family doctor, to help him express a sense of hopelessness. Williams is called upon during a midnight visit, to inform the two Givens brothers (aged fourteen and twelve) that their mother is dying from carcinoma of the pancreas. The doctor performs magnificently. He begins with some preliminary symbolic gestures. He deposits his brandy on the mantel, he goes over to the window to look out into the night, he polishes his spectacles and he finally asks the boys to sit down.

> Ben and Aidan perched on the sofa. Their father wouldn't look at them. Dr Williams lowered himself to the edge of the rocker . . . 'Your father has asked me to talk to you,' he said, 'because it's hard for him to do it himself.' 'That's okay,' said Aidan. 'Your mother can't be cured,' said the doctor. 'That's what we found out over in Spokane. She has a tumor, a cancer of the pancreas. There is nothing we can do to cure her.' 'But you're a doctor,' Ben said. Dr Williams fingered his chin. 'A doctor isn't a magician . . . if I was, I'd cure your mother.' 'What do you mean you can't cure her?' 'I mean I'm just a man with a little learning and some medicines in an old black bag. I can't stop cancer of the pancreas.' 'Yes you can. You have to.' Ben's father raised his head . . . 'There's no point in arguing with Dr Williams,' he said. 'You hush now, Ben.' Ben turned his face to the floor. 'I thought you were a good doctor,' he whispered.[106]

The perfect bedside manner

Henry James' Sir Luke Strett,[107] 'the greatest of London doctors', is one of the most impressive physicians in fictional literature. Unlike Balzac's saintly Dr Benassis,[108] who has secluded himself in an isolated French village (*see* p. 40), Sir Luke practices in a fashionable part of London where his activities are likely to come under intense scrutiny from his peers. 'Sir Luke' contrasts sharply with 'Sir Mark', the other titled Englishman in *The Wings of the Dove*.[107] Mark, the aristocrat, is shallow, idle, scheming and vicious. Luke, the scientific, hard-working professional man, remains totally uncorrupted by his success. Even during his first brief consultation with Milly Theale he is a source of inspiration to her, 'so crystal-clean the great empty cup of attention that he set between them on the table'.[109]

Sir Luke is aware of Milly's poor prognosis and succeeds in conveying this information to his patient while at the same time making her feel better.[110] He avoids 'professional heartiness, mere bedside manner, which she would have disliked'.[109] He shows himself to be 'interested, on her behalf in other questions beside the question of what was the matter with her'.[109] The nature of Milly Theale's fatal illness (? anorexia nervosa, ?? inflammatory bowel disease) is not revealed. She is 'slim, constantly pale, delicately haggard', she is 'suddenly taken ill', she develops an 'upset',[111] which threatens to delay her European trip and, towards the end, she 'turns her face to the wall'.[112] Against this background, we see Sir Luke travel halfway across Europe because of 'a huge interest' in the case of the American heiress as well as 'a huge fee'.[112] He keeps his part of the bargain by spending long hours at Milly's bedside and by expressing some hope even at the terminal stage.[112]

Sir Luke is an extraordinarily powerful priestly figure, 'a great, grave, charming man' looking 'half like a general and half like a bishop'.[109] Milly, after her first brief consultation, feels 'as if I had been on my knees to the priest. I've confessed and I've been absolved'.[109] Naturally, this wonderful man's knowledge and interests extend to subjects other than medicine. 'If he hadn't been a great surgeon he might . . . have been a great judge . . . of the beautiful.'[112] Almost uniquely among fictional physicians, Sir Luke Strett has the facility of making his patients (or at least one particular patient) want to help him with 'his' problem even if it turns out to be insoluble.[110] Milly even thinks in terms of a role reversal between patient and physician. 'What was he . . . but patient, what was she but physician from the moment she embraced the necessity of saving him alarms.'[112]

Sir Luke's power is felt not only by his impressionable and gentle patient but also by Merton Densher, journalist and ambiguous friend of the dying girl.[112] Without saying a word about Milly's condition, Sir Luke makes Merton feel more comfortable, simply by 'the breadth of his shoulders'. Sir Luke 'knew what mattered and what didn't' and he makes 'odd things natural'. Even the symbolically inclement weather improves after Sir Luke's arrival. 'He'll stay to the end,' declares Densher, 'he's magnificent.'[112]

Summary

While some fictional physicians conduct themselves suitably towards their patients, many do not. Doctors are inappropriately optimistic, their mode of speech and gestures appear histrionic, and some of their remarks and questions are useless and mischievous. Despite a thin superficial layer of compassion, patients are treated insensitively or insincerely or both. Remarkably, around a deathbed, this annoying behavior becomes less obtrusive. Writers of fiction generally use the term 'bedside manner' pejoratively.

References

1   *Punch* (1884) 15 March, p. 121.
2   Herrick R (1900) *The Web of Life*. Macmillan, London, p. 7.
3   Illych I (1976) *Limits to Medicine*. Penguin, Harmondsworth, 1990.
4   Stoeckle JD (1987) *Encounters Between Patients and Doctors*. MIT Press, Cambridge, MA, pp. 1–129.

5   Simpson JA and Weiner ESC (eds) (1989) *Oxford English Dictionary*, vol. 2. Clarendon Press, Oxford, p. 53.

6   Plato (4th century BC) *Gorgias*. Translated by Lamb WRM. Loeb's Classical Library, Heinemann, London, 1967, p. 291.

7   Yedidia MJ, Gillespie CC, Kachur E, Schwartz MD, Ockene J, Chepaitis AE, Snyder CW, Lazare A and Lipkin M (2003) Effect of communication training on medical student performance. *JAMA*. **290**: 1157–65.

8   Shem S (1978) *The House of God*. Richard Marek, New York, pp. 43–4.

9   Molière JBP (1666) The Physician in Spite of Himself. Translated by Waller AR. In: *The Plays of Molière*, vol. 5. John Grant, Edinburgh, 1926, pp. 154–5.

10   Lacy J (1672) *The Dumb Lady or The Farrier Made Physician*. Thomas Dring, London, p. 13.

11   Thompson M (1949) *The Cry and the Covenant*. Pan Books, London, 1969, p. 123.

12   Flannery MC (2001) The white coat: A symbol of science and medicine as a male pursuit. *Thyroid*. **11**: 947–51.

13   Dunn JJ, Lee TH, Percelay JM, Fitz JG and Goldman L (1987) Patient and house officer attitude on physician attire and etiquette. *JAMA*. **257**: 65–8.

14   Gledhill JA, Warner JP and King M (1997) Psychiatrists and their patients: views on forms of dress and address. *Brit J Psych*. **171**: 228–32.

15   Ellis AE (1958) *The Rack*. Penguin Books, London, 1988, p. 62.

16   Bernhard T (1978) Breath – A Decision. In: Bernhard T (1985) *Gathering Evidence*. Translated by McLintock D. Alfred A Knopf, New York, pp. 240–1.

17   Beauvoir S de (1964) *A Very Easy Death*. Translated by O'Brian P. Andre Deutsch and Weidenfeld and Nicolson, London, 1966.

18   Green G (1956) *The Last Angry Man*. Charles Scribner's Sons, New York.

19   Ibid., p. 188.

20   McKinstry B (1990) Should general practitioners call patients by their first names? *Brit Med J*. **301**: 795–6.

21   Gledhill JA, Warner JP and King M (1997) Psychiatrists and their patients: views on forms of dress and address. *Brit J Psych*. **171**: 228–32.

22   Chandler R (1953) *The Long Good-Bye*. Pan, London, 1979, pp. 102–3.

23   Osler W (1889) *Aequanimitas*. HK Lewis, London, 1920, p. 5.

24   Bennett A (1923) *Riceyman Steps*. Cassell, London, 1947, pp. 245–64.

25   Crichton M (Jeffery Hudson, pseudonym) (1968) *A Case of Need*. Signet, New York, 1969, p. 51.

26   Osler W (1903–5) *Aphorisms*. Bean RB and Bean WB (eds). Charles C Thomas, Springfield, IL, 1961, Aphorism 268, p. 130.

27   Edson M (1993) *Wit*. Faber and Faber, New York, 1999, pp. 55–7.

28   Pasternak B (1957) *Doctor Zhivago*. Translated by Hayward M and Harari M. Pantheon, New York, 1958, pp. 67–9.

29   Stafford J (1953) *The Interior Castle*. Harcourt Brace and Company, New York, p. 202.

30   McCullers C (1953) *Clock Without Hands*. Houghton Mifflin, Boston, MA, 1963, pp. 61–3.

31 Levenkron S (1997) *The Luckiest Girl in the World*. Scribner, New York, p. 73.

32 Thompson M (1955) *Not as a Stranger*. Michael Joseph, London. pp. 275–7.

33 Mauriac F (1925) *The Desert of Love*. Translated by Hopkins G. Eyre and Spottiswoode, London, 1949, p. 63.

34 Stafford J, op. cit., p. 198.

35 Ibid., p. 205.

36 Ibid., pp. 208–17.

37 Ibid., p. 206.

38 Franzen J (2001) *The Corrections*, Fourth Estate, London, 2002, p. 364.

39 Malègue J (1932) *Augustin, ou, Le maître est là*, vol. 2. Spes, Paris, 1935, pp. 380–5.

40 Lurie A (1974) *The War Between the Tates*. Heinemann, London, pp. 115–17.

41 Irving J (1985) *Cider House Rules*. Bantam Books, New York, 1986, pp. 55–67.

42 Cronin AJ (1937) *The Citadel*. Gollancz, London, p. 95.

43 Malègue J, op. cit., vol. 2.

44 Ibid., pp. 216–30.

45 Hellerstein D (1986) Touching. In: Hellerstein D. *Battles of Life and Death*. Houghton Mifflin, Boston, MA, pp. 69–73.

46 Cheever S (1987) *Doctors and Women*. Methuen, London, 1988.

47 Ibid., pp. 43–5.

48 Richardson S (1747–8) The History of Clarissa Harlowe. In: Stephen L (ed.) *The Works of Samuel Richardson*, vol. 7. Henry Sotheran, London, 1883, p. 378.

49 Ibid., p. 398.

50 Drabble M (1965) *The Millstone*. Weidenfeld and Nicolson, London, pp. 138–43.

51 Selzer R (1979) In Praise of Senescence. In: Selzer R. *Confessions of a Knife*. Simon and Schuster, New York, pp. 100–10.

52 Frede R (1960) *The Interns*. Corgi, London, 1965, p. 59.

53 Dix J (1846) *Pen and Ink Sketches of Poets, Preachers, and Politicians*. David Bogue, London, pp. 174–81.

54 Richardson HH (1917–29) *The Fortunes of Richard Mahony*. Penguin, London, 1990, pp. 273–4.

55 Zola E (1887) *The Earth*. Translated by Parmee D. Penguin, Harmondsworth, 1980, pp. 395–6.

56 Ibid., p. 486.

57 Daudet LA (1894) *Les Morticoles*. Fasquelle, Paris, 1956, pp. 258–9.

58 Simenon G (1941) The Country Doctor. Translated by Ellenbogen E. In: Simenon G (1980) *The White Horse Inn and Other Novels*. Hamish Hamilton, London, pp. 198–205.

59 Young FB (1938) *Dr Bradley Remembers*. Heinemann, London, pp. 242–5.

60 Cozzens JG (1933) *The Last Adam*. Harcourt Brace and Company, New York.

61 Ibid., p. 66.

62 Ibid., p. 42.

63 Ibid., p. 35.

64 Ibid., pp. 285–6.

65 Ibid., pp. 150–2.

66 Ibid., p. 232.

67 Ibid., p. 215.

68 Ibid., pp. 251–5.

69 Ibid., p. 298.

70 Ibid., p. 106.

71 Alcott LM (1863) Hospital Sketches. In: Showalter E (ed.) (1988) *Alternative Alcott*. Rutgers University Press, New Brunswick, pp. 26–39.

72 Wambaugh J (1985) *The Secrets of Harry Bright*. Sphere Books, London, 1987, p. 93.

73 Sava G (1979) *No Man is Perfect*. Robert Hale, London, p. 39.

74 Kipling R (1932) The Tender Achilles. In: Kipling R. *Limits and Renewals*. Macmillan, London, pp. 343–67.

75 Auden WH (1936) Miss Gee. In: Auden WH (1970) *Selection by the Author*. Penguin, Harmondsworth, pp. 43–5.

76 Davies R (1951) A Mixture of Frailties. In: Davies R (1986) *The Salterton Trilogy*. Penguin, London, pp. 717–25.

77 Puzo M (1968) *The Godfather*. Fawcett, Greenwich, CN, pp. 45–6.

78 Hierocles and Philagrius (3rd century AD) *The Philogelos*. Translated by Baldwin B. Gieben, Amsterdam, 1983, p. 34.

79 Wadd W (Unus Quorum, pseudonym) (1827) *Nugae Canorae: Or Epitaphian Mementos (in Stone Cutters' Verse) of the Medici Family of Modern Times*. JB Nichols, London, p. 7.

80 Ellis AE, op. cit., pp. 354–5.

81 Rhinehart L (1971) *The Dice Man*. Panther Books, London, 1975, pp. 37–42.

82 Lee H (1960) *To Kill a Mockingbird*. Popular Library, New York, 1962, pp. 82–3.

83 Rinehart MR (1935) *The Doctor*. Farrar and Rinehart, New York, pp. 99–100.

84 Kipling R, op. cit., p. 349.

85 Bennett A (1908) *The Old Wives' Tale*. Hodder and Stoughton, London, 1964, pp. 461–3.

86 Young FB, op. cit., pp. 14–16.

87 Spark M (1959) *Memento Mori*. Reprint Society, London, 1965, pp. 69–70.

88 Amis K (1974) *Ending Up*. Jonathan Cape, London, pp. 8–10.

89 Ibid., pp. 76–80.

90 Ibid., pp. 161–3.

91 Ibid., pp. 84–5.

92 Simenon G (1950) The Heart of a Man. In: *The Second Simenon Omnibus*. Hamish Hamilton, London, 1974, pp. 151–60.

93 Cao Xue Qin (also spelt Tsao Hsueh Chin) (1791) *The Story of the Stone* (also known as *The Dream of the Red Chamber*). Translated by Hawkes D. Penguin, Harmondsworth, UK, 1973, pp. 217–28.

94 Ellis AE, op. cit., p. 140.

95 Van Der Meersch M (1943) *Bodies and Souls*. Translated by Wilkins E. William Kimber, London, 1953, p. 36.

96 Mann T (1901) *Buddenbrooks*. Translated by Lowe-Porter HT. Penguin, Harmondsworth, 1957, pp. 429–39.

97 Aesop (approx 570 BC) *The Complete Fables*. Translated by Temple O and Temple R. Penguin, London, 1998, p. 184.

98 Doyle AC (1894) Behind the Times. In: Doyle AC (1934) *Round the Red Lamp*. John Murray, London, pp. 1–8.

99 Williams WC (1938) Dance Pseudomacabre. In: Williams WC (1984) *The Doctor Stories*. New Directions, New York, pp. 88–91.

100 Martineau H (1839) *Deerbrook*. Virago Press, London, 1983, p. 44.

101 Percy W (1987) *The Thanatos Syndrome*. Farrar, Straus and Giroux, New York, p. 363.

102 Leavitt D (1989) *Equal Affections*. Penguin, London.

103 Ibid., p. 29.

104 Ibid., pp. 173–4.

105 Dreiser T (1919) The Country Doctor. In: Dreiser T (1930) *Twelve Men*. Constable, London, pp. 102–22.

106 Guterson D (1999) *East of the Mountains*. Bloomsbury, London, pp. 74–5.

107 James H (1902) *The Wings of the Dove*. Signet Classics, New York, 1964.

108 Balzac H de (1833) *The Country Doctor*. Translated by Marriage E. Dent, London, 1923.

109 James H, op. cit., pp. 165–70.

110 Ibid., p. 304.

111 Ibid., pp. 81–97.

112 Ibid., pp. 400–37.

CHAPTER 4

The history and physical examination; investigations; the diagnosis

In real life, the patients or the patients' relatives tell the doctor their stories, helped along or interrupted by the doctor's questions. Some of these questions, such as 'How long since you first noticed this?' simply seek to clarify the patients' statements, others like 'Has anyone in the family had similar problems?' have diagnostic implications. The patients provide the answers, which are duly committed to paper or to some electronic device. During the physical examination the doctor inspects, palpates, moves limbs, takes measurements and again records his findings. Unlike court proceedings, details of medical interrogations and examinations are, with few exceptions,[1] not described in fictional literature.* Most novelists, dramatists and short-story writers evidently consider such details uninteresting or scatological and, instead of providing clinical information, emphasize the negative aspects of the doctor–patient relationship: routine questions and procedures that seem entirely innocuous to a physician may appear as mindless exercises or even tortures to a patient, especially if their purpose is not adequately explained.

Satisfactory medical histories

A few truncated medical interviews appear not to arouse any resentment in the writer or the fictional patient. Samuel Warren in *A Slight Cold*[2] provides a brief interrogation of a patient with incipient pneumonia. 'Are you thirsty at all? Any catching in the side when you breathe? Any cough?' The patient's answers are not recorded but they evidently alarm the doctor sufficiently to make him write a prescription for 'tartarized antimony'. The medication is of no avail and 'Captain C' dies a few days later.[2] Dr Sevier,[3] who is making a house call, 'sat down in a chair, continuing his direct questions. The answers were all bad'.[3] The nature of the questions such as 'does it hurt you to urinate?' or 'have you been passing blood from the back passage?' and the 'bad' answers are not revealed. Waldo Yorke, the weak male character in *Doctor*

---

* Even when gruesome details (such as the performance of an episotomy) are supplied, they tend to involve treatment rather than the patient's medical history.

Zay,[4] who finds himself under the care of a female physician (Dr Zay Lloyd) after sustaining an ankle injury, is asked a series of professional questions which he cannot connect with his injury but which he does not resent. She

> required his age, his habits, family history and other items not immediately connected in the patient's mind with a dislocated ankle.[4]

Among Chekhov's slovenly, disgruntled and incompetent doctors one finds occasional characters whose behavior suggests, at least for a while, that the practice of medicine is more than a cruel joke. In *An Awkward Business*[5] the reader is given a very brief glimpse into an outpatient clinic at a Russian country hospital towards the end of the nineteenth century. Young Dr Gregory Ovchinnikov, who copes on his own with the entire spectrum of medical disorders, and 'processes' forty-five sick people in one morning,[5] is about to see a new patient.

> 'Anna Spiridonovna,' the doctor called. A young peasant woman in a red dress entered the surgery and said a prayer before the icon. 'What's troubling you?' the doctor asked. Glancing mistrustfully at the door through which she had come and at the door to the dispensary, the woman approached the doctor. 'I don't have no children,' she whispered.[5]

We do not hear what other questions are asked and we are not told the details of Anna Spiridonovna's physical examination or the treatment prescribed for her infertility.

The interview between a psychiatrist and a delusional patient in Drabble's *The Radiant Way*[6] is recorded in more detail.

> 'And these voices,' Liz asked of the patient sitting before her, 'what do they sound like? Is it a man's voice or a woman's voice? Or both?' Silence. Liz scribbled on her pad, auditory hallucinations . . . 'Sometimes,' the patient tentatively volunteers at last, leaning forward confidentially, speaking in a low, soft voice, 'they are music.' And he smiles as though imparting something precious . . . 'And what worries me is this . . . The advice they give me, I have to do it but it is bad. Bad things.' . . . 'Do you do what they say, the voices? Even when you think it is bad?' A pause. 'The voices are good. It is me that is bad.'[6]

Mona Van Duyn's intern,[7] who comes across as a thorough and only faintly ridiculous little man, asks a series of questions that appear disconnected and irrelevant to the patient. He has been taught to take a full history, so he makes enquiries about

> Bowel movements, chickenpox, the date of one's first menstruation,
> The number of pillows one sleeps on, postnasal drip.

He performs a complete physical examination. He promises the patient that he will leave no stone unturned to achieve a diagnostic label.

> 'Don't worry, if there's anything going on here,' the interne says,
> 'We'll find it. I myself have lots of ideas.'

He comes back the next day for another specimen.

> 'A little more blood, I'm on the trail.' He'll go far,
> My interne.[7]

Enquiries concerning sexual activities vary according to the patient's social status (*see* Chapter 10). Dr Stephen Maturin, Captain Jack Aubrey's friend, confidant and physician,[8] who behaves in a thoroughly professional manner when the Captain consults him about his depression, and who is quite capable of telling the Captain the unembellished truth (*see* p. 217), becomes remarkably circumspect when enquiring about sexual activity. Instead of using 'normal' terminology, he asks whether Aubrey has engaged in 'any commerce with Venus' at the ship's last port of call (Sydney).[8]

The interrogation of Larry Ward by Dr George Bull in Cozzens' *The Last Adam*[9] also concerns sexually transmitted disorders but the interview occurs under entirely different conditions. Larry, a handsome young man, who looks after the 'farm animals and gasoline motors' of one of the town's wealthy families, has known Dr Bull all his life. The boy, who has indeed had 'commerce with Venus', feels awful (he actually has typhoid fever), and does not know how to begin. The year is 1933.

> Larry clasped both hands together swallowing. He shifted in his chair. Finally he said, hushed: 'I think I got something, Doc.' 'Oh you do, do you? Well what have you got?' Larry gulped again, wordless and George Bull snorted. 'Uh, huh,' he agreed. 'Well don't get in a sweat. This isn't the YMCA . . . Been fooling with Betty Peters?' 'No, I . . . guess it must have been Charlotte Slade, Doc. She's the only one.' 'Well, she's certainly starting young.'[9]

The physical examination consists of 'a short arm inspection' and the doctor concludes (erroneously) there is nothing wrong with Larry other than a guilty conscience. He goes on to give the young man a lecture.

> 'Once is an accident; might happen to anyone. But if it goes on and by any chance I see her start swelling, this town'll be too hot for you not married to her. That'll be five dollars just to help you remember.'[9]

The patient evidently regards the encounter as satisfactory even though the ultimate outcome is disastrous.

Resentment of the doctor's questions

In contrast to these relatively gentle interviews, the elicitation of some medical histories engenders considerable resentment in the patient, the reader or both. Judge Clane in *Clock Without Hands*[10] becomes very angry when he recalls his interrogation at Johns Hopkins Hospital, which forced him to face the facts concerning his eating habits.

> When Dr Hume asked if I overate I assured him I ate just an ordinary amount. Then his questions chiseled finer. He asked, for instance, how many biscuits I had at a meal and I said 'Just the ordinary amount.' Chiseling in closer, in the way that doctors do, he inquired what was the 'ordinary amount.' When I told him 'Just a dozen or two' I felt right then and there I had met my Waterloo.[10]

Similarly, Anne Sexton's *Unknown Girl in the Maternity Ward*[11] has no doubt put up with the usual barrage of questions ('Is this your first pregnancy?' 'Have you had a blood transfusion?' 'When was your last menstrual period?'). After yet another interrogation she cries out:

> 'The doctors are enamel. They want to know the facts'[11]

implying that these white, hard, sterile and impenetrable people may be asking the 'correct' questions but that like enamel (? chipped enamel) they and their questions are far removed from what really matters.

Another 'enamel' character torments Professor Vivian Bearing, Margaret Edson's heroine, who suffers from terminal metastatic ovarian carcinoma.[12] The professor has already been thoroughly evaluated in her physician's office but, after her admission to hospital, she is obliged to tell her story again, to answer the same questions and to undergo a further pelvic examination, this time at the hands of a research fellow.[13] Edson emphasizes the mindless nature of the 'structured' questionnaire, which becomes particularly degrading when administered as part of a 'protocol' by an insensitive young man.

> 'How old are you?' 'Fifty.' 'Are you married?' 'No.' 'Are your parents living?' 'No.' 'How and when did they die?'[13]

The professor has to endure this form of torture for another forty questions, which include such gems as:

> 'Are you having sexual relations?' 'Not at the moment.' 'Are you pre- or post-menopausal?' 'Pre.' 'When was the first day of your last period?'[13]

All this useless material will no doubt be fed into a computer in the hope that that a 'cancer research' publication will emerge.

The incompetent Dr Armand Petrov in Lightman's *The Diagnosis*,[14] who is resented for his disorganization and his inefficiency, is also particularly inept at taking a medical history. Having kept Bill Chalmers for an hour and a quarter in the waiting room and another thirteen minutes (in his underpants) in an examination cubicle (*see* Chapter 2), Petrov now tries, unsuccessfully, to take a history and perform a physical examination at the same time.[15]

> Suddenly there was a knock and the door opened and closed. Dr Petrov was in the room, flying about and talking in a blur, small silver instruments dangling from his pockets. The doctor immediately set to work hammering different parts of Bill's body. When did the numbness begin? Any weakness in the hands or arms? Had he been suffering from

headaches? Was his appetite strong? 'I'll be right back.' The doctor vanished.

Petrov does not return, and the patient is told, after peeping out of the door and summoning a nurse, to get dressed and see the doctor in another room.[15] Chalmers' interview with a psychiatrist is equally frustrating.[16] The doctor asks irrelevant questions about Bill's parents, his marriage and his only child, as if any of these topics could have the slightest bearing on Bill's peripheral neuropathy. To make matters worse, he takes two unrelated phone calls during Bill's scheduled time (*see* p. 55).

Patients may exaggerate their symptoms, especially in order to obtain a medical certificate stating they are unfit for work (*see* p. 232), but deliberate attempts to mislead doctors are rare, and even more rarely succeed. An example of this 'general rule' is to be found in *Dr Phillips: a Maida Vale idyll*,[17] where Charles Doveton consults Dr Benjamin Phillips, ostensibly because of a sore elbow, but in reality to discover the identity of a woman who emerged from the doctor's office some minutes earlier. The doctor, who 'saw no trace of disease in the arm but much embarrassment and uneasiness in the face', becomes suspicious and asks,

> in his gravest professional manner . . . 'When did you first begin to grow nervous about your arm?' A rosy flush mounted to Charlie Doveton's cheek as he replied: 'Oh just now, . . . I mean, a long time ago . . . I don't know! . . . I say, Doctor, I want to ask you something.' The doctor rose. At last the young man seemed coming to the point.[17]

Similarly, the device of asking a doctor for medical information ostensibly on behalf of a third party seldom deceives fictional physicians. Alejandro Stern, Scott Turow's masterful trial lawyer,[18] is afraid he may have acquired genital herpes and asks his son, Dr Peter Stern, for information

> on behalf of someone with a need to know. . . . 'If one is exposed . . . how long before the disease appears?' Peter waited. 'Look Dad . . . do you think you have herpes?'[18]

The physical examination

As every medical student is taught, the process of observing a patient for objective physical signs occurs in two stages. Some abnormalities, such as obesity, short stature, a limp, abnormal movements and inappropriate behavior, are discoverable without the patients' consent and without their awareness that they are being scrutinized diagnostically. Blood pressure measurement, palpation and more invasive procedures require the patient's tacit or formal permission.

Wilkie Collins' *The Moonstone*[19] contains a convincing description of a doctor who recognizes that a patient's companion is sick, though the actual signs are not revealed. Lady Julia Verinder has taken her apparently hysterical daughter to London to see a 'medical man' who is also an old family friend.

> After prescribing for Rachel, he said he wished to speak to me privately in another room. I expected, of course, to receive some special direction for the management of my daughter's health. To my surprise he took me gravely by the hand and said. 'I have been looking at you . . . with a professional as well as a personal interest. You are, I am afraid, far more urgently in need of medical advice than your daughter.' He put some questions to me which I was at first inclined to treat lightly enough, until I observed that my answers distressed him.[19]

A formal examination is arranged for the next day though the signs are again not disclosed (*see* Chapter 5).

Chekhov, in *A Case History*,[20] provides more clinical details. Dr Korolyov has been summoned urgently to a small industrial town to see Liza Lyalikov, the only daughter and heiress of a local factory proprietor. Liza suffers from what sounds like chronic depression with panic attacks, but the doctor notices something unexpected. The patient has an 'outsize lower jaw . . . [and] large cold ungainly hands'. These signs of acromegaly, possibly with hypothyroidism, which would nowadays become the focus of investigations and intervention, denote the presence of a disease that was untreatable in 1898, and are not discussed with the patient. Korolyov and Liza part friends.[20]

Charles Marsden, Eugene O'Neill's fussy, middle-aged, homosexual writer,[21] develops an instant aversion to Dr Edmund Darrell, a neurologist, mainly because he suspects that the young doctor is scrutinizing him.

> Marsden (thinking sneeringly) 'Amusing these young doctors . . . perspire with the effort to appear cool! . . . Giving me the fishy diagnosing eye they practice at medical school.'

Marsden's resentment is not entirely groundless. Darrell's 'probing, examining look' has convinced him that Marsden is 'one of those poor devils who spend their lives trying not to discover which sex they belong to'.[21]

The formal elicitation of physical signs, which requires the patient's consent and cooperation, is described by Plato.[22] A doctor,

> who is enquiring into the health . . . of [a patient] . . . looks at his face and at the tips of his fingers and then he says: 'Uncover your chest and back to me that I may have a better view.'[22]

There is no hint of any resentment on the part of this examinee at being asked to disrobe. In more modern literature, the physical examination, essentially an attempt to gather evidence, has acquired additional connotations. Some patients and even some doctors perceive it as a therapeutic measure ('a good overhaul'), others as an indecent assault* ('feeling me all over'), and yet others, as a meaningless ritual.

Leo Tolstoy, who seems pathologically obsessed with the 'licentiousness' of the physical examination, makes one of his characters complain bitterly about his wife's physicians 'who cynically undressed her and felt her all over,[23] for which I had to

---

* Erotic encounters and fantasies engendered by the physical examination are described (*see* Book IV) but the procedure has been so thoroughly sanitized that such events are relatively rare.

thank them and pay them money' (*see* pp 25–6). Similarly, Venice Harpenden in Arlen's *The Green Hat*,[24] who believes she is sterile, refuses to see a doctor, partly because she considers the physical examination a meaningless hocus pocus (*see* p. 195).

> 'Do you actually think that I've got to go to some dud doctor and have him poking about all over me before I know what's *me*?'[24]

According to Tolstoy, the physical examination is not only an exercise in lewdness; it is also employed when the doctor is convinced of its futility. Ivan Illych's doctor, who is well aware that Ivan is dying

> begins with a most serious face to examine the patient, feeling his pulse and taking his temperature and then begins the . . . auscultation. Ivan Ilych knows quite well that all this is nonsense and pure deception . . . but he submits to it all.[25]

Hans Castorp's examination by Dr Behrens (the 'Hofrat'), which elicits only mild resentment, is one of the most detailed in fictional literature.[26] Hans, who has been visiting his tuberculous cousin at the sanatorium, has developed a fever, and decides that he requires medical attention. The young men bump into the doctor and, after a few pleasantries, Hans announces that he is unwell.

> 'You don't say!' Behrens cried out. I suppose you think you are telling me news? Do you think I've no eyes in my head?

An appointment is made during this casual encounter for Hans to accompany his cousin, who is scheduled for an examination the next day. The two are examined in each other's presence.[26]

First comes the inspection:

> The Hofrat . . . looked at him sharply – not in the face, as one man looks at another, but at his body; turned him around, as one would an inanimate object, and looked at his back.

Then comes the percussion:

> [Behrens] tapped from the wrist, using the powerful middle finger of his right hand as a hammer, and the left as a support.

During the auscultation Behrens directs Hans to take deep breaths and to cough and he calls out technical terms like 'vesicular' and 'rhonchi' to his assistant, who acts as scribe.[26]

Malègue, who is somewhat dismissive of percussion of the chest, describes the process (inaccurately) as 'little ritual taps with one hand knocking against the fingers of the other'[27] ('les petits coups rituels frappés par une main sur les phalanges de l'autre'), implying that the procedure is a useless exercise.

Auscultation of the chest may be equally futile. Paul Hasleman, a teenager in Conrad Aiken's *Silent Snow, Secret Snow*,[28] has developed hallucinations, presumably due to schizophrenia. Despite his psychotic state, the boy retains sufficient insight to understand that Doctor Howells, who has been summoned because of his 'curious absent-mindedness', is approaching the problem from the wrong angle. He

> stood before the doctor under the lamp, and submitted silently to the usual thumpings and tappings. 'Now will you please say Ah!' 'Ah.' 'Now again please, if you don't mind.' 'Ah.' 'Say it slowly and hold it if you can.' 'Ah-h h-h-h-h-.' 'Good.' How silly all this was. As if it had anything to do with his throat! Or his heart. Or lungs.[28]

Doctor Howells' attempts at eliciting psychological problems are equally clumsy and ineffectual.

> 'Now Paul – I would like very much to ask you a question or two. You will answer them, won't you – you know I am an old friend of yours, eh?' . . . His back was thumped twice by the doctor's fat fist – then the doctor was grinning at him with false amiability . . . 'I would like to know is there anything that worries you?'

Paul terminates the interview by claiming all these questions have given him a headache; he runs off to his room and abandons himself to his fantasies.[28]

The stethoscope, the principal badge of office of the contemporary doctor, is lampooned by one of the inmates in Ellis' tuberculosis sanatorium.[29] A noisy party in the room of one of the patients is enlivened by the arrival of the clown of the institution, carrying an assortment of 'medical' instruments including a rusty saw, a pair of pliers, a barometer and a piece of hosepipe which serves as a 'stethoscope'. One end of this tube is placed against the chest of a young female patient, while the clown stares 'lasciviously down the other'.[29] When Dr Vernet, the senior physician, arrives and attempts to restore order and decorum, the clown briefly interrupts the proceedings by creeping up behind Vernet and quietly giving him the hosepipe examination. The physician, who is also the medical administrator, swings around, takes in the scene at a glance, manages to control his temper and leads the clown back to his own room.[29]

In contrast to these infidels and scoffers, Francis Brett Young's Dr John Bradley[30] still believes in percussion and auscultation. After he has taken his patient's pulse and temperature:

> his face . . . became set with a quiet intensity . . . There was a ruthlessness in the fine old hands that percussed and palpated, lingering here and there in the process when sound or sensation seemed to differ from the normal. 'Say ninety-nine,' he said. 'Not like that! Don't whisper it. Your voice is all right.'[30]

The vaginal examination 'first with a rubber gloved finger then with a cold metal instrument'[31] obviously has the potential to provoke discomfort, anxiety and a variety of other emotions. Clara, the young wife of the elderly *Honorary Consul*,[32] who has worked in a South American whorehouse, refuses to undergo a physical examination during her initial encounter with Dr Plarr, but relents when the doctor assures her that he will not perform a vaginal examination.[32]

Remarkably, the standard neurological examination is also portrayed, in several works, as a threatening and dehumanizing procedure.[14] Simenon's hemiplegic and aphasic René Maugras[33] watches suspiciously as the neurology professor

> muttered to himself rather than to his patient as he went up to the bed: 'Let's see what's been happening!' . . . [He] took a little hammer from his pocket and tapped Maugras' knees and elbows with it, after which he scratched the soles of his feet with a sharp instrument. He repeated the process two or three times with a look of interest that seemed considerably greater than his interest in Maugras.[33]

Burgess' Edwin Spindrift, PhD (Linguistics), cuckold and assistant professor in one of the British Colonial Universities,[34] also finds the neurological examination a hateful experience. Spindrift, who suffers from some unidentified intra-cranial lesion, fails to establish rapport with his neurologist who makes him feel like a poorly performing competitor at a quiz session.

> 'And what is this smell?' asked Dr Railton. He thrust a sort of inkwell under Edwin's nose. 'I may be wrong, but I should say peppermint.' He awaited the quiz-master's gong . . . 'You are wrong, I'm afraid,' said Dr Railton. 'Lavender.' Gong. But he was still in the round. 'And this?' 'Probably something citrous.' 'Wrong again. Terribly wrong. Cloves.' There was a tone of moral indictment in the gentle voice . . . 'Not so good, is it? Not at all good' . . . Dr Railton pounced with a tuning fork. He brought it sizzling like a poker, up to Edwin's right cheek. 'Can you feel that?' 'Middle C.' 'No, no, can you feel it?' 'Oh yes.' Dr Railton looked grim, allowing Edwin no triumph. He got in quickly with: 'How would you define spiral?'[34]

Later in the course of the examination when Edwin fails to walk in a straight line, Railton 'boyishly laughed and play-punched Edwin on the chest, tousled his hair and tried to break off a piece of his shoulder' in an unsuccessful attempt to put him at ease.[34]

Worse is in store for Arthur Kopit's Mrs Emily Stilson,[35] who has been admitted to hospital suffering from a stroke and who is terrified by the doctor's 'routine' questions. Mrs Stilson has severe dysphasia, and believes she is now being subjected to a variety of tortures.

> Can you feel this? Can you feel this? Name something that grows on trees. Who fixes teeth? What room do you cook in? What year is this?

When the doctor asks her to repeat the simple phrase 'We live across the street from the school', Mrs Stilson answers in nonsense poetry: 'Malacats on the forturay are the kesterfats of the romancers',[35] with the implication that this meaningless response is entirely appropriate to the occasion. In the grotesque tortures inflicted on Schneiderman's sick doctor,[36] the neurological examination constitutes the central event:

they hammered his limbs, needled his skin and twisted his testes. They
scraped the soles of his feet, rattled his head with tuning forks, stood him
up and knocked him down.[36]

Schneiderman offers a partial explanation for the perception that the neurologist
and his tools of trade constitute a threat. For patients with symptoms and signs of
nervous system disorders there is always one diagnostic option: they are mad.[36]

On the other hand, the neurological examination of President (in exile) Manuel
Villegas by Professor Grandval of the University of Paris[37] is described as a gentle
and civilized event. Dr Ernesto Castillo, who presents the account in the first person,
is treated like a very junior medical student by the God-Professor, though he is
allowed to stay and act as interpreter.

> The moment Villegas entered the room, Professor Grandval became a
> totally different man – smiling, soft-spoken, gentle and infinitely cour-
> teous. And Villegas responded. Except that neither could speak the
> other's language very well, they were within minutes behaving like two
> old friends. To establish that sort of relationship with a patient, I . . .
> would need hours or days – or an eternity. Except when I was called
> upon to interpret, they ignored me. The questioning began almost
> imperceptibly, a smooth continuation, so it seemed, of the initial
> politeness but it was very thorough. How often did the [speech] difficulty
> occur? When, mostly? What time of day? How long to recover? . . . Was
> there any numbness? Twitching? . . . How about the arms and legs? After
> about half an hour the physical examination began. Again very thor-
> ough. Finally Professor Grandval said to the patient: 'I want to take some
> small sections of muscle . . . It won't hurt because I will give you . . .
> injections like your dentist does.' . . . Another forty minutes and it was
> over . . . 'That is all,' said Professor Grandval . . . Villegas sat up. 'What
> do you think, Professor?' . . . 'There are several possibilities, Monsieur,'
> he said blandly. 'As soon as I have been able to form an opinion, I will let
> Dr Castillo know, it may take several days.'[37]

The Professor concludes that Villegas has amyotrophic lateral sclerosis but the true
nature of the disease is not revealed to the patient (*see* pp 137–8).

Junior doctors feel uncomfortable with patients who complain of multiple
symptoms but lack any objective findings. Scott Fitzgerald's *One Interne*[38] is not
a good story. The plot is tortuous and contrived, while the behavior of the sick
intern (Dr William Tulliver V) is so bizarre that it might have come out of one of
Molière's comedies. However, before he is taken ill, Tulliver is a very credible intern,
especially with his first patient who complains of multiple symptoms.

> 'My head aches, my bones ache, I can't sleep, I don't eat. I've got fever' . . .
> The thermometer registered no fever and Dr Tulliver's diligent search for
> physical signs went unrewarded.

Neither Tulliver nor his fellow intern have been trained to deal with these kinds of
cases 'who aren't cases' and both would have preferred 'something more clearly

defined'.[38] The patient's reaction to Dr Tulliver's 'diligent search for physical signs' is not recorded.

Resentment as the result of the examination is widespread and varied. Virginia Woolf in *Mrs Dalloway*[39] expresses a great deal of hostility towards Sir William Bradshaw, the prominent London psychiatrist, who behaves in a thoroughly professional manner. He 'never hurried his patients', 'he gave [them] three-quarters of an hour' and he even asks 'if Mrs Warren Smith was quite sure she had no more questions'. Clarissa Dalloway, no doubt speaking for Virginia Woolf, finds this professionalism offensive. She describes Sir William Bradshaw as

> a great doctor yet to her obscurely evil, without sex or lust, extremely polite to women but capable of some indescribable outrage – forcing your soul, that was it.[39]

Rosenbaum's chief character,[40] a doctor with cancer of the larynx, is now a patient in a university hospital where, after forty years of medical practice, he is given 'a taste of his own medicine'. In particular, he has to put up with perfunctory and repetitive interviews such as his own patients no doubt had to endure over the years. The doctor is scheduled to undergo a biopsy of his larynx later in the day.

> The resident came in, took my history, listened to my heart and lungs, felt my neck and belly and asked if I needed a sedative. 'No,' I told him. He smiled and left. Now the anesthesiologist came in and asked the same questions . . . did I smoke? Did I drink? Was I allergic? – And he listened to my heart and lungs.[40]

The doctor-patient is not impressed by this parody of a physical examination. 'All they're doing is going through the motions. In case I die under anesthesia, they can prove to the lawyers in a malpractice suit that they had examined me.'[40]

Some patients are so angry that they resent prudent and even obligatory clinical procedures. They do not see the point of being questioned about their past and family histories[41] but they may be equally resentful when what they consider appropriate questions are omitted.[42] Maugin, the famous actor, who knows he smells of cheap wine (*see* pp 87–8), resents Dr Biguet, who asks no questions about wine or other forms of alcohol. Presumably, Maugin's drinking habits are common knowledge and the doctor can see no point in asking rhetorical questions.[42]

Patients may complain that the sphygmomanometer cuff is too tight and that the 'enormous pressure' gives them a pain in the arm,[43] but they are just as likely to protest when on a particular occasion the doctor neglects to take their blood pressure.[44] Even the creation and maintenance of accurate records, which are considered essential to good clinical practice, may give rise to resentment. 'Do you know', asks one of Frede's nurses rhetorically, 'how much distance doctors put between themselves and patients by writing things down?'[45] Ken Harrison, the angry and suicidal quadriplegic in *Whose Life Is It Anyway*,[46] expresses himself more vigorously.

> 'You . . . doctors with your so-called professionalism which is nothing more than a series of verbal tricks to prevent you relating to patients as human beings . . . I say something offensive about you and you turn your

professional cheek . . . If you were treating me as human, you would tell me to bugger off.'[46]

Hand-washing

After the examination, while the patients are getting dressed, doctors generally wash their hands. In Carson McCullers' *Clock Without Hands*,[47] JT Malone, who is still lying on the examination couch, resents this activity. Dr Hayden 'washing his hands at the Corner wash-basin . . . offended Malone',[47] presumably because hand-washing calls to mind the symbol for the abandonment of responsibility.[48]* The washbasin, which also occurs in Auden's *Miss Gee*,[50] constitutes, to the doctor, an elementary means for maintaining cleanliness and hygiene. To Malone and to Ivan Illych,[51] who resent the entire medical profession, the hand-washing act transforms the doctor from an 'artisan' who lays hands on sick people in order to help them, to a member of the scientific community who lays hands on patients in order to study them. He becomes part of the 'research bureaucracy' to whom patients are statistics regardless of the clinical outcome.[51]

The hand-washing scene in *The Doctor from Dunmore*[52] is not the sole reason for Dr Fitzwilliam's' unpopularity among the villagers on the island of 'Innisheen'. He is a wealthy member of the Protestant 'establishment', while they can barely afford 'the price of a decent pair o' britches to wear to Mass on Sunday'.[52] He demands an enormous fee for coming over from the mainland (*see* p. 28). He rudely interrupts the local bone-setter who wants to tell him about the 'blessed water from St Colum's well' and what it had done for 'Mick Corrigan, God rest his soul'. The doctor is not interested in the villagers' superstitions or their economic circumstances. Instead, he asks for hot water, soap, a clean towel 'if you have one',[52] and he ostentatiously washes his hands before examining the patient. When he disappears into the sick room, a villager remarks: 'Wouldn't that old fella provoke a saint?' One of the neighbors responds: 'He's enough to provoke the whole twelve apostles'.[52]

Tests

After a visit to the doctor or a doctor's visit to a patient, tests may be ordered to help solve diagnostic problems. To the doctors, such investigations provide a brief respite before they have to come out into the open with a diagnosis and a management plan. Patient with no discernible pathology but with multiple organic symptoms readily accept recommendations for repeated tests, which support their belief that someone will one day discover the 'true' nature of their disease. Chronic residents of institutions are more skeptical. They know that tests are sometimes unpleasant ('a flashy show of cold steel and frightful bloodshed'[53]), frequently inconclusive and rarely useful in their management. These hardened veterans, who do not anticipate any improvement in their conditions, are particularly suspicious of new residents

---

* The hand-washing ritual and its symbolic significance are discussed in detail by Richard Selzer.[49]

who repeat tests that have already been performed by their predecessors. Mr Klippelfeil,* a 'world famous professor of helminthology' and now an inpatient on the neurology service of the Paradiso Veterans Administration Hospital, has a biopsy-proven brain tumor but worries that the new resident will order further tests including a further biopsy. One of the other patients warns him: 'Every doc wants a piece of tumor for himself'.[54]

Paul Davenant, of 'Les Alpes' sanatorium, whose pulmonary tuberculosis refuses to respond to any of the treatment modalities available at the time, is submitted to a number of investigations,[55–57] all of them unpleasant and none of them of the slightest value in diagnosis, prognosis or treatment. His bronchogram is a form of torture, which nearly ends in disaster,[55] the painful bone marrow examination, via a sternal puncture,[56] frightens him and on one occasion he has spend an entire day in the laboratory 'undergoing tests which made him retch physically and mentally'.[57]

Bill Chalmers' tests, forty years later, are more sophisticated and less distressing but equally useless.[58,59] Bill, who suffers from a progressive and ultimately fatal form of peripheral neuropathy, is subjected to a CT scan, an MRI examination, a series of biochemical and electro-physiological tests[58] and a PET procedure,[59] all of them justifiable in an undiagnosed neurological case, but none of them contributory. Towards the terminal stage of the illness, Chalmers' wife wants him to go back to the hospital where the doctors will no doubt 'order another round of examinations for him',[60] but Bill has had enough and refuses to have further tests or treatment.

Diagnosis

Since the days of Hippocrates, physicians trained in the discipline of Western medicine have found it necessary to 'give the ill[ness] . . . a name',[61] regardless of whether they can cure it or not (*see* p. 123). Mere phenomenological accounts such as are found in the Bible[62] are considered insufficient, and some sort of label is required, even though it may simply consist of a synonym for the patient's symptoms. Hippocrates himself, after accurately documenting the course of a fatal disease, feels impelled to diagnose 'phrenitis',[63] whatever that term may have meant to him. Dr Medhurst, not one of the most distinguished disciples of Hippocrates,[64] uses outlandish diagnostic terms, largely to bamboozle his patients, who do not appreciate a 'what's in a name?' attitude. Even sophisticated college graduates require 'trademarks' for their ailments. Polly Andrews, the most likeable member of McCarthy's Vassar *Group*[65] finds it outrageous that her boyfriend, who has been seeing a psychoanalyst on a regular basis, has never been given a diagnosis.

> If you went to a doctor with a rash . . . wouldn't you feel entitled to know whether he thought you had measles or prickly heat?[65]

Over the years several myths concerning diagnoses have found their way into the literature, some of them persisting to this day. Towards the end of the nineteenth and the early part of the twentieth centuries when diagnosis was regarded as a kind of a bridge problem,[66] or a crossword puzzle with a few scanty clues and the answer

---

* *See* footnote p. 207.

provided in the post-mortem room the next day,[67,68] finding the cause of a patient's symptoms and putting a name to it was considered akin to crime detection. Dorothy Sayers' 'Lord Peter Wimsey',[66] in a flippant mood, asks Dr Hartman

> 'How d'you do it? . . . Is there a regular set of symptoms for each disease like calling a club to show your partner to go to no trumps? You don't just say: This fellow's got a pimple on his nose therefore he has fatty degeneration of the heart?' 'I hope not,' said the doctor dryly. 'Or is it more like getting a clue to a crime?' went on Peter. 'You see something, a room or a body . . . all knocked about . . . and there's a damn sight of symptoms of something wrong and you've just got to pick out the ones which tell the story?' 'That's more like it,' said Dr Hartman. 'Some symptoms are significant in themselves, like the condition of the gums in scurvy . . .'[66]

At this point, Dr Hartman's explanations of 'soft' and 'hard' clinical signs are interrupted by a shrill scream emanating from an upstairs apartment, where a murder is being committed. During the subsequent criminal investigation Dr Hartman's diagnostic abilities prove totally inadequate. His medical training has conditioned him to believe that he is being told the truth – Wimsey and his servant know better. More seriously, the doctor is apt to form hypotheses and 'he only sees the facts which fit in with his theory'.[69]

Also around the end of the nineteenth century, and well into the twentieth, the ability to arrive at a diagnosis was considered a special gift, acquired in somewhat mysterious circumstances by only a handful of physicians. Dr Benjamin Phillips, *The Idyll of Maida Vale*[70]

> had the gift of diagnosis. He gave the lie to the saying that 'a rapid diagnosis is a wrong diagnosis.' He could read life or death on a patient's face with unerring instinct.[70]

Proust accepts and perpetuates the myth of the uncanny diagnostician[71,72] (whose reputation is almost certainly based on a few lucky guesses and an ability to intimidate his colleagues). Proust's Dr Cottard has convinced himself, his colleagues, and his patients that he possesses this mysterious gift. According to Proust, diagnostic acumen

> does not imply superiority in the other departments of the intellect, and a person of the utmost vulgarity, . . . who is without the slightest intellectual curiosity, may perfectly well possess it.[72]

Cottard becomes internationally famous and his increasingly dogmatic pronunciamentos assume the status of holy writ.

> Everyone praised . . . the penetration, the unerring judgment of his diagnoses.[71]

Helen Ashton's Dr Richard Gaunt[73] is similarly portrayed as a man with a very limited intellect, who nonetheless possessed the gift of diagnosis.

> He had been a man of many small generalizations and proverbs, no friend to professional novelties, accustomed to work by rule of thumb.

Somehow, this totally unscientific character who would have regarded any new concept with grave suspicion, has become, like a birdwatcher,

> an uncannily clever but utterly unreasoning master of diagnosis.[73]

A third misconception is the notion that provided the 'correct' test is performed it is always possible, by an orderly process of logical reasoning, to arrive at a diagnosis. Conversely, without a diagnosis there can be no rational treatment.

> Confronted with symptoms which may be those of three or four different complaints it is . . . [the physician's] judgment that must decide with which, despite the more or less similar appearance of them all, he has to deal.[72]

Proust does not seem to understand and contemporary health administrators certainly do not understand that arriving at a diagnosis is often a messy process, with bits of evidence emerging and being discarded while the patients improve or deteriorate and while they receive treatment. Some symptom complexes remain unclassifiable so that the patient has to be managed without a label. Well-trained physicians take this uncertainty principle for granted. 'Healing . . . is not a science' was one of the messages transmitted by Dr George Augustus Auden to his son Wystan Hugh.[74]

The imprecision inherent in medical practice, and the ability to make rational decisions and recommendations in the absence of exact data, forms almost the core of the physician's profession. Weir Mitchell[75] is one of the few writers to articulate the fact that some physicians see this imprecision as a challenge rather than a source of frustration. When the Fairthorne sisters discuss the idealized Dr Sydney Archer, one of them expresses the view that Archer 'has too much intellect for the professional uncertainties of medicine'.[75] Archer himself disagrees. He admits the uncertainty, but he adds, 'that is part of the interest'.[76] On the other hand, Lightman's Bill Chalmers, who has an undiagnosed disorder, falls into the hands of physicians who cannot distinguish between the luggage and the label and who aggravate rather than relieve his anguish.[14]

Diagnostic success stories

Several stories by physician/authors describe the sense of achievement that may follow the establishment of a 'correct' diagnosis. Cronin's *The Citadel*[77] contains a convincing account of a physician who examines a previously placid coalminer, whose behavior has altered in recent weeks. Dr Andrew Manson, the medical hero, who handles the situation competently and sympathetically, reaches the diagnosis by the traditional inductive method.[77]

> There must be a reason, Manson thought doggedly . . . Staring at the swollen features before him, puzzling . . . for some solution of the

conundrum, he instinctively reached out and touched the swollen face . . .
All at once . . . a terminal vibrated in his brain . . . It was myxedema . . .
Temperature – it was subnormal. Methodically he finished the examina-
tion fighting back each successive wave of elation.[77]

A less dramatic diagnostic success comes to Dr Jay Reese who practices 'bread-and-
butter' pediatrics[78] (*see* p. 146), and who finds that occasional diagnostic challenges
add flavor to his routine activities. A boy with an itchy, painful rash over the upper
part of his trunk is discovered to suffer from an allergic reaction to gypsy moth
larvae after running 'shirtless through chest high grass'. Dr Reese's lady friend is full
of admiration.

> 'You're a good detective,' she said. 'I like the way you look for clues. I
> like the way you enjoy it when you find them.' 'Me too. It's the best thing
> I do. It's the only fun really except when kids hug me and get better.'[78]

A correct diagnosis may provide a sense of accomplishment even at a post-mortem
examination, without the doctor appearing particularly heartless. Pasternak in
Doctor Zhivago[79] describes the case of

> a woman [who] had died . . . in the surgical ward. Yurii Andreievich
> [Zhivago] had diagnosed echinococcus of the liver but everyone thought
> he was wrong. An autopsy was to be made today but the . . . [pathologist]
> was a habitual drunkard and you never could tell how careful he would
> be . . . [Later that day] standing by the window, the flabby elderly . . .
> [pathologist] was holding up a jar with some opaque liquid . . . 'Everyone
> is impressed – echinococcus it was.'[79]

Obviously, diagnostic problems are more difficult when they occur on the 'production line' of the emergency room, and the only person to solve them is a very
junior intern. Somerset Maugham's Philip Carey[80] has to deal with a predicament
faced by generations of young house officers: should inebriated individuals and
potential malingerers be offered the scarce hospital resources designated for
'genuinely' sick people?

> The wards were crowded and the house surgeon was faced with a
> dilemma when patients were brought in by the police; if they were sent
> on to the station and died there, disagreeable things were said in the
> papers; and it was very difficult sometimes to tell if a man was dying or
> drunk.[80]

Ravin takes up this theme towards the end of the twentieth century. Dr William
Ryan, an intern working in the emergency department of a New York hospital in the
1980s, has to cope with challenges very similar to those described by Somerset
Maugham seventy years earlier. He has to pick 'the dangerously ill out of all the flus,
earaches, feeling dizzys and feeling terribles who present . . . themselves to the ER
door'. . . . Dr Ryan even scores a diagnostic success.

> The real delight was admitting an ostensible turkey who proved to be genuinely sick, like the lady with the clot in her lung. She had a few risk factors but not much of a story. Ryan admitted her on . . . 'clinical acumen' . . . Her lung scan showed a big pulmonary embolus. It was so big, the nuclear medicine man didn't even hedge his report, as he almost always did.[81]

Dr Ryan's jargon and his sentiments (especially the term 'turkey') are classical 'Internese', but the sense of triumph at having scored a hit can be appreciated and confirmed by any physician who has ever worked in an Emergency Department.

Doctors who spend insufficient time evaluating their patient's stories may miss vital clues,[82] and there are several accounts by doctor/authors of 'near-misses'.[83–85] In Ravin's *Seven North*,[83] a Mrs Waterhouse presents to Dr Benjamin Abrams with very vague symptoms. She is tired, she cries for no reason and Dr Abrams is on the point of asking her whether she has considered a visit to a psychiatrist. However, there are some unusual features suggestive of Addison's disease. 'I felt very pleased with myself, catching that diagnosis, but then I considered how very close I'd come to missing it.'[83] Dr Steven Rushton's sense of triumph at having correctly diagnosed a patient's perforated duodenal ulcer ('half his breakfast floating around . . . in his peritoneal cavity . . . on top of two pints of brown ale'[84]) is tempered by the realization that the admission to hospital was a stroke of luck. The patient, James McNair, has been complaining of severe abdominal pain for years, multiple tests have been negative 'and the experts had unanimously concluded that his symptoms were entirely psychogenic'.[84] On this particular occasion, Dr Rushton, who is in a hurry, refers McNair to hospital because it seems the easiest means of getting rid of a patient with a convoluted, time-consuming history. 'I knew that it had been a case of getting him out of my hair and that the dividing line between triumph and disaster had been, in this case, paper-thin.'[84]

Another near miss is described by Huyler in *Sugar*.[85] A two-year-old black girl has been brought into the Accident and Emergency Department because earlier that evening, the child was staring into space several times. It is ten o'clock on a Friday night, there are half a dozen patients waiting and the resident, as well as the child's parents, are getting impatient. There is no significant medical history, the physical examination is completely normal and the little girl is scampering around the room happily. The resident is on the point of sending the family home, when, as an afterthought, he inquires whether the child 'might have gotten into someone's medications'. It turns out that the grandmother is taking oral hypoglycemic agents and that the little girl's blood sugar is low. 'I felt . . . terrified by what I had almost missed. One question.'[85]

The professional sense of accomplishment that follows an astute diagnosis or a successful treatment has nothing to do with the fee or the patient's gratitude. It comes from the feeling that, for once, one of the doctor's works has turned out 'artistically correct'.

> [There are] conflicts between diseases and physicians . . . of which physicians alone have any knowledge and whose reward in cases of success is never found in the paltry price of their labors nor indeed under the patient's roof but in the sweet gratification . . . bestowed upon true artists by the satisfaction they feel . . . in having accomplished a worthy work.[86]

Summary

The history and physical examination are regarded by most physicians as the backbone of clinical medicine, and referred to affectionately by habitual patients as a 'good overhaul'. However, detailed and intrusive questions, especially if repeated, have the potential to evoke antagonism, so that a simple question relating to the family history may elicit an angry response. The tongue depressor, the percussion hammer and the sphygmomanometer may be viewed as instruments of torture. Patients are particularly resentful of what they perceive as mindless, repetitive procedures. The establishment of a diagnosis is not an orderly process like a judgement after a trial and in many patients no firm diagnosis is ever made.

References

1 Hellerstein D (1986) *Battles of Life and Death*. Houghton Mifflin, Boston, MA.

2 Warren S (1832) A Slight Cold. In: Warren S. *Diary of a Late Physician*, vol. 2. Blackwood, Edinburgh, pp. 201–22.

3 Cable GW (1885) *Dr Sevier*. James R Osgood and Company, Boston, MA, pp. 7–19.

4 Phelps ES (1882) *Doctor Zay*. Feminist Press, New York, 1987, pp. 51–2.

5 Chekhov AP (1888) An Awkward Business. In: *The Oxford Chekhov*, vol. 4. Translated by Hingley R. Oxford University Press, London, 1980, pp. 99–115.

6 Drabble M (1987) *The Radiant Way*. Weidenfeld and Nicolson, London, pp. 132–3.

7 Van Duyn M (1959) In the Hospital for Tests. In: Van Duyn M. *To See to Take*. Atheneum, New York, 1971, pp. 45–7.

8 O'Brian P (1992) *The Truelove*. WW Norton, New York, pp. 15–35.

9 Cozzens JG (1933) *The Last Adam*. Harcourt Brace and Company, New York, pp. 164–6.

10 McCullers C (1953) *Clock Without Hands*. Houghton Mifflin, Boston, MA, 1963, pp. 61–3.

11 Sexton A (1960) Unknown Girl in the Maternity Ward. In: Sexton A. *To Bedlam and Part Way Back*. Houghton Mifflin, Boston, MA, p. 34.

12 Edson M (1993) *Wit*. Faber and Faber, New York, 1999.

13 Ibid., pp. 23–7.

14 Lightman A (2000) *The Diagnosis*. Pantheon Books, New York.

15 Ibid., pp. 116–17.

16 Ibid., pp. 200–1.

17 Danby F (Julia Frankau) (1887) *Dr Phillips: a Maida Vale idyll*. Garland Publishing, New York, 1984, pp. 32–4.

18 Turow S (1990) *The Burden of Proof*. Warner Books, New York, 1991, p. 180.

19 Collins W (1868) *The Moonstone*. Perennial Classics, Harper and Row, New York, 1965, pp. 211–12.

20 Chekhov AP (1898) A Case History. In: *The Oxford Chekhov*, vol. 9. Translated by Hingley R. Oxford University Press, London, 1975, pp. 69–78.

21 O'Neill E (1928) Strange Interlude. In: O'Neill E (1988) *Complete Plays*, vol. 2. Library of America, New York, p. 660.

22 Plato (4th century BC) *Protagoras*. Translated by Jowett B. In: Buchanan S (ed.) (1979) *The Portable Plato*. Penguin, Harmondsworth, p. 103.

23 Tolstoy L (1891) The Kreutzer Sonata. Translated by Maude A. In: Simmons EJ (ed.) (1966) *Leo Tolstoy, Short Novels*, vol. 2. Modern Library, Random House, New York, pp. 148–9.

24 Arlen M (1924) *The Green Hat*. George H Doran, New York, p. 221.

25 Tolstoy L (1886) The Death of Ivan Ilych. Translated by Maude L and Maude AC. In: Simmons EJ (ed.) (1966) *Leo Tolstoy, Short Novels*, vol. 2. Modern Library, Random House, New York, pp. 47–9.

26 Mann T (1924) *The Magic Mountain*. Translated by Lowe-Porter HT. Penguin, Harmondsworth, 1960, pp. 174–81.

27 Malègue J (1932) *Augustin, ou, Le maître est là*, vol. 2. Spes, Paris, 1935, pp. 380–5.

28 Aiken C (1932) Silent Snow, Secret Snow. In: Aiken C (1982) *Collected Short Stories*. Schocken Books, New York, pp. 216–35.

29 Ellis AE (1958) *The Rack*. Penguin, London, 1988, pp. 173–5.

30 Young FB (1938) *Dr Bradley Remembers*. Heinemann, London, pp. 14–16.

31 O'Brien E (1965) *August Is A Wicked Month*. Jonathan Cape, London, pp. 219–20.

32 Greene G (1973) *The Honorary Consul*. Simon and Schuster, New York, p. 83.

33 Simenon G (1963) *The Patient*. Translated by Stewart J. Hamish Hamilton, London, pp. 33–4.

34 Burgess A (1960) *The Doctor is Sick*. Heinemann, London, 1968, pp. 1–3.

35 Kopit A (1978) *Wings*. Hill and Wang, New York, pp. 29–41.

36 Schneiderman LJ (1972) *Sea Nymphs by the Hour*. Authors Guild Backinprint.Com, Lincoln, NE, 2000, p. 174.

37 Ambler E (1974) *Doctor Frigo*. Fontana Collins, Glasgow, 1976, pp. 132–3.

38 Fitzgerald FS (1935) One Interne. In: Fitzgerald FS. *Taps at Reveille*. Charles Scribner's Sons, New York, pp. 294–313.

39 Woolf V (1925) *Mrs Dalloway*. Zodiac Press, London, 1947, pp. 104–13.

40 Rosenbaum EE (1988) *The Doctor* (also titled *A Taste Of My Own Medicine*). Ivy Books, New York, 1991, p. 37.

41 Cobb IS (1915) Speaking of Operations. In: Zevin ED (ed.) (1945) *Cobb's Cavalcade*. World Publishing Company, Cleveland, OH, 1945, pp. 17–37.

42 Simenon G (1950) The Heart of a Man. Translated by Varèse L. In: *The Second Simenon Omnibus*. Hamish Hamilton, London, 1974, pp. 151–62.

43 Oates JC (1971) The Metamorphosis. In: Oates JC (1972) *Marriages and Infidelities*. Vanguard Press, New York, p. 372.

44 Pym B (1980) *A Few Green Leaves*. EP Dutton, New York, pp. 2–17.

45 Frede R (1985) *The Nurses*. WH Allen, London, 1986, p. 86.

46 Clark B (1972) *Whose Life Is It Anyway*. Amber Lane Press, Ashover, UK, 1978, p. 34.

47 McCullers C, op. cit., p. 5.

48 The Bible (1st century AD) Revised Standard Version. Oxford University Press, New York, 1977, Matthew, 27: 24.

49 Selzer R (1985) My Brother Shaman. In: Jones AH (ed.) *Literature and Medicine*, vol. 2. Johns Hopkins University Press, Baltimore, MD, pp. 41–4.

50 Auden WH (1936) Miss Gee. In: Auden WH (1970) *Selections by the Author*. Penguin, Harmondsworth, pp. 43–5.

51 Illich I (1976) *Limits to Medicine*. Penguin, London, 1990, pp. 254–5.

52 Dillon TP and Leary N (1940) The Doctor from Dunmore. In: Fowler HG (1957) *Curtain Up*. Melbourne University Press, Carlton, Victoria, Australia, pp. 126–34.

53 Schneiderman LJ, op. cit., p. 18.

54 Ibid., p. 11.

55 Ellis AE, op. cit., pp. 62–6.

56 Ibid., pp. 83–4.

57 Ibid., p. 258.

58 Lightman A, op. cit., pp. 180–2.

59 Ibid., p. 324.

60 Ibid., p. 367.

61 Arnold M (1867) A Wish. In: Tinker CB and Lowry HF (eds) (1966) *Arnold Poetical Works*. Oxford University Press, London, pp. 249–51.

62 The Bible (approx. 4th century BC) Revised Standard Version, Oxford University Press, New York, 1977, II Chronicles, 21: 18–19.

63 Hippocrates (5th century BC) Epidemics III, Case VIII. Translated by Jones WHS. *Loeb's Classical Library*, vol. 1. Heinemann, London, 1923, p. 233.

64 Young FB, op. cit., pp. 242–5.

65 McCarthy M (1954) *The Group*. Signet, New York, 1963, p. 284.

66 Sayers DL (1928) The Vindictive Story of the Footsteps that Ran. In: *Lord Peter Views the Body*. Gollancz, London, 1979, p. 167.

67 Bashford HH (1911) *The Corner of Harley Street: being some familiar correspondence of Peter Harding MD*. Constable, London, 1913, p. 14.

68 Williams WC (1934) Jean Beicke. In: Williams WC (1984) *The Doctor Stories*. New Directions, New York, pp. 69–77.

69 Sayers DL, op. cit., pp. 168–80.

70 Danby F (Julia Frankau), op. cit., p. 71.

71 Proust M (1913–22) *Remembrance of Things Past*, vol. 1. Translated by Scott-Moncrieff CK and Kilmartin T. Penguin, Harmondsworth, 1985, p. 467.

72 Ibid., p. 536.

73 Ashton H (1930) *Doctor Serocold*. Penguin, London, 1936, p. 10.

74 Auden WH (1972) The Art of Healing, In Memoriam David Protetch MD. In: Auden WH. *Epistle to a Godson and Other Poems*. Faber and Faber, London, pp. 13–15.

75 Mitchell SW (1901) *Circumstance*. Century Company, New York, 1902, p. 48.

76 Ibid., p. 42.

77 Cronin AJ (1937) *The Citadel*. Gollancz, London, p. 68.

78 Busch F (1984) Rise and Fall. In: Busch F. *Too Late American Boyhood Blues*. David R Godine, Boston, MA, p. 26.

79 Pasternak B (1957) *Doctor Zhivago*. Translated by Hayward M and Harari M. Pantheon, New York, 1958, pp. 102–5.

80 Maugham WS (1915) *Of Human Bondage*. Signet Classics, New York, 1991, p. 521.

81 Ravin N (1981) *MD*. Delacorte Press/Seymour Lawrence, New York, p. 333.

82 Baron RJ (1985) An introduction to medical phenomenology: I can't hear you while I'm listening. *Ann Int Med*. **103**: 606–11.

83 Ravin N (1985) *Seven North*. EP Dutton/Seymour Lawrence, New York, pp. 110–16.

84 Russell R (1985) *While You're Here, Doctor*. Souvenir Press, London, pp. 109–15.

85 Huyler F (1999) Sugar. In: Huyler F. *The Blood of Strangers*. University of California Press, Berkeley, CA, pp. 127–31.

86 Balzac H de (1840) *Pierrette*. Translated by Ives GB. George Barrie and Sons, Philadelphia, PA, 1897, pp. 215–16.

CHAPTER 5

Explanations; the medium and the message; the truth

To write prescriptions is easy but to come to an understanding with people is hard.[1]

Doctor, doctor come here quick
Doctor, doctor I feel sick.
Doctor, doctor, will I die?
No, dear child, do not cry.[2]

The nature of the problem

When the physical examination is over, the findings have been recorded and the performance of tests can no longer be used as an excuse for procrastination, doctors are expected to provide the sick person or a responsible family member with appropriate explanations. In particular, they have to answer questions concerning the nature and expected duration of the patient's illness, and the likelihood or otherwise of a recovery. However, as soon as the doctor begins to speak, he is faced by major and perennial communication problems relating both to the language and the contents of his message: how should technical information be conveyed? How much bad news should be disclosed? Patients have an aversion to medical jargon, but they like what they see as 'Mickey Mouse' language even less. Different educational standards prevail, so that what constitutes advanced medical terminology to one individual is regarded as childish patter by another. Many patients want detailed answers to their questions, but lack the background to understand even the most basic physiological concepts. They ask for the truth but do not necessarily profit from the revelation of all the unpleasant details. What is the appropriate method of dealing with these predicaments?

There are no 'right' answers, but one of the difficulties is clearly identified by George Eliot's Dr Tertius Lydgate,[3] who has 'the medical accomplishment of looking perfectly grave, whatever nonsense was talked to him'.

Lydgate's conversation with Dorothea Brooke on hospitals and therapeutic principles has been less than satisfactory.

'She is a good creature . . . but a little too earnest,' he thought. 'It is troublesome to talk to such women. They are always wanting reasons yet they are too ignorant to understand the merits of any question.'[3]

Carossa's *Doctor Gion*[4] fails miserably when he tries to explain the concept of red and white blood cells to 'Emerence', a simple servant girl who suffers from acute myeloid leukemia. Emerence has never looked down a microscope, and cannot grasp the idea of blood cells. At the end of the session she asks:

'If I were to eat red beetroot or to drink red wine wouldn't that help?' [The doctor] felt as if he had made a mistake somewhere.[4]

Unsuitable terminology; medical jargon

Medical jargon has impressed and annoyed lay members of the community since classical times. Pliny, in his diatribe against the medical profession,[5] implies that unscrupulous physicians use incomprehensible medical terms to impress gullible patients and that the technique works well.

Our . . . foolish . . . countrymen . . . have less confidence and trust in those things which concern their life and health if they be intelligible . . . than in others which they understand never a whit.[5]

Semi-Latin medical phrases have been employed and ridiculed for centuries. In Middleton's restoration comedy *Anything for a Quiet Life*,[6] Ralph, who is suffering from a penile chancre, is visiting Sweetball, a barber-surgeon. Ralph wants to get back to his shop but Sweetball tries to convince him that the situation is serious and that a 'business as usual' attitude is inappropriate. He uses Latin terms to reinforce his arguments.

Barber: You must have a little patience when you are a patient. If preputium (the foreskin) be not too much perished you shall lapse a little.
Ralph: What's that sir?
Barber: Marry if there be exulceration (an ulcer) between preputium and glans, by my faith the whole penis may be endangered as far as the os pubis (pubic bone).
Ralph: What's this you talk on sir?
Barber: If they be gangrened once, testiculi (testicles), vesica (bladder) and all may run to mortification.[6]

In the eighteenth century Henry Fielding similarly makes fun of Tom Jones' surgeon[7] who uses Latin terms when simple English would have been quite adequate.

The os or bone very plainly appeared through the aperture of the vulnus or wound . . . I apprehended immediate mortification.[7]

All of this is quite incomprehensible to Fielding's Lieutenant, who also resents the surgeon's evasiveness. In answer to direct questions as to whether Tom's life is in danger, the doctor replies 'who is there among us who . . . can be said to be out of danger?'[7]

One hundred years later, doctors no longer introduce Latin words into their conversations but they still write 'omni mane' instead of 'every morning' on their prescription pads,[8] while some of their secret hieroglyphics 'would not have misbecome the tomb of Cheops'.[8] They use a polysyllabic terminology, which makes them sound like an article out of a quarterly journal,[9] and they are fond of the double negative, employed in medical jargon to this day. Behavioral disturbances in a young man, declares Dr Wycherley in Reade's *Hard Cash*,[9] may constitute 'precursory indications of incipient disease of the cerebro-psychical organs'. The patient's depressive symptoms are 'not unaccompanied' by withdrawn behavior. Reade offers two explanations for Wycherley's tendency to use jargon. One of them restates Pliny's view:[5] 'This foible earned him the admiration of fools; and that is as invaluable as they are innumerable.'[9] The other relates to Wycherley's method of conveying bad news. 'He rarely irritated a fellow creature', and his kind of circumlocution is obviously less emotive than a simple statement like 'the boy is going mad'. Neither Reade nor Pliny seems to consider that medical terminology is used during doctors' training and in conversations between colleagues, and that the failure to switch from one language to another may simply reflect a lack of linguistic talent.

The scientific terms describing human disease processes continue to give rise to annoyance. Matthew Arnold in *A Wish*[10] prays that when he lies on his deathbed he will be spared the irritating gibberish of the smart diagnostician:

> Spare me the whispering, crowded room
> The friends who come, and gape and go,
> The ceremonious air of gloom –
> All, which makes death a hideous show.
> Nor bring to see me cease to live
> Some doctor full of phrase and fame,
> To shake his sapient head and give
> The ill he cannot cure a name.[10]

Wells' young doctor who treats 'Uncle Ponderevo' in his final illness is described in just four adjectives: 'Mysterious . . . technical . . . modern . . . unhelpful.'[11] Even in the second half of the twentieth century, patients complain about the doctors' obscure and outlandish vocabulary. In Wouk's *Youngblood Hawke*,[12] several members of the Hawke family are waiting outside the delivery room for the birth of a baby who, they believe, may have inherited its father's total alopecia (it had not). These people, who are terrified, have to put up with an intern who 'seemed about sixteen years old', who talks in 'medical school jargon' and whose only professional accomplishment consists of the way he wears his stethoscope round his neck. The expectant father waits until the youthful doctor has left before he complains 'It's a funny thing how hard it is to get a straight answer from a doctor.'[12]

Leon Daudet, who dislikes most aspects of clinical practice, finds medical terms particularly distasteful. Some simply restate the patient's complaint in a foreign language, while others are designed to hide the physician's ignorance. The patient who complains of a sore tongue and is told by his doctor that he has 'glossitis' is simply being informed, with the help of a Greek word, that he has a sore tongue.

> A patient asked Doctor Boridan one day 'What's the matter with me?' and stuck out his tongue, which was swollen and red. 'How do you say tongue in Greek?' asked the imperturbable doctor. 'Gloss' replied the other. 'Well, my friend, you've got glossitis.'[13]

According to Daudet, the traditional term 'hemophilia' is worse. Its semantics are ridiculous and it fails to explain the pathophysiology of the disease.

> 'This ill-chosen expression indicates that the patient loves blood whereas in fact he experiences excessive blood loss . . . The quacks use the most extraordinary expressions derived from Greek or Latin . . . in order to hide their ignorance.'[13]

Of course, Daudet knew nothing about the blood-clotting cascade and it is doubtful that he would have approved of a contemporary physician talking to a distraught mother in terms of amino-acid sequences of Factor VIII or the long arm of the X chromosome.

Walker Percy[14] criticizes the inappropriateness rather than the etymology of medical terms. The euphemisms employed by the medical profession to describe fat individuals, including 'big', 'stout', 'heavy' and 'obese', all annoy Percy who concludes that 'physicians have an unerring knack for the wrong word'.[14] In *The Moviegoer*,[15] Percy makes the hero, John Bickerson Bolling, son of a doctor and mature medical student, declare that he feels 'unspeakably depressed by . . . the sad little analogies doctors like to use'.[15]

Oversimplification

The doctor's failure to use medical terminology may also cause patients to become annoyed. The main medical character in Mann's *Magic Mountain*,[16] Hofrat Behrens, provides two of his patients with simplistic explanations 'in non-technical language out of regard for their lay minds',[16] and the gifted young men evidently resent this patronizing attitude.

Similarly, Frank Wilson, the intelligent and irascible retired civil engineer in David Williamson's *Travelling North*,[17] dislikes the primitive explanations provided by Dr Saul Morgenstein, who practices in a small Queensland town. The doctor is not particularly conversant with the pharmacology of glyceryl trinitrate and digoxin, his explanations lack credibility, and the patient objects:

> Frank: Just exactly how do the tablets I'm taking at present operate and how do they differ from the other prescriptions available?
> Saul: The Trinitrin* relieves the immediate symptoms and the Lanoxin tones up your heartstrings.

---

* The efforts by pharmaceutical companies to promote proprietary rather than generic names for particular compounds have been so successful that twentieth-century fictional physicians rarely use generic terms. They prescribe 'Sintron'[18] and 'Elavil'[19] much the same way as doctors in the real world prescribe 'Viagra' rather than sildenafil. In due course the drugs may become obsolete and the brand names unrecognizable.

> Frank: Saul, I hope you don't feel I'm being excessively demanding, but
> I'm starting to find the level of your medical explanations a little
> . . . unsatisfactory.
> Saul: You don't need to know the details.
> Frank: Listen Saul, I'm the one who's going to die of this condition, not
> you, so if you don't mind, I'll decide what I need to know and
> what I don't.[17]

Frank wins this particular battle and walks out of Morgenstein's office with an armful of medical and pharmacological text books.[17] However, another argument between Morgenstein and Frank Wilson[20] ends in a tactical victory for the doctor. On this occasion Wilson complains of impotence:

> Frank: I haven't told you the whole truth, Saul. There's another reason
> I'm . . . depressed.
> Saul: What's that?
> Frank: I can't manage to do something I've always managed to do and
> it's giving me a bloody . . . inferiority complex.
> Saul: Frank, you are nearly seventy-six, you have a weak heart, you
> had, I suspect, more than your fair share of erotic satisfaction in
> life, so for heaven's sake grow old gracefully.[20]

This time, Williamson's sympathies are clearly with the physician even though Saul's stale 'grow old gracefully' and his therapeutic approach to a patient with impotence are hardly 'correct' from the clinical point of view.

After fifteen years, Alison Lurie's Professor Brian Tate[21] still resents his wife's obstetrician, 'a cautious prissy man' who had advised her to 'avoid intercourse' during the last trimester of her first pregnancy. It is not clear whether Professor Tate resents the advice itself or the old-fashioned language which he apparently considered out of place at the time and which still rankles now. Danielle Zimmern, another of Lurie's characters, complains bitterly about Dr Bunch who 'never tells anyone anything . . . He doesn't talk to you at all if he can help it'. Her friend Erica Tate agrees and adds: 'What's worse, he never listens to you.' Danielle compares Dr Bunch unfavorably with a veterinarian who recently treated her dog 'like a person' while Dr Bunch 'treats me like an animal'.[21]

In a subsequent scene in *The War Between The Tates*,[22] Dr Bunch gives a clear display of his propensity to think and express himself in out-of-date clichés, and his inability to listen to his patients. Erica Tate, whose husband has impregnated one of his graduate students, phones Dr Bunch for advice concerning the availability of abortion services for a 'friend' (the year is 1969). Dr Bunch immediately assumes that Erica is phoning on her own behalf.

> Believe me, I've seen many cases of this kind, and in my experience these
> late children, these 'little afterthoughts' as I call them, are often . . . the
> greatest source of satisfaction . . . to both parents.

Doctor Bunch refuses to believe that Erica is not pregnant and offers to write her 'a little prescription' for a tranquilizer[22] (*see* p. 76).

Bad news

More important than the choice of words is the content of the doctor's explanation. Endless debates have failed to provide a definitive answer to the question of whether sick individuals should be provided with full details on the subject of their illnesses. Should an anxious patient be told about an incidentally discovered abnormality when no effective treatment is available or necessary? How insistently should a doctor berate patients concerning their self-destructive habits, when his advice will almost certainly fall on deaf ears? Does the doctor's obligation towards his patient completely override the specific request by family members that crucial information be withheld?

Some patients obviously want full details, favorable or otherwise. According to Harriett Martineau,[23] dying patients want 'to have their trouble lightened to them ... not by using any deceit ... but by simply treating their case as a matter of fact'.[23] Wilkie Collins' Lady Verinder, who is serendipitously discovered to suffer from 'insidious heart disease'[24] (*see* pp 103–4) and given a poor prognosis, is not at all resentful about 'the real situation [being] made known to [her]'. When the doctors tell her 'she may live for some months' or 'die before another day ha[s] passed over [her] head', she reacts by 'set[ting her] worldly affairs in order'.[24]

One of the most memorable scenes in *Middlemarch*[25] describes the consultation between the Reverend Edward Casaubon, who suffers from ischemic heart disease, and his physician, Dr Tertius Lydgate. When Casaubon asks whether his symptoms are 'those of a fatal disease' and requests 'the truth without reservation', the doctor suddenly realizes that 'here was a man who . . . for the first time found himself looking in the eyes of death' and in whose mind 'the commonplace "we must all die" [was being transformed into] the acute consciousness "I must die – and soon"'. Dr Lydgate is determined not to be 'tempted into momentous prophes[ies and] gratuitous prediction[s]',[26] and goes on to provide Casaubon with scientifically accurate information, conveyed in what are probably the correct terms for this particular patient.

> 'Death from this disease is often sudden. At the same time no such result can be predicted. Your condition may be consistent with a tolerably comfortable life for another fifteen years or even more.'[25]

Had Lydgate been less contemptuous of Casaubon's 'researches', which he knows will never amount to anything, he might have mitigated his verdict with a little unscientific optimism like: 'I have a hunch that in your case the outcome will be favorable.' (In the event, it was not.)

Dr Ezra Wendell, the central character in Weir Mitchell's *In War Time*,[27,28] is particularly inept when it comes to providing information and reassurance to Edward Morton, a young man suffering from progressive leg weakness (? multiple sclerosis). Edward wants to know what to expect.

> 'Shall I lose all use of my legs?' 'No, I think not.' 'Will my head suffer? Shall I lose my mind?' 'No, that doesn't often happen in these troubles.' ... 'There is, I suppose, not the faintest chance that I shall ever be well enough to sit on a horse?' 'Hardly, I think but while there's life there's

> hope.' Wendell was ashamed of this stupid commonplace of consolation but, in truth, he did not know what to say.[27]

Edward, who prefers outdoor activities to intellectual pursuits, and who entertains hopes of joining the army,[28] is devastated.

> 'And to think of all the healthy-legged idiots who can go to the front . . . Oh doctor . . . it's hard!' 'Yes,' replied Wendell, 'it is hard!' and so saying regretted the distinctness with which he had answered the young man's straightforward queries. He had left himself none of the usual vaguely consolatory doubts on which the over-questioned doctor is apt to fall back.[27]

It is unlikely that a thirty-year-old general practitioner (in the 1860s) could have guessed the nature of Edward's condition, let alone provided the young man with a rational prognosis. However, no matter what his thoughts on the disease, Wendell's answers are clearly wrong. To the question that signifies 'Will I finish in a wheelchair?' the answer should have been 'Definitely not'. The question 'Will I go mad?' should also have been answered with a firm negative. Even the horse-riding question could have been handled more appropriately. There is not a hint about appropriate alternative activities even though, in fact, Dr Wendell subsequently made the young invalid's life more endurable by interesting him in 'books, botany and the microscope'.[29]

By contrast, Dr Coutras in Somerset Maugham's *The Moon and Sixpence*[30] uses the brutally honest approach to convey disastrous news to Charles Strickland, and, in the case of this particular patient, the technique proves entirely appropriate. Strickland, the reclusive and irascible artist, who lives in a hut seven kilometers from the nearest Tahitian village, suffers from a shocking, untreatable illness of which he is yet unaware. He is not seeking medical advice, but his 'native woman' and her family recognize the signs of lepromatous leprosy and summon Dr Coutras. The doctor, 'shrewd, hearty and good-natured . . . had delivered sentence of death on many men' and does not waste time on pleasantries and unimportant details.

> 'Look at yourself in the glass,' he told Strickland. Strickland gave him a glance, smiled and went over to a cheap mirror in a little wooden frame that hung on the wall. 'Well?' 'Do you not see a strange change in your face? . . . Mon pauvre ami, must I tell you that you have a terrible disease?' 'I?' 'When you look at yourself in the glass you see the typical appearance of the leper.' 'You are jesting,' said Strickland. 'I wish to God I were.' 'Do you intend to tell me that I have leprosy?' 'Unfortunately there can be no doubt about it.' . . . 'How long do you think I can last?' 'Who knows? Sometimes the disease continues for twenty years. It is a mercy when it runs its course quickly.'[30]

Strickland takes his death sentence with stoical courage. He

> went to his easel and looked reflectively at the picture that stood on it. 'You have had a long journey. It is fitting that the bearer of important tidings should be rewarded. Take this picture. It means nothing to you now but it may be that one day you will be glad to have it.'[30]

Dr Coutras feels that it would be absurd to offer expressions of regret in the face of such a terrible catastrophe and he takes his leave.

> It was with a heavy heart that I drove back to . . . Papeete.[30]

WH Auden declares[31] that if he were dying he would expect his physician

> To say so, not insult me
> With soothing fictions.[31]

How typical are such individuals? Over the centuries, doctors have coped with this dilemma by employing a 'Need to Know' approach, which was formulated very precisely by Oliver Wendell Holmes in his address to a graduating class of medical students in 1871:

> Your patient has no more right to all the truth than he has to all the medicine in your saddlebags . . . He should get only just so much as is good for him.[32]

When the prognosis is poor or the diagnosis obscure, Holmes strongly advises his young medical audience to embark on a deliberate process of deception or obfuscation. If the patient suffers from cancer of the lung, 'tell him he has asthmatic symptoms'. If the problem consists of an unexplained back pain, 'I have known the term "spinal irritation" serve well on such occasions.'[32]

The unnamed doctor in Guibert's *To the Friend who did not Save my Life*,[33] who takes care of patients with AIDS, uses an intermediate approach when it comes to informing a patient about the mortal nature of his illness. He

> does not tell the patient the truth straight out but . . . gives him the means and the opportunity . . . to figure it out for himself, which also allows him to remain blessedly ignorant if that's what he wants.[33]

The problem of truthful explanations becomes particularly treacherous when family members ask whether a patient with a terminal illness is in any immediate danger and how much longer he can be expected to live.

> This was the kind of question the doctor hated. If you said a patient couldn't live another month, the family prepared itself for a bereavement and if then the patient lived on, they visited the medical attendant with the resentment they felt at having tormented themselves before it was necessary. On the other hand, if you said the patient might live a year and he died in a week, the family said you did not know your business.[34]

Generations of medical students have been taught never to give precise time frames in this context, and, to this day, doctors are reluctant to provide accurate survival estimates,[35] though patients' families continue to come up with statements like 'The doctor gave him six months to live'.

Doctors as incorrigible liars; false optimism

The paternalistic style, which is currently considered obsolete, was widely employed and resented, with many patients suspecting that significant facts were being withheld from them and that important information was being conveyed between members of the profession in secret or at least behind the backs of the most concerned individuals. Suspicions concerning the habitual mendacity of doctors were expressed by Petrarch,[36] with feelings of mistrust persisting into relatively recent times. Bulwer-Lytton in *What Will He Do With It*[37] makes Mayor Josiah Hartopp declare that even 'first-rate' doctors provide misinformation as a matter of policy.

> Doctors always exaggerate in order to get more credit for the cure . . . Tis the way with doctors to talk cheerfully if one is in danger and to look solemn if there is nothing to fear.[37]

One of Choromanski's characters believes that doctors are so used to lying to their patients that they become totally incapable of telling the truth.[38]

> The doctor is always telling the patients lies. It must become a habit with him even in . . . [his] private life.[38]

Choromanski goes on to provide an example of a doctor's habitual dishonesty.[39] Dr Tamten, who is having a clandestine affair with a married woman, is on his way to the X-ray department when he is accosted in the corridor by one of his patients.

> The patient on crutches limped after him [and] . . . asked nervously: 'Doctor, is it true it's not getting worse? Why is there water on the knee?' Tamten tapped him on the shoulder with his usual fixed smile as he said 'A trifle, a trifle . . . Everything's fine.'[39]

As soon as the patient is out of earshot, Tamten remarks to his assistant: 'Probably have to amputate that poor fellow's leg'.[39]

In a fanciful story perpetuating the myth that the medical profession is collectively engaged in a conspiracy to conceal the truth, Hecht[40] wonders

> whether the secrecy with which the [medical] fraternity surrounds its gatherings is designed to keep the layman from discovering how much it knows or how much it doesn't know.[40]

'Professional heartiness'[41] (*see* p. 93) and dishonest optimism at the bedside may generate profound anger, disbelief or amused contempt, depending on the setting. The syndrome is described in Aesop's Fables,[42] where it engenders a feeling of helplessness.

> A sick man, who was questioned about his health by the doctor, replied that he was sweating heavily. 'That is good,' said the doctor. Then he

asked him the next time how he was feeling, and the patient said he had
been shivering so much that he was badly shaken up. 'That's also good,'
said the doctor. Then he called on the man a third time and asked how he
was. He replied that he had had diarrhea. 'That's good too,' said the
doctor and went on his way. Then one of the sick man's parents came to
visit him and asked how he was. 'I'm dying of good symptoms,' he
replied.[42]

Leo Tolstoy, in one of his greatest short stories,[43] describes a physician whose
inappropriate use of a cheerful attitude totally destroys his credibility. The patient is
an intelligent professional man (Ivan Illych) who suffers from a terminal illness
(? pancreatic cancer).

> Now there is a ring at the door bell. Perhaps it is the doctor? It is. He
> comes in fresh, healthy, plump and cheerful with that look on his face
> that seems to say: 'There now, you're in a panic about something but
> we'll arrange it all for you directly.' The doctor knows this expression is
> out of place here, but he has put it on once and for all and can't take it off
> – like a man who has put on a frock coat in the morning to pay a round
> of calls. The doctor rubs his hand vigorously and reassuringly. 'Brr! How
> cold it is . . . just let me warm myself,' he says as if it were only a matter
> of waiting till he was warm and then he would put everything right.[43]

The physician's hypocritical behavior is extended to the patient's wife, who
complains that Ivan

> doesn't take his medicine at the proper time . . . and lies in a position that
> is no doubt bad for him . . . The doctor smiled with a contemptuous
> affability that said: what's to be done? These sick people do have foolish
> fancies of that kind but we must forgive them.[43]

The false optimism at the deathbed of Oscar Thibault,[44] which is described from the
doctor's point of view, seems slightly more effective. Dr Antoine Thibault is caring
for his father who is dying from hypernephroma of his remaining kidney. He comes
each day,

> often twice a day and at each visit, indefatigably – as though he were
> renewing a dressing on a wound – he racked his brains to conjure up new
> arguments, logical, if insincere . . .[44]

Antoine's attempts at originality are not very successful. On each occasion he repeats

> in the same tone of certitude, the self same words of comfort. 'What can
> you expect, father! Your digestive organs aren't what they were when
> you were a young man and they've been pestered . . . with drugs . . . for at
> least eight months.'[44]

Hemingway's enthusiastic rehabilitation doctor, who considers a 'positive' attitude
more important than credibility,[45] provokes grim disbelief in one of his charges and

derision in another. The action takes place in a Milan hospital where patients with war injuries and congenital deformities exercise on fancy equipment.

> The doctor came up to the machine where I was sitting and said: 'What did you like best to do before the war? Did you practice a sport?' I said, 'Yes, football.' 'Good,' he said. 'You will be able to play football again better than ever.'[45]

This prediction is, of course, quite unrealistic.

> My knee did not bend and the leg dropped straight down from the knee to the ankle without a calf and the machine was to bend the knee and make it move as in riding a tricycle. But it did not bend yet and, instead, the machine lurched when it came to the bending part.[45]

The doctor repeats his good tidings:

> 'You are a fortunate young man. You will play football again like a champion.' In the next machine was a major who had a little hand like a baby's. He winked at me when the doctor examined his hand, which was between two leather straps that bounced up and down and flapped the stiff fingers and said, 'And will I too play football, captain-doctor?'[45]

The major is not impressed by the rehabilitation doctor's zeal, and declares that he has no confidence in the entire program.[45]

Somerset Maugham's Dr Tyrrell[46] displays his false optimism in the setting of an outpatient clinic where poor patients are treated free of charge.

> From commerce with students and poor people, Dr Tyrrell had the patronizing air, and from dealing always with the sick he had the healthy man's jovial condescension, which some consultants achieve as the professional manner. He made the patient feel like a boy confronted by a jolly school master; his illness was an absurd piece of naughtiness which amused rather than irritated.[46]

Dr Tyrrell arrives at the clinic

> with quick movements and a breezy manner. He reminded one slightly of a clown leaping into an arena of a circus with the cry: Here we are again. His air seemed to indicate: What's all this nonsense about being ill? I'll soon put that right.[46]

Harmful truths

The abandonment of the 'Holmesian' principles[32] and too-generous helpings of the truth have caused several fictional physicians to be deserted by their clientele. Here is

Axel Munthe[47] berating his friend and colleague Dr Norstrom who has just lost a patient after telling him 'the truth':

> 'Why did you tell the Russian professor . . . that he had angina pectoris? Why did you explain to him all the symptoms of his fatal disease?' 'He insisted upon knowing the truth. I had to tell him or he would not have obeyed me' . . . 'He told you a lie when he [said] he wanted to know everything and that he was not afraid of death. Nobody wants to know how ill he is, everybody is afraid of death . . . This man now is far worse. His existence is paralyzed by fear, it is all your fault.'[47]

The practice of Dr Norstrom, the compulsive truth-teller, is not flourishing while his disgruntled patients flock to Dr Munthe for comfort and lies.[47]

The inability or unwillingness to dissemble lands Dr Richard Mahony in trouble on more than one occasion. Mahony, whose bedside manner is discussed on page 79, is shown the door by a leading citizen of the town after the doctor advises him to 'keep the sherry decanter out of [his wife's] reach'.[48] Another time, Mahony

> had poor little Amelia Grindle up in arms by telling her that her sickly first-born would mentally never be quite like other children. To everyone else this had been plain from the outset; but Amelia had suspected nothing, having . . . no idea when a baby ought to begin to take notice . . . Richard said it was better for [Amelia] to face the truth betimes, than to spend her life vainly hoping and fretting. [While aware that] doctors must always wrap the truth up in silver paper, [Mahony, nevertheless] set such store by truth and principle, that he did not . . . care . . . whether he offended people or not . . . Once on a time he had been noted for his tact. It was sad to see it leaving him in the lurch.[48]

Simenon's Dr Elie Bergelon[49] does not specifically advocate withholding the truth, but he expresses considerable doubts about the therapeutic value of providing a label for a patient's complaints. He certainly does not share Dr Medhurst's view[50] that an outlandish diagnosis impresses the patients, and that the more unpronounceable the name, the better they will feel (*see* pp 80 and 111). On the contrary, the doctor's verdict that a set of symptoms indicates the presence of a particular disease may actually be counter-productive.

> 'Have you had any pain or discomfort recently?' he would ask his patients. 'I think so. Every now and then, especially when I wake up in the morning, a sort of dull ache in my chest.' 'How long has this been going on?' For him, these were routine questions, part of the daily round. For them, those few minutes spent in his consulting room after they had waited their turn on the little chairs upholstered in green velvet in the waiting room, represented a decisive turning point. Symptoms, which until then had been nothing more than barely noticeable twinges, were identified by name and suddenly the patient was someone suffering from an illness.[49]

Judge Clane and JT Malone, the two main characters in McCullers' *Clock Without Hands*,[51] both express considerable resentment against their respective physicians who reveal too many unfavorable clinical details, and tell them what they do not wish to hear. The judge suffers from type II diabetes mellitus; Malone has chronic myeloid leukemia. Judge Clane complains:

> 'I hate it, God damn it, when doctors presume to tell me the so-called truth. I was so angry meditating about that diet problem, I might have then and there had a stroke.' 'No it's not right,' Malone assented. He had asked for the truth, but in asking had asked only for reassurance. How could he dream that an ordinary case of spring fever could be a fatal disease? He had wanted sympathy and reassurance and he got a death warrant. 'Doctors, by God, washing their hands, looking out windows, fiddling with dreadful things while you are stretched out on a table.'[51]

William Wharton in *Dad*[52] makes one of his characters complain bitterly about a physician who insists on telling a patient the truth, even though family members have specifically requested that the patient be deceived. Dr Santana, the urologist who is treating 'Dad' Tremont for transitional cell carcinoma of the bladder

> must have skipped all his classes in bedside manner.[52]

The patient's son, John Tremont, who holds a PhD in psychology, has previously warned Dr Santana about 'Dad's' mental state, his dependency and his modesty ('just someone manipulating his penis is a big shock'[52]) and has been told not to worry. Now comes the debriefing session.

> I'm buttoning [Dad's] shirt [after the initial office cystoscopy] when Dr Santana comes back in. He has a clipboard in his hand. 'Well, Mr Tremont we'll have to look at that.' Dad stares at Santana, then at me; his voice quavers. 'What does he mean, Johnny; look? I thought he just looked.' Dad turns towards the doctor. 'I mean I'll have to schedule you for surgery, Mr Tremont.' . . . I'm standing behind Dad, signaling like crazy; Santana is ignoring me. Dad looks around for reassurance and I try to smile . . . 'Yes, there are some small growths in there and we'll need to excise them. We'll go in through the penile canal the way we did today. We won't do any real surgery. Don't you worry Mr Tremont, there's nothing to it.' Big deal. Not to worry. Dad's already halfway worrying himself to death.[52]

When the histological results are available a few days later, John Tremont Junior again meets up with Dr Santana, who informs him that the bladder tumors are malignant and that 'Dad' will require chemotherapy. Tremont, who has decided to lie to his father about the true nature of his condition, pleads with the urologist to support him.

> 'Please, whatever you do Dr Santana, don't tell my father. He's terribly anxious and frightened.' 'Come Mr Tremont, you'd be surprised what these old people can take. Their children tend to underestimate older people.' His attitude worries me. He doesn't seem to understand or want

to understand. 'Doctor this is not so in this case. My father's deathly frightened.' . . . 'Mr Tremont, this was a relatively simple excision; it hardly qualifies as an operation.' I repeat, as forcefully as I can, how I'd appreciate it if he would hold off telling Dad he has cancer. I thought he was listening.[52]

Dr Santana considers he has an 'ethical obligation' to be open with the patient and he disregards the son's advice. The old man reacts to the news by rapidly becoming uncommunicative and incontinent and Dr Santana is blamed for 'Dad's' deterioration.[52]

Young Dr Jim Wyatt, the hero of *Bright Scalpel*,[53] loses a patient after truthfully admitting his ignorance and aggravating this confession with a particularly inept remark. 'I made the mistake of telling the lady that if I could cure chronic asthma I wouldn't be here in Maywood.' The patient, despite her membership of Jim's father's church, calls in a different doctor for her next asthma attack.[53]

One of the worst offenders against the rule of not providing a patient with harmful information is Lightman's Dr Armand Petrov,[54] who is attempting to diagnose an obscure form of peripheral neuropathy. Bill Chalmers, the patient, wants to know the nature of his problem, while Petrov tries to prevaricate.

'It could be any number of things. We begin by ruling things out.' 'Like what?' Petrov was silent. 'What should we be ruling out?'[54]

When he can no longer evade Bill's direct questions, the doctor behaves like a medical student who has partially memorized a list, which he now regurgitates 'untouched by human mind'.

'Numbness can be caused by a metabolic deficiency, such as lack of vitamin B_{12}. Numbness can also be caused by lead poisoning or a viral infection. You could have something very rare such as leprosy.'[54]

Petrov obviously lacks the common sense to keep quiet about a disease like leprosy, which even he, in his ignorance, realizes is rare in the Boston area. The very mention of the name can do nothing for the patient other than frighten him, possibly as a punishment for asking too many questions.[54] Petrov's medical behavior produces in the patient and the reader, a degree of antipathy almost reminiscent of Pliny[5] or Petrarch.[36] Like Pliny's physicians,[5] Petrov, whose name, choice of words and mannerisms suggest an 'alien' origin, represents the evil foreign physicians, who are torturing the local citizens.

Withholding information

If 'Dad' Tremont[52] and Bill Chalmers[54] receive too many clinical details, Arnold Bennett's *Lord Raingo*[55] complains that he does not get enough. Indeed, Bennett illustrates brilliantly that at times it is almost impossible for a physician to gauge the 'right' amount of information to provide to an intelligent and aggressive patient suffering from a fatal illness.[55] Samuel Raingo, a member of the British government, becomes dangerously ill at the height of his career and dies of a combination of a lung infection and long-standing valvular heart disease, despite the efforts of the most prominent physicians available at the time. His medical treatment is absolutely correct (for 1918) but, throughout his illness, Raingo feels that he is a victim of a conspiracy and that he is being given catch phrases rather than the truth.

> Doctor Heddle (the local doctor) came earlier than usual and took his temperature and sounded him and listened to his arcana (sic) and variously examined him all afresh. No information was given to the patient. 'What is my temperature?' he asked, crossly impatient. 'Well,' said Dr Heddle, 'I've known worse.' 'Damn it all!' Sam broke out. 'Can't I know my own temperature?' He felt savage, despite weakness. 'One hundred and two,' answered the doctor cornered, intimidated, beaten.[55]

Sir Arthur Tappitt, Lord Raingo's London internist, is more subtle.[55] He informs his VIP patient, who has developed an empyema, that 'fluid [has accumulated] in [his] pleural cavity' and that a drainage procedure is indicated. He adds confidentially:

> 'Mind you, I wouldn't gossip with every patient like this.' 'That's his stock phrase,' thought the politician who wanted more details. 'Then it's pleurisy I've got, eh?' 'Yes if you want labels.' 'And what about pericarditis?' asked Sam who was busy recalling old fragments of hearsay concerning pneumonia. 'What's that?' 'The pericardium is the cavity that the heart lies in. It's a sack. If it's affected too, then people who like labels would be justified in saying you had pericarditis.' 'And have I?' 'Not necessarily.' 'And when shall you do the operation?'[55]

The drainage procedure is performed that afternoon[55] but Lord Raingo does not improve. He tries to read cabinet papers but finds that he cannot concentrate. His son Geoffrey asks Sir Arthur whether it is in order for the distinguished patient to work a bit.

> 'Certainly! If he feels like it. And doesn't overdo it.' Sam detected the insincerity in the benevolent tones as infallibly as though he had been the reader of all hearts. He could almost see Sir Arthur wink at Geoffrey, almost hear him whispering: 'Doesn't matter much what he does now. Let him follow his fancy.' So morbid and sensitive was his imagination.[55]

Brian Casey, the sixteen-year-old high-school student and poliomyelitis victim in Sheed's *People Will Always Be Kind*,[56] also resents being kept in the dark. Brian's legs are obviously not going to recover but Dr Samson who has 'taken care' of Brian throughout his illness has decided to withhold this information.

> Dr Samson . . . peeped under the packs and nodded. What did he see? He asked Brian to flex his right knee. Brian couldn't but the doctor nodded again anyway. 'How does it look, Doc?' he asked. 'Very good. No sign of atrophy,' said Dr Samson. 'Yeah, but is there any sign of life?' The Doctor smiled. 'Don't be in such a hurry. These things take time.' You see, you see? He said I'm going to get better. Brian wasn't sure whether to

press the inquiry and shoot for more specific assurances. OK – shoot. 'What would you say the chances are, Doc?' Samson . . . straightened up and swung into a man-to-man match. 'Brian, I can't give you odds.' (The year is 1945, and the chances of recovery, as Dr Samson subsequently explains to Brian's father, much less than fifty per cent.) 'People are working night and day on this thing. And your own spirit could make a big difference.' Ten years in medical school to learn that? . . . Fighting spirit indeed. If they were relying on that, the game was up.[56]

Brian's father, Kevin Casey, is even more antagonistic towards Dr Samson and, quite unjustifiably, blames him for the poor outcome. In Kevin's case, the situation is aggravated by sectarian overtones and by the realization that his son's condition is incurable, but most of his anger stems from the doctor's inability to convey bad news.

That morning, before picking Brian up, Kevin had talked with Dr Samson . . . Samson had been his usual evasive self, squirting smoke screens of 'wait and see's' and 'early to tell's' but when he saw that Kevin would settle only for the worst he said 'unless science comes up with something, his chances are only fair.' God, he hated people like Samson. There was a sense of no Irish need apply about him. 'There should be some sign of life now, Mr Casey. The arms seem to be all right' . . . [but] then he launched into a stream of Latin names, glibius flatulus, ponderus maximus, not Latin a Catholic would use, indicating that Brian's legs were a wasteland where no life would stir again.[56]

Dr Samson's advice to let Brian discover the truth gradually may be clinically correct but it evokes further ill feelings in Brian's father.

'I wouldn't tell your wife about this,' said Dr Samson. 'What about my son?' 'Why tell him? He'll get used to his condition in a year or two and he won't mind knowing then.' If Samson had his way no one would ever be told anything. Everyone would pass through life knowing nothing at all, caressed by lies. His only medicine was anesthesia. 'You don't trust my son, is that it?' Kevin said as pleasantly as possible. 'You don't think he's strong enough for the truth?' 'Few people are. Remember, Brian is only a boy of what? Sixteen? Precocious in some ways. But don't be misled by that. It will take all the courage he has, to face it when he has to.' Please, Doctor, spare us your wisdom, OK? You have utterly failed to help us professionally. In fact you have done nothing at all so far as I can see. So do not lecture us on how to live . . . Kevin felt for a mad moment that the doctor was to blame for the whole thing; his sly evasions, his passivity had held Brian in check for precious weeks.[56]

The gynecologist in Boris Pasternak's *Doctor Zhivago*[57] carries this attitude one step further – he gives no explanations at all.

He . . . always responded to questions by shrugging his shoulders and staring at the ceiling. These silent gestures were meant to suggest that, whatever the advances of science there were more things in heaven and earth, friend Horatio, than science ever dreamt on (sic).[57]

Ken Harrison, the quadriplegic sculptor in Clark's *Whose Life Is It Anyway*,[58] complains angrily about physicians who ration information and hand it out in small installments.

> Doctors dole out information like a kosher butcher giving out pork sausages[58]

whereas the patients want to understand all the aspects of their ailments. Of course, it is highly unlikely that Mr Harrison would have found a complete lecture on the physiology of the transsected cervical cord less traumatic, particularly if the implications for his own lifestyle were explained in detail immediately after admission, rather than gradually as he discovered them.

Another type of patient is represented by Joan Green, a thirty-four-year-old patient at the 'Whipple Cancer Hospital', who has osteogenic sarcoma with pulmonary metastases and pleural effusions,[59] and is not certain whether she wants more of the truth or less. Here she is interrogating Dr William Ryan who is less than three months into his internship.[60]

> 'About my outlook, so to speak . . . I guess in a way, I really don't want to know, not everything you know. That is, I want to know and I don't want to know too much.' 'It's hard to tell only part of the truth,' said Ryan . . . Mrs Green . . . start[ed] to cry. 'I'm asking what to expect, if there's any hope at all?' 'There's always hope. As far as what to expect, more tests more scans . . .' 'Oh, I don't mean that. Where is the tumor now? . . . Is it in my lungs? Is it everywhere?' 'It's not everywhere. It's in your lungs,' said Ryan. 'My God,' Mrs Green sighed . . . 'It's gone from my leg to my lungs. Where else? Where next?' 'As far as we know, just the lungs.' 'As far as you know?' 'I can only tell what I know.' 'But you imply it could be anywhere!' 'Could be isn't meaningful. I could have a tumor too.'

Mrs Green had several further questions, none of which Ryan is able to answer satisfactorily, but he manages to shift the focus a little.[59]

Deception

Straightforward, consistent deception is occasionally condoned, possibly because it assumes a desire on the part of the patients to let themselves be deluded or because the alternative option appears even worse. Dr Ernesto Castillo's patient, President (in exile) Don Manuel Villegas, has amyotrophic lateral sclerosis (*see* p. 108). There is no effective treatment and Villegas will therefore be receiving 'supportive therapy'.[61] A French Intelligence Agent interrogates Dr Castillo about the meaning of this term while Castillo's girl friend, Elizabeth, is listening in. The doctor explains:

'In this . . . [case, "supportive therapy"] is merely a euphemism for deceit . . . It could take various forms. Prescribing massage and giving him useless injections would be one. Telling the patient he's feeling better and persuading him to believe you would be another. Or, if that doesn't work, you tell him he must be patient and give his medications a chance. You can explain what a unique clinical picture he represents and talk vaguely about a new drug that's being developed . . . Naturally you dose him with sedatives and anti-depressants as required. And when he starts to go downhill fast, as you have always known he will, you give him a perplexed look and say "we're not looking as well as we should today – we must do something about that." So then you give him something to make him think he feels better for a few hours. That is supportive therapy for Monsieur Villegas.' 'Monstrous,' said Elizabeth angrily. 'Are all doctors as bad as this?' I bridled. 'Well I could always march in, stand at the end of his bed and say, "Sorry, my friend, you have amyotrophic lateral sclerosis and it's incurable, so just lie back and suffer."'[61]

Dr Salter, who 'looked more like a hard-bitten horse dealer than Hartscombe's leading GP',[62] brazenly deceives his patients whenever he considers this strategy indicated. While non-urgent complaints are treated 'with the medicine he trusted most, the passage of time',[63] additional measures are employed for acute emergencies.

He could quieten a child with a broken arm or a woman with a crushed finger by producing what he called a special pain-killing pill flown in from America which he kept in a small paper in his waistcoat pocket.[64]

When Fred Simcox (the son of the local minister) asks what this potent medication contains, he is told:

'It's a rare drug known as an Extra Strong Mint.' 'You're an old fraud,' Fred Simcox told him. 'Of course, I'm just like your father. It's faith, thats what we are both after.'[64]

The entire medical consultation may be an act of deception if the doctor is asked 'to drop in by accident'. The person arranging the 'chance' visit is usually a close relative who wants the request to remain secret especially if the patient suffers from psychiatric problems. In Warren's *Preparing for the House*,[65] the doctor not only 'drops in', but also conspires with the wife of the unwitting, hypomanic patient to procure a sedative ('five and twenty drops of laudanum'), which she proposes to 'slip into his wine at dinner'. Of course, the two are acting in the patient's best interest in trying to prevent him from making a fool of himself by making what would have been a rambling speech in the British House of Commons.[65]

Summary

The debriefing of a patient, especially when the news is bad or unclear, is one of the most difficult tasks confronting a physician. There is no single 'correct' method but several approaches are manifestly wrong and give rise to deep resentment. A few fictional authors suggest that the pendulum has swung too far in the direction of 'patient autonomy'[66] and that the paternalistic approach may sometimes be more appropriate.

References

1   Kafka F (1919) A Country Doctor. In: Kafka F (1978) *Wedding Preparations (in the Country) and Other Stories*. Translated by Muir W and Muir E. Penguin, Harmondsworth, pp. 119–24.

2   Anonymous (1978) Doctor, Doctor, Come Here Quick. In: Turner I, Factor J and Lowenstein W. *Cinderella Dressed in Yella*. Heinemann Educational, Richmond, Australia, p. 15.

3   Eliot G (1871–2) *Middlemarch*. Penguin, London, 1988, pp. 118–20.

4   Carossa H (1931) *Doctor Gion*. Translated by Scott AN. Robert O Ballou, New York, 1933, p. 16.

5   Pliny the Elder (Gaius Plinius Secundus) (1st century AD) *Natural History*, Book 29. Translated by Holland P. Southern Illinois University Press, 1962, pp. 294–7.

6   Middleton T (1662) Anything for a Quiet Life. In: Bullen AH (ed.) (1885) *The Works of Thomas Middleton*, vol. V, Act II, Scene 4. JC Nimmo, London, pp. 281–2.

7   Fielding H (1749) The History of Tom Jones – A Foundling. In: Stephen S (ed.) (1882) *The Works of Henry Fielding*, vol. 1. Smith Elder, London, pp. 359–93.

8   Reade C (1863) *Hard Cash*. Chatto and Windus, London, 1894, pp. 32–3.

9   Ibid., pp. 210–11.

10 Arnold M (1867) *A Wish*. In: Tinker CB and Lowry HF (eds) (1966) Arnold Poetical Works, Oxford University Press, London, pp. 249–51.

11 Wells HG (1909) *Tono Bungay*. Ernest Benn, London, 1926, p. 409.

12 Wouk H (1962) *Youngblood Hawke*. Doubleday and Co., New York, pp. 330–1.

13 Daudet LA (1894) *Les Morticoles*. Fasquelle, Paris, 1956, p. 115.

14 Percy W (1987) *The Thanatos Syndrome*. Farrar Straus Giroux, New York, p. 13.

15 Percy W (1961) *The Moviegoer*. Noonday Press, New York, 1977, pp. 152–4.

16 Mann T (1924) *The Magic Mountain*. Translated by Lowe-Porter HT. Penguin, Harmondsworth, 1960, p. 219.

17 Williamson D (1980) *Travelling North*. Currency Press, Sydney, p. 51.

18 Simenon G (1963) *The Patient*. Translated by Stewart J. Hamish Hamilton, London, pp. 33–4.

19 Wharton W (1981) *Dad*. Alfred A Knopf, New York, pp. 159–62.

20 Williamson D, op. cit., pp. 46–7.

21 Lurie A (1974) *The War Between the Tates*. Heinemann, London, pp. 57–70.

22 Ibid., pp. 115–17.

23 Martineau H (1839) *Deerbrook*. Virago Press, London, 1983, p. 44.

24 Collins W (1868) *The Moonstone*. Perennial Classics, Harper and Row, New York, 1965, pp. 211–12.

25 Eliot G, op. cit., pp. 459–61.

26 Ibid., p. 321.

27 Mitchell SW (1885) *In War Time*. Century Company, New York, 1913, pp. 98–103.

28 Ibid., p. 163.

29 Ibid., p. 371.

30 Maugham WS (1919) *The Moon and Sixpence*. Penguin, Harmondsworth, 1953, pp. 198–203.

31 Auden WH (1972) The Art of Healing. In Memoriam David Protetch MD. In: Auden WH. *Epistle to a Godson and Other Poems*. Faber and Faber, London, pp. 13–15.

32 Holmes OW (1871) The Young Practitioner. In: Holmes OW (1892) *Medical Essays 1842–1882*, vol. 9. Holmes Works, Houghton Mifflin, Boston, MA, pp. 370–95.

33 Guibert H (1990) *To the Friend who did not Save my Life*. Translated by Coverdale L. Quartet Books, London, 1991, pp. 23–5.

34 Maugham WS (1915) *Of Human Bondage*. Signet Classics, New York, 1991, pp. 595–6.

35 Lamont EB and Christakis NA (2001) Prognostic disclosure to patients with cancer near the end of life. *Ann Int Med*. **134**: 1096–105.

36 Petrarch F (1355) Invective Contra Medicum. In: *Petrarch, Works*, vol. 2. Gregg Press, Ridgewood, NJ, 1965, 1200–33 (Latin).

37 Bulwer-Lytton EGE (Pisistratus Caxton, pseudonym) (1859) *What Will He Do With It*, vol. 1. Routledge and Sons, London, undated, p. 211.

38 Choromanski M (1932) *Jealousy and Medicine*. Translated by Arthurton-Barker E. New Directions, Norfolk, CT, 1964, p. 20.

39 Ibid., p. 38.

40 Hecht B (1959) Miracle of the Fifteen Murderers. In: *A Treasury of Ben Hecht*. Crown Publishers, New York, pp. 189–203.

41 James H (1902) *The Wings of the Dove*, Chapter XII. Signet Classics, New York, 1964, p. 169.

42 Aesop (approx. 570 BC) *The Complete Fables*. Translated by Temple O and Temple R. Penguin, London, 1998, p. 184.

43 Tolstoy L (1886) The Death of Ivan Illych. Translated by Maude L and Maude AC. In: Simmons EJ (ed.) (1966) *Leo Tolstoy, Short Novels*, vol. 2. Random House, New York, pp. 47–9.

44 Martin du Gard R (1922–9) *The Thibaults*. Translated by Gilbert S. John Lane The Bodley Head, London, 1939, p. 529.

45 Hemingway E (1927) In Another Country. In: *The Complete Short Stories of Ernest Hemingway*. Scribner Paperback Edition, Simon and Schuster, New York, 1998, pp. 206–10.

46 Maugham WS (1915) *Of Human Bondage*. Signet Classics, New York, 1991, pp. 438–42.

47   Munthe A (1929) *The Story of San Michele*. John Murray, London, 1950, p. 176.

48   Richardson HH (1917–29) *The Fortunes of Richard Mahony*. Penguin, London, 1990, pp. 304–10.

49   Simenon G (1941) The Country Doctor. In: Simenon G (1980) *The White Horse Inn and Other Novels*. Translated by Ellenbogen E. Hamish Hamilton, London, pp. 198–205.

50   Young FB (1938) *Dr Bradley Remembers*. Heinemann, London, pp. 242–5.

51   McCullers C (1953) *Clock Without Hands*. Houghton Mifflin, Boston, MA, 1963, pp. 61–3.

52   Wharton W (1981) *Dad*. Alfred A Knopf, New York, pp. 104–18.

53   Seifert E (1941) *Bright Scalpel*. Aeonian Press Inc., New York, 1973, p. 10.

54   Lightman A (2000) *The Diagnosis*. Pantheon Press, New York, pp. 119–20.

55   Bennett A (1926) Lord Raingo. In: *The Arnold Bennett Omnibus Book*. Books for Libraries Press, Plainview, New York, 1975, pp. 372–410.

56   Sheed W (1973) *People Will Always Be Kind*. Weidenfeld and Nicolson, London, pp. 27–37.

57   Pasternak B (1957) *Doctor Zhivago*. Translated by Hayward M and Harari M. Pantheon, New York, 1958, p. 102.

58   Clark B (1972) *Whose Life Is It Anyway*. Amber Lane Press, Ashover, UK, 1978, p. 52.

59   Ravin N (1981) *MD*. Delacorte Press/Seymour Lawrence, New York, pp. 66–7.

60   Ibid., pp. 155–7.

61   Ambler E (1974) *Doctor Frigo*. Fontana Collins, Glasgow, 1976, pp. 163–4.

62   Mortimer J (1985) *Paradise Postponed*. Penguin, Harmondsworth, 1986, p. 47.

63   Ibid., p. 140.

64   Ibid., p. 113.

65   Warren S (1832) Preparing for the House. In: Warren S. *Diary of a Late Physician*, vol. 1. Blackwood, Edinburgh, pp. 86–95.

66   Ingelfinger FJ (1980) Arrogance. *N Engl J Med*. 303: 1507–11.

CHAPTER 6

Treatment: successes and failures

Wonderful little, when all is said
Wonderful little our fathers knew.
Half their remedies cured you dead,
Most of their teaching was quite untrue.

Yet when the sickness was sore in the land
And neither planet nor herb assuaged
They took their lives in their lancet hand
And oh what a wonderful war they waged.[1]

The doctor as healer

A great many crocodile tears have been shed over the disappearance of the horse and buggy doctors with their 'holistic' approach and their capacity for treating patients as human beings. The specialists who have replaced them, it is claimed, combine technical ability with business acumen, and treat diseases rather than people. This superficial analysis ignores the most important skill that helps doctors deal with sick individuals – familiarity with sickness. This familiarity transcends time, place and methods of medical training, and is only partially dependent on available therapeutic agents. Whether compassionate or callous, erudite or ignorant, specialist or generalist, medical persons are better able than the lay public to tell the difference between serious and trivial problems. They can distinguish a living person from a corpse. At the other end of life, despite the clumsiness and clownishness of professional brethren like Dr Slop (who knocks out three of his own front teeth with a pair of obstetrical forceps[2]), medical individuals are generally aware of whether or not the birth of a baby is imminent. Above all, persons with even a scrap of medical training do not wring their hands or run away at the sight of injuries. A story dating from the second century AD, and reminiscent of the parable of the Good Samaritan, depicts the essence of medical behavior during an emergency.[3]

Galen's friend and travelling companion, in a fit of temper, has inflicted severe head injuries on two of his servants, and then run off because of a sense of guilt and shame and because he becomes frightened of 'the great quantity of blood that was flowing'. The doctor, who is not afraid of blood, remains behind, treats the injured men and escorts them back to Athens.[3]

Another aspect of the doctors' training and experience that stands them in good stead in their role as healers is their tolerance. Physicians are used to stupid, self-destructive and perverse individuals; they have seen and heard it all before, and they express neither astonishment nor horror when confronted with yet another example of 'deviant' behavior. They have been trained to avoid moralistic attitudes and recriminations which impede the rational management of sick people. Mauriac's Dr Paul Courrèges,[4] despite his flaws (he is about to commit a major breach of medical ethics – *see* Book II, Chapter 1), remains absolutely professional in his acceptance of human follies:

> There was no secret of the human heart to which he had not been made privy, and, as a result, his tolerance where his fellow men were concerned, was almost unlimited.[4]

Crighton's Dr Lewis Carr,[5] another flawed character, displays the 'correct' attitude towards 'evildoers' despite his self-serving political activities and his tendency to gossip:

> A doctor can't . . . make value judgments. We clean up after . . . bad drivers and mean drunks . . .[but] it isn't our job to slap anybody's hand and give them a lecture on driving or alcohol.[5]

Yet another medical characteristic relates to doctors' deeply ingrained conviction that when medical calamities occur, it is their obligation to help the sick. Kipling's Nicholas Culpeper,[1] a seventeenth-century physician-astrologer, who knew little apart from the passage of planets and cold water cures, refuses to leave a plague-stricken village even when he has the opportunity to escape. 'The plague was here . . . what else could I have done?'[1]

To doctors, 'helping the sick' generally means intervention rather than reassurance. They administer treatment regardless of the desires or the needs of the community, and, at times, regardless of the desires or the needs of the patients. They see themselves as maintenance men rather than philosophers and any self-doubts concerning the usefulness of their therapeutic activities are rapidly suppressed. When Paul Davenant, the tuberculous hero in Ellis' *The Rack*,[6] becomes despondent, expresses a death wish and wonders whether any further treatment is worthwhile, his doctor has no such qualms:

> Ought I to try and keep you alive if you have no very great wish to live? I don't know, monsieur, and I don't very much care. Perhaps you would be better dead; perhaps we would all be better dead. Issues like these I leave to more exalted intellects than my own. We are here a breakdown factory and I am the mécanicien chef. What is given to me broken, I try to repair. And no questions.[6]

Patients, in general, expect and want doctors to intervene:

> When your child is ill or your wife dying . . . what you want is comfort, reassurance, something to clutch at were it but a straw. This, the doctor

brings you. You have a wildly urgent feeling that something must be done; and the doctor does something.[7]

The 'rough and ready cure'; repetitive tasks

Most forms of medical intervention do not involve spectacular, life-saving procedures.[8] The patients' problems are generally of a minor and transient nature so that it is impossible to determine whether the ensuing recovery occurs as the result of, in spite of or regardless of the treatment. Nevertheless, many doctors, in the most varied settings, enjoy simple monotonous therapeutic activities, which give them, as well as the patients, a feeling of accomplishment. Here are two of the doctors in *Kings Row*[9] arguing about the tedious nature and the inconsequentiality of medical treatment. Dr Maughs, the old physician, declares:

> There's a lot of poppycock written and talked about the nobility of a doctor's work. You hear that mostly from somebody who's not practicing medicine and never did. It's monotonous and most times commonplace. Same things – bad colds, stomach-aches, constipation and the like. Seldom interesting.[9]

Dr Parris Mitchell, the youthful medical hero, agrees but retains his enthusiasm. 'Stomach-ache and constipation – but you do something about it, day after day.'[9] Intellectual tours de force or surgical extravaganzas are not required to provide Dr Steven Rushton,[10] an English general practitioner, with a sense of fulfillment. He gets pleasure from simple 'menial' tasks such as removing sutures, syringing ears and dealing with nosebleeds, which make 'almost no intellectual demands' on him. The immediate benefits reported by the patient[10] give Rushton a sense of superiority over his academic colleagues who write articles that appear in medical journals but fail to cure the sick people in his waiting room.[11]

Similarly, 'Doctor' Iannis in *Captain Corelli's Mandolin*,[12] who has received no formal medical training, but acts as physician as well as veterinarian and dentist on a Greek island, derives a great deal of satisfaction from his work. On the opening page of the book, de Bernières provides a very credible account of a day in the life of a general practitioner.*

> [Iannis] had enjoyed a satisfactory day in which none of his patients had died or got any worse. He had attended a surprisingly easy calving, lanced one abscess, extracted a molar, dosed one lady of easy virtue with Salvarsan [and] performed one unpleasant but spectacularly fruitful enema.[12]

He also 'produced a miracle' by extracting a foreign body from the ear of one of the townspeople. Iannis, who possesses the 'right' mixture of confidence and self-doubt,

---

* Helen Ashton[13] describes a satisfying day in the life of a general practitioner whose activities are more complex than those of Dr Iannis[12] and include the delivery of a baby and attendance at a death-bed.

behaves impeccably throughout his medical career and, as far as one can gather, his therapeutic activities result in little or no harm.[12]

Unlike Iannis, Dr Jay Reese[14] has received a regular medical education. A board-certified pediatrician in an office practice, Reese has days when he is thoroughly contented, despite the apparently insignificant and monotonous nature of the work.

> [Reese] came to his clinic early and worked without a break . . . He treated a plantar wart, and he gave children allergy shots and he tested their urine and he swabbed at crimson throats. He stared down over tongues and under uvulae to ferret where diseases hid. The kids looked up and he looked down and while they gagged over his tongue depressor he made gagging noises back at them so they watered at the eyes and retched and giggled at once. He was happy all day.[14]

Even the angry Dr Samuel Abelman,[15] whose practice is falling apart, derives some pleasure from this aspect of his work. One of his colleagues remarks, almost incredulously:

> He gets a kid off a sickbed, he lances a boil, he lowers a fever, hell, he prescribes kaopectate and stops a guy from crapping his brains out – he enjoys all that.[15]

Unfortunately, when a particular task becomes too repetitive, the doctor may develop professional boredom and emotional blunting. In the 1940s, attending to a rape victim is considered one of the doctor's noble and tragic assignments.

> He asked no questions; his physicians eyes seeing Dyanna's ravaged body read the essential facts of what had happened. . . . Parris Mitchell worked swiftly and efficiently . . . After he had snapped shut his bag he turned to Aunt Carrie. 'She'll sleep now.'[16]

By the 1990s, sexual assault centres have been established in all major cities, but the routine nature of looking after the injured women has made Dr Mara Fox lose whatever compassion she may have felt when she took on the job[17] (*see* Book II, Chapter 4).

The prescription: pharmaceutical representatives

An essential part of the 'rough and ready cure' is the prescription. Henry James' Dr Austin Sloper, whose clientele consists largely of wealthy women with non-organic complaints,[18] despite his scholarly attitude and his attention to details

> always ordered you to take something. Though he was felt to be extremely thorough, he was not uncomfortably theoretic; and if he sometimes explained matters rather more minutely than might seem of use to the patient he never went so far . . . as to trust to the explanation

alone but always left behind him an inscrutable prescription. There were some doctors that left the prescription without offering any explanation at all; and he did not belong to that class either, which was after all the most vulgar . . . I hasten to add that he was not the least of a charlatan. He was a thoroughly honest man . . . and had none of the little tricks and pretensions of second rate reputations.[18]

To some patients, the doctor's prescription is the most important part of the consultation, equivalent or superior to receiving communion in church.

There was nothing in churchgoing to equal the triumphant moment when you came out of the surgery clutching the ritual scrap of paper.[19]

Remarkably, the influence of the pharmaceutical industry on prescribing habits, which in recent years has provoked some adverse comment,[20] is hardly discussed. Every contemporary Western doctor, whether in private practice or on the staff of a hospital, has received visits from representatives of drug manufacturers, and yet these visitors scarcely receive a mention in fictional literature. Busch describes 'the loud false laughter of a drug salesman',[21] but as Mary Rinehart had pointed out four decades earlier, the term 'salesman' is inappropriate. 'He was not a salesman, he was a giver of largess.'[22] In the early part of the twentieth century the 'free' samples consisted largely of purgatives (euphemistically referred to as liver pills) and baby food. After World War I the detailers distributed 'hypnotics and sedatives required by the jazz period'.[23] In the 1950s it was vitamins and antibiotics.[24] The drug representatives also bring instructional material such as weight charts[22] and they give promotional lecturettes, talking 'quickly and to the point'.[22] For some isolated doctors the pseudo-scientific patter of pharmaceutical sales representatives was, until recently, the main source of postgraduate education.[25] The use of proprietary rather than generic names for drugs is discussed on p. 124.

Detailed lifestyle changes

In the days before efficacious therapeutic agents became available, physicians concerned themselves with minutiae of lifestyle changes to an extent that appears quite bizarre to a modern reader. Patients are forbidden to sing[26] or to write.[27] Detailed instructions are issued concerning the avoidance of particular foods or activities.[28] There is not the slightest evidence that any such prohibitions are beneficial, but the 'orders' presumably keep the patients away from physical stress, emotional trauma and alcohol, and assure them of the doctor's interest in their cases.

In a story published less than one hundred years ago[28] one of Dr Harding's patients, a trial lawyer, feels 'pumped out, uncertain, [and] doubtful each morning if . . . [he] can get through the day without breaking down'. Harding has examined this man in the past and considers him 'physically sound'. Both the doctor and the patient are 'disbeliever[s] in drugs' so, instead of a harmless prescription, the patient receives detailed instructions on what to eat, what to read, when to go to bed and when to walk in the street during the four days before his next appearance in court. Only one newspaper is allowed

> and that of an unsensational character. . . . For twenty-four hours you must live on milk and milk alone, no matter how hungry you may become. . . . For breakfast, upon the second [day], have a bowl of bread and milk. Lunch in bed on some sole or plaice, followed by a rice pudding and some stewed fruit. Rise at three, spend an hour in the garden if the day is warm enough, and have tea at half-past four . . . accompanied by two boiled eggs . . . Have a warm bath, followed by a cold sponge down at seven o'clock when you must retire to bed.[28]

Dr Harding's orders for the next two days are less restrictive but equally detailed, and include permission to drink 'some home-brewed ale' on the fourth day.[28] The doctor's orders are carried out to the letter, followed by the patient's full recovery.[29]

Dawson's Dr John Selkirk, an uncharacteristically judgemental and moralistic member of the profession, even manages to cure a dying woman by restoring to her the affections of her wayward husband.[30] Selkirk, who knows John and Mary Carson personally, is aware of the tensions between them: Mary has been unable to follow her husband in his climb up the social ladder, so that he has become interested in another woman who is better educated and more intelligent than his wife.

> Early next morning there came a hurried message from Carson saying that his wife was very ill. I went at once and found all the signs of typhoid fever. It was a month since I had seen Mary Carson. The month had wrought dreadful havoc with her. She was very weak, depressed and full of a quiet despair about herself . . . She said with a dreary smile 'Doctor, you will do what you can for me I know, but you must not count on me to make an effort to live. I don't want to get better. . . . I am a drag upon . . . my husband . . . and a hindrance. He will find someone else.' I looked on that frail suffering creature entering on the grim conflict for her life without desire of life and I found it in my heart to curse Carson . . . I went downstairs to the library where Carson was awaiting me. He was walking up and down, deadly pale and betraying every symptom of extreme emotion. 'Well Doctor?' he said hoarsely. 'Carson,' I said, 'sit down. I have something to say to you.' He threw up his hands with a gesture of infinite despair and broke into choked vehement speech. 'I know what you are going to say . . . Mary is dying and you've come to tell me I've killed her. Oh, I've been a fool, a brute – God help me. My offence is gross; there is no extenuation; doctor, I lay my heart bare to you; she asked for the bread of love; I gave her stones. I seem to have walked in a dream and I wake to loathe myself.'[30]

The melodrama continues, leaving the early twenty-first-century reader to wonder whether patients and patients' relatives really spoke and behaved in this theatrical fashion one hundred years ago. The story ends happily. After much self-recrimination, the errant husband comes to realize that if he can convince his wife that he still loves her, she may be saved. Carson 'washed her feet with his tears and wiped them with the hairs of his head . . . The desire for life . . . returned to her because love had come back'.[30]

On the other hand, Dr Stirling's[31] recommendations to Constance Povey for changes in her lifestyle are not a success. Despite his erudition and his communication skills[31] (*see* p. 85), Stirling commits an error of judgement when he prescribes travel for a woman who has lived in the same house in 'Bursley' all her life. At the age of sixty, Constance, notwithstanding her native shrewdness and considerable wealth, is a woman of extremely circumscribed education and interests. The thought of travel fills her with alarm while trips to foreign countries are quite unthinkable. When she consults Dr Stirling for sciatic pain aggravated by 'the act of sneezing',[32] the doctor does not restrict his activities to the relief of pain; he also tries to brighten up her way of life. 'Why doesn't she go out and about and enjoy herself?[33] . . . Why doesn't she go to some seaside place and live in a hotel?' The doctor's own tastes intrude. He would love to live in a hotel 'among jolly people. Parties. Games. Excursions'.[33] At such an establishment, Stirling would no doubt win all the trophies at the Edwardian equivalent of 'Trivial Pursuit'. For Constance this kind of life is quite unacceptable. She takes the doctor's advice and goes to stay at a hotel in a 'spa' town for a few weeks but becomes homesick for her old and inconvenient house and expresses considerable resentment towards the doctor and his inappropriate suggestions.[34]

Therapeutic triumphs

Jimmy Kildare[35] and his clones[36] are to be found in many hospital romances, films and television serials. These 'medical cowboys'[36] usually act the part of the 'good guys' heroically fighting the forces of darkness and ignorance, and mostly coming out victorious. They are erudite diagnosticians, skillful and innovative surgeons and compassionate obstetricians. They provide instant cures for major psychiatric problems. Here is a surgeon from Elizabeth Seifert's *Bachelor Doctor*:[37]

> Capped, gowned and masked he would stand beside the [operating] table and begin to work silently on the problem which he had already studied and solved, doing the work he had previously planned, his hand sure, his voice clear – a doctor. And only a doctor.[37]

Robert Merrick in Lloyd Douglas' *Magnificent Obsession*, a typical medical miracle worker, begins his adult life as a very convincing playboy.[38] After an improbable Pauline conversion, Merrick decides on a career change and turns into (what else?) a brain surgeon. Within a few weeks of graduation he has invented an electrocautery apparatus,[39] which he uses to restore his future wife's eyesight.[40]

Tennessee Williams' hypochondriacal Alma Winemiller,[41] a daughter of the manse, becomes ecstatic when discussing the powers of the medical profession with young Dr John Buchanan:

> To be a doctor. And deal with these mysteries under the microscope lens . . . I think it is more religious than being a priest! There is so much suffering in the world it actually makes one sick to think about it . . . But

a physician! Oh my! With his magnificent gifts and training what a joy it must be to know that he is equipped and appointed to bring relief to all of this fearful suffering.[41]

While Tennessee Williams, Dr Buchanan and the audience are likely to regard these schoolgirl gushings as ludicrous and pathetic, Alma's faith in medical doctors is clearly genuine.[41]

Kildare and his successors rarely have to deal with chronic or untreatable illnesses, with hopelessly retarded children or with patients who get worse instead of better. Shem's cynical and grotesque *House of God*[42] and Dooling's Gothic *Critical Care*,[43] with their medical caricatures, are obviously part of a reaction against the genre of 'Medical Westerns'.[36]

However, some major therapeutic successes are to be found in more serious works of fiction. Leon Daudet's *Les Morticoles*,[44] while principally a satire against the Paris teaching hospitals of the 1890s, contains a realistic account of a heroic, life-saving procedure. When a tracheostomy becomes blocked and no suction apparatus is available, Dr Misnard places his mouth over the opening ('appliqua ses lèvres sur la plaie') and sucks out the pus and the infected necrotic material ('la sanie et les détritus funestes'). He is then able to reinsert the cannula, and the patient, who had been in extremis, starts to breathe again. The assistants, the nurse and the patients in the adjacent beds are full of excitement at having witnessed this triumph over death ('domptant la mort') and the patient's wife, who is present throughout the procedure, tries to embrace Dr Misnard. He seems embarrassed by all this enthusiasm and disappears ('mais lui semblait gêné par ces expansions et disparut'), but dies of the same disease (presumably diptheria) two days later.[44]

Another act of self-sacrifice, which results in the successful delivery of a forty-year-old primipara, is described by Don Marquis.[45] Dr Stewart who 'was born . . . the same year the British burned the White House in Washington' has practiced medicine

> nearer sixty than fifty years. Nobody ever heard him say anything about loving . . . [his patients]. Nor did anybody hear the word 'service', so popular since, from his lips.[45]

But neither the floods nor his own illness could stop the dying old man attending the confinement of Myra Tucker, whom he had himself delivered forty years earlier. Dr Stewart's young colleague, Dr Hastings, who drives a 'horseless carriage', has declined to attend because he has a broken leg, but when he becomes worried the old man might not make it, he changes his mind and rides his horse to the isolated farmhouse. The baby is delivered successfully but Dr Stewart dies on a sofa in the living room. Just before his death

> [Dr Stewart] sat fully upright on the couch and spoke loudly – spoke as a commanding general might in brevetting a younger officer for gallantry on a field of battle with pride and authority and affection in his tones: 'By God boy,' he said, 'you're a doctor.' He sighed a long deep sigh and relaxed. . . . He was leaving his people in good hands.[45]

The successful resuscitation of an apparently stillborn baby constitutes one of the highlights of *The Citadel*.[46] Martin du Gard's Dr Antoine Thibault performs an emergency ligation of a torn femoral artery on a round dining room table.[47] During the procedure he raps out orders to his hastily recruited assistants who obey 'like soldiers under fire'. They hold retractors, administer chloroform and run off to obtain supplies while he cuts, clips and ties. The child survives and at the end of the procedure one of the assistants

> gazed at Antoine with spellbound awe – the look that Martha may have given the Savior when Lazarus rose from the tomb.[47]

While the account of Antoine Thibault's surgical adventure[47] has been debased by multiple subsequent such descriptions in works of 'light' literature, the story of his success in relieving the anguish of a guilt-ridden father of a handicapped child[48] remains one of the great passages in medical fiction and is cited in full. Monsieur Ernst, a teacher, who has married late in life, has fathered a single child, a little boy who suffers from an unidentified 'speech disorder' (? autism). The appointment to see Dr Antoine Thibault has been made for the little boy, but the father precedes his family into the doctor's office and unburdens himself. Many years earlier, he had been treated for syphilis. Might the child's problems be due to the 'sins of the father'? The doctor's response is prompt and unequivocal.

> 'What possible connection can there be between that . . . little misfortune of yours which was taken in hand at once and completely cured and your little boy's infirmity which will very likely pass away quite soon? . . . If I have grasped your meaning, my dear sir, your scruples do you credit, but speaking as a professional man let me tell you quite frankly that from the scientific point of view they're simply . . . ludicrous.' . . . Antoine now deliberately introduced new hypotheses. 'Was the child . . .[premature]?' Monsieur Ernst blinked at Antoine; the question took him by surprise. 'What? . . . [premature?] . . . No!' 'Was it a difficult labor?' 'Very much so.' 'Forceps used?' 'Yes.' 'Ah . . . that, I should say, explains quite a lot.' Then to cut things short he added 'Well let's have a look at our little patient,' and began to move towards the waiting room. But then the child's father stepped quickly forward and clutched Antoine's arm. 'Is that true doctor? Is it really true? You're not saying it just to . . . Doctor, will you give me your word for it? Your word of honor?' Antoine swung round him and saw a look of entreaty, of famished hunger to believe, mingled with boundless gratitude. The joy that surged across him was that which follows only on a successful effort or a good deed well done. The child? Well he would see what he could do. Meanwhile where the man before him was concerned, his duty was plain: at all costs he must lift the load of anguish from that tormented soul. He let his gaze sink into the others eyes, and answered in a deep and emphatic voice 'I give you my word of honor!' After a moment's silence he opened the door. In the other room he saw an elderly lady in black and a playful little scamp with curly brown hair whom she was trying to keep quiet, penning him between her knees . . . There was a sad and gentle beauty in her careworn features that went straight to Antoine's heart . . . 'Would you mind coming this way?'[48]

The language strikes the modern reader as sentimental, while the conclusions may be factually incorrect. However, from a therapeutic perspective, the doctor's declaration is absolutely right, its effect on the anguished father dramatic and the old-fashioned sense of achievement well deserved.

Treatment failures: incurable conditions

When the patient fails to improve, deteriorates or dies, the doctor's 'bad' treatment is likely to be criticized. If the disease proves incurable, comments are made about the 'obviously' futile attempts at intervention even though, at the time the treatment was administered, the 'incurability' was by no means obvious. Dr Adam Stanton, the priestly and incorruptible surgeon in *All the King's Men*,[49] is diminished by his failure to cure Tom Stark, the Governor's son. Tom becomes quadriplegic during a football game when his spinal cord is damaged beyond recovery.[50] While the attempted decompression operation is entirely justified from the medical point of view, its failure constitutes a major milestone on the road towards Stanton's destruction. More than half a century later, the doctors looking after Bill Chalmers[51] attempt to improve his progressive peripheral neuropathy with plasmapheresis – a reasonable measure in these circumstances.[51] Unfortunately, in Bill's case, the procedure is not a success and the memory of

> his blood flowing through the clear plastic tube into the machine and back to the blue vein in his arm

fills him with a final sensation of impotent fury at the purposelessness of it all.[52]

Feminist writers express intense anti-medical sentiments especially when the doctor is male, the patient female and the disease untreatable. Mary Moody Schwartz in Yglesias' *How She Died*[53] has developed breast cancer during her second pregnancy at the age of twenty-six. Mary, the daughter of a convicted atom bomb spy and agitator for 'left wing' causes, is angry about her surgeon's fast voice, about the treatment she has received and is about to receive, and about the doctor's unwillingness to spell out her hopeless prognosis. 'They cure one thing and make you sick with another.'[53]

If more than one therapeutic modality is available, the doctor is censured for selecting the wrong one. Failed surgical treatment is blamed on the doctor's incompetence or inexperience while unforeseen complications are attributed to lack of care and attention.

Treatment failures: non-compliance

One scenario provides the doctor with an excuse for a poor outcome – patient non-compliance. Antonia, in *The Tales of Hoffman*, whose doctor has give orders that she is not to sing, disobeys and dies.[26] The *Lady of the Camellias*,[27] whose doctor has forbidden her 'to touch a pen', writes a note to her former lover and pays the appropriate penalty. The asthmatic Marcel,[54] who ignores Professor Cottard's dietary restrictions, continues to wheeze until his parents make him follow the doctor's dietary instructions to the letter.

The unnamed doctor in Brieux' *Damaged Goods*[55] who is faced with a non-compliant patient may strike modern readers as pompous, judgemental and theatrical, but he is the true hero of the play and he acts at all times like a model physician, combining 'correct' medical advice with discretion and compassion. He tries hard to persuade George Dupont, who recently contracted syphilis and who is engaged to be married, to break off his engagement so as not to risk infecting his wife and future children. George promises to come back the following week and, in the meantime, to think things over. The doctor realizes he has failed.

> 'No, I shall not see you next week and what is more, you will not think it
> over. You came here knowing what you had, with the express intention
> of not acting by my advice unless it agreed with your wishes.'[55]

The doctor expresses a sense of guilt at not being able to prevent the misery awaiting George and other men who act like him. 'I am almost afraid of not having been persuasive enough. I feel as though . . . I were the cause of their misery.' When the inevitable happens and the Duponts produce a syphilitic infant, the doctor tells the parents that he is morally and legally obliged to warn the wet nurse about the dangers involved in breast-feeding this infant. Madame Dupont Senior, the child's grandmother, declares that she is prepared to 'lose her soul to save the child', and that she will pay the nurse a large sum of money so as to make her stay, but the doctor is adamant: 'I shall not allow you to take that responsibility . . . I shall speak to the nurse and give her the fullest particulars which I am convinced you have not done.' Despite his apparent harshness, the doctor is capable of considerable compassion and, in the end, he manages to restore some family harmony.[55]

Another non-compliant patient is described by Arnold Bennett in *Riceyman Steps*.[56] Henry Earlforward, the eccentric, miserly bookseller, who is unable to swallow any food, refuses to go into hospital. While Dr Raste is explaining the situation to Mrs Earlforward on the landing outside the bedroom

> they both saw the bedroom door open and the lank figure of the patient
> in his blue-gray nightshirt emerge . . . 'It's not the slightest use you two
> standing chattering there,' Henry muttered bitterly, 'I'm not going into a
> hospital so you may as well know it.'[56] . . . 'Better get back to bed,
> Mr Earlforward.' said the doctor rather grimly and coldly. 'I'm going
> back to bed. I don't need you or anyone else to tell me I oughtn't to be
> out here'. . . . And he limped back to bed triumphant.[56]

A few days later, Earlforward's intransigence and Raste's inflexibility result in a rupture of the doctor–patient relationship.[57] Raste, who has gone to considerable trouble to make all the arrangements, is now emotionally committed to Earlforward's hospitalization and unable to accept the patient's refusal. 'You'll have to be put under observation, watched for a bit and X-rayed. You can't possibly be nursed properly here', argues the doctor.

> 'I won't go to the hospital,' Mr Earlforward coldly interrupted him. 'I
> don't mind having a private nurse here. But I won't go to the hospital.' . . .
> Dr Raste in addition to being exasperated . . . had now positively
> determined to get him into the hospital and it was this resolve that had

prompted him to give special attention to Mr Earlforward's case, disorganizing all his general work in favor of it. He could not allow himself to be beaten by the inexplicable caprice of a patient . . . [Earlforward had] convinced himself that he would prefer anything, even death to incarceration in a great hospital . . . with its rows of beds . . . the semi-military bearing of the nurses, the wholesaleness of the affair, the absence of privacy, the complete subjection of the helpless patients, the inelasticity of regulations . . . 'I don't think I'll go into a hospital,' he said quietly turning his face away. The words were mild, the resolution invincible . . . The doctor crossed over to look at him in the face. Their eyes met in fierce hostility. The doctor was beaten. 'Very well,' said he with bitter calm. 'If you won't, you won't. There is nothing else for me to do here. I must ask you to be good enough to get another adviser. And . . . please remember that if the worst comes to the worst. I shall certainly refuse to give a certificate.' 'A certificate, sir?' Elsie (the housekeeper) faltered. 'Yes. A certificate of the cause of death. There would have to be an inquest,' he explained with implacable and calculated cruelty. But Mr Earlforward only laughed – a short dry sardonic laugh. . . . The doctor with the pompous solemnity of a little man conscious of rectitude slowly picked up his hat from the chest of drawers. 'But what am I to do?' Elsie appealed. 'My good woman, I don't know. I wish I did. I've done what I could; and I can't take the private affairs of all Clerkenwell on my shoulders. I've other urgent cases to attend to.' With a faint snigger which his will was too late to suppress . . . the doctor walked majestically out of the room.[57]

Earlforward dies after a hematemesis a few days later, and, at autopsy, a cancer is found at the gastro-esophageal junction.[58]

Dr Raste constitutes somewhat of an exception – most doctors have learnt to regard their patients' non-compliance as part of the illness or at least to treat it as a complication rather than a personal insult. 'Oh forgive me!' says one of Dr Tom Thurnell's patients in Kingsley's *Two Years Ago*.[59] 'Oh if I'd minded what you said.' Recriminations are not part of Thurnell's repertoire: 'Never mind what might have been, let's feel your pulse'.[59] Similarly, Tom Evans, Dr Andrew Manson's patient in *The Citadel*,[60] who has more faith in the district nurse than in Manson, dispenses with the doctor's services. When the nurse applies contaminated 'carron oil' to Evans' scalded elbow, which inevitably becomes infected and then stiff, Andrew shows no sign of 'I told you so' satisfaction. On the contrary, 'he muttered an expression of regret. He had no rancor against Evans, only a sense of sadness'.[60]

Treatment failures: lack of attention to the patient's complaints and suggestions

Patients who deteriorate after capriciously refusing or neglecting to follow their doctor's recommendations simply reinforce the doctor's perceived power and omniscience. On the other hand, when fictional patients form the opinion (rightly or wrongly) that their treatment is inappropriate, the authors generally take the side of the patient. This scenario is particularly likely to occur when insecure physicians feel uncomfortable with patients' diagnostic or therapeutic suggestions, which are regarded as 'attacks on . . . [their] own prerogative of superior intelligence'.[61]

George ['Monk'] Webber in Thomas Wolfe's *The Web and the Rock*,[62] who has been admitted to Dr ['Geheimrat'] Becker's clinic in Munich after sustaining scalp lacerations in a drunken fight, dislikes the Geheimrat at first sight. The doctor whose 'brutal fingers probed and pressed and sponged' looks and behaves like a caricature of an ugly German. Becker, a surly character, has

> short thick fingers . . . hairy hands . . . [a] bullet head . . . [a] stiff clipped brush of a gray-black moustache, [a] bald skull with an ugly edge of shaved blue skin and [a] coarse pleated face scarred with old dueling wounds . . . At the first . . . Monk believed that there was another smaller wound . . . at the back of his head which the doctor had not seen. But his fame was so great, his manner so authoritative and his speech to Monk when he had mentioned it, so gruff and so contemptuous, that Monk had said no further word, yielding to the man's authority.[62]

That night there is a scene in the hospital when the Mother Superior confirms that there is another wound. Monk demands to see the Geheimrat immediately.

> Shaking with a feeling of outrage and insult, Monk shouted loudly down the hall; 'Geheimrat Becker! . . . Becker . . . Where is Becker? . . . I want Becker . . . Geheimrat Becker – Geheimrat Becker –' jeeringly 'great Geheimrat Becker – are you there?' His face a map of outraged decency, . . . [the hospital orderly] took Monk by the arm and whispered: 'Quiet. . . . Are you mad? . . . The Herr Geheimrat Becker is not here.' 'Not here?' Monk stared unbelievingly into the square face. 'Not here?' 'Nein,' implacably, 'not here.' The limping butcher was not here! – In his own slaughter pen! The shaven butcher with his scarred face, his shaven head, his creased neck – was not here! – Where he was born to be, to limp along these halls, to probe thick fingers at a wound . . . to hurl himself upon the maimed and wounded of the earth, to force them roughly back upon a table as he had forced Monk back and then to take their flesh and bones into his keeping, to press, probe, squeeze with brutal fingers and if necessary to chisel open their skulls . . . even to cut down to the living convolutions of man's thought.[62]

After some further outbursts Monk is finally induced by the hospital staff to go back to his bed. Wolfe evidently believes that the patient, whose opinion has been ignored, is entitled to his expression of outrage even though he punishes innocent bystanders rather than the perpetrator.

Hemingway's flawed ambulance surgeons in *God Rest You Merry, Gentlemen*[63] are not as repulsive or as arrogant as Dr Becker,[62] but neither of them listens to the psychotic young man who asks to be castrated as a 'cure' for his masturbation and both fail to recognize the danger signals. Doc Fischer, the Jewish gambler and abortionist, tries to convince the boy that his 'lust' is natural. 'It's a sin against purity', replies the patient. Doc Wilcox, the drunkard, tells the young man to 'go and . . . .' 'When you talk like that I don't hear you,' the boy said with dignity.

In the end the two of them fail to take appropriate steps to prevent the disaster, and the young man mutilates himself.[63]

Another doctor who ignores his patient's complaint is Updike's Dr Pennypacker, whose fields of endeavor include the ear, the nose and the throat as well as the eyes. When Clyde Behn consults Pennypacker for a twitching eyelid,[64] the doctor treats him for various other 'problems', which do not bother Clyde at all. He remembers the doctor as

> an aloof administrator of expensive humiliations. In the third grade he had made Clyde wear glasses. Later, he annually cleaned, with a shrill push of hot water, wax from Clyde's ears and once had thrust two copper straws up Clyde's nostrils in a futile attempt to purge his sinuses.[64]

The various treatment failures in the past used to make Clyde feel unworthy for not responding to the doctor's futile and mindless ministrations, and the pattern is repeated on this occasion.[64] The consultation begins inauspiciously with the contrived friendliness of a voluptuous receptionist.

> The top half of a Dutch door at the other end of the room opened and framed in the square, Pennypacker's secretary turned the bright disc of her face toward him. 'Mr Behn?' she asked in a chiming voice. 'Dr Pennypacker will be back from lunch in a minute.'

When the doctor arrives 'the petite secretary-nurse, switching like a pendulum, led him through the sanctums'. Pennypacker 'a tall stooped man with mottled cheekbones and an air of suppressed anger' who filled

> his little rooms with waiting patients and wander[ed] from one to another like a dungeon keeper[64]

ignores the twitch, takes away Clyde's horn-rimmed glasses and prescribes metal frames. He comes up with a non-diagnosis of 'middle-aged eyes' and produces a bottle of eyedrops to stop eyelashes falling out. When Clyde asks: 'Will it cure the tic?' Pennypacker impatiently snapped, 'the tic is caused by muscular fatigue' and having 'violated' his eyes, shows him out of the office barely able to see.[64]

Buzacott's Lisa Pembroke,[65] a delinquent suffering from an advanced malignancy which is obviously not responding to chemotherapy, wants to stop taking medications. She can see no point in the medical staff persisting with their efforts for the sake of 'doing something'. Her wishes are ignored, leaving her to express contempt and hatred for her physicians in her diary:

> Some time later I come back to consciousness. It's time for this pill or that pill. Some injection maybe. It doesn't matter really. It keeps them happy. Still, I tell them I don't want it. They think I'm scared so they treat me like a schoolgirl . . . I just ignore them.[65]

'Muzil', the homosexual writer and art critic,[66] expresses considerable hostility towards physicians who instead of treating their AIDS patients' respiratory and gastro-intestinal problems prescribe antidepressants for them. He fumes: 'They're so fed up with their patients' phlegm and diarrhea that they start dabbling in psychoanalysis and come up with the most outrageous diagnoses'.[66]

Treatment failures: medical incompetence

Instances of medical incompetence, even those resulting in major disasters, may be reported factually and without resentment, especially if the authors have had medical training or, like Gustave Flaubert and Ernest Hemingway, come from medical families. Dr Charles Bovary, who has no surgical training and no common sense, handles a clubfoot operation and the postoperative management so badly that the leg becomes gangrenous and has to be amputated.[67] Curiously, Dr Bovary, the perpetrator, is portrayed as a victim rather than a villain (*see* p. 247). Catherine Barkley's Cesarean section in *A Farewell to Arms*[68] ends with a dead infant and a dead mother. Her lover, Frederic Henry, is stunned but there are no recriminations or resentful remarks about what should have been done. The doctor offers to drive Frederic home.

> 'No thank you. I am going to stay here a while.' 'I know there is nothing to say. I cannot tell you –' 'No' I said. 'There is nothing to say.' . . . 'It was the only thing to do,' he said. 'The operation proved –' 'I do not want to talk about it,' I said.[68]

Even Dr Charles Ivory in Cronin's *The Citadel*,[69] who incises rather than ligates a vascular lesion during an abdominal operation, and causes the patient to bleed to death on the operating table, provokes resentment against a bad system rather than a bad doctor. After the patient's death, Ivory tells the distraught widow (who is grateful for this condescension) that 'no power on earth could have saved him'[69] and the matter goes no further.

While these ancient disasters would nowadays be followed by appropriate inquiries, there is no contemporary shortage of calamities due to medical incompetence or inexperience, and, to some extent, such tragedies are inevitable.[70]

Treatment failures: the wrong choice

Decisions that have to be made on the basis of incomplete evidence may prove, in retrospect, to have been incorrect. In a medical setting this may mean a major catastrophe.

Samuel Beckett's Dr Nye[71] has to face up to such a problem. Nye, a flawed character, suffers not only from depression but also from several behavior problems, which he attributes to some 'trivial and intimate' childhood incident involving his nanny.[71] He practices as an internist, performing routine chores such as ordering 'a Wasserman's test on an old schoolfellow' or seeing hospital patients whose conditions vary little from day to day. However, he has sufficient insight to realize, when confronted by a boy with bilateral tuberculous empyemas, that, on this occasion, he cannot dither around. A choice has to be made on the basis of inadequate evidence.

> The point had been reached where he must decide whether to . . . [recommend an operation] at once or hold his hand a little longer. It was a decision that lay outside the scope of his science because from the strictly pathological point of view there was as much to be urged on the one side as on the other. Nevertheless it had to be made and at once, and by him.[71]

Dr Nye recommends surgery and the boy dies.

Solemn Oath, by Hannah Alexander, is a somewhat contrived story written around a religious theme, though the physician/author demonstrates a detailed knowledge of contemporary medical dilemmas. Fifteen-year-old Shannon Becker, 'uncomfortable with her rapidly burgeoning female contours', wants a prescription for an oral contraceptive because she is contemplating sex with 'Lance', a somewhat older high-school student, who 'thought I was weird because I was still a virgin'.[72] Dr Mercy Richmond, Shannon's family doctor, avoids moralistic attitudes, but briefly hesitates before deciding which is the lesser evil. Should she, by implication, condone this child's entry into the 'meat market' or would it be better to refuse prescribing the 'pill' and risk a pregnancy? Dr Richmond's tactic of threatening Shannon with sexually transmitted diseases and the side effects of estrogens to frighten her into temporary abstinence is not a success. Lance tells his classmates that Shannon is vacillating and an associate lout rapes her.[72]

The doctor with the one-track mind

The older literature is replete with accounts of single-minded doctors who know only one diagnosis or one kind of treatment, which they apply, with varying degrees of success, to all-comers. Regardless of the nature of their misconceptions which range from harmless crackpot theories to lethal forms of intervention, doctors afflicted by this problem are ignorant of statistics, their speculations concerning the pathogenesis of disease are laughable and their tedious therapeutic repertoire involves agents that are obsolete, harmful or both. Surprisingly, some elements of this syndrome persist into the twenty-first century and not only among practitioners of 'alternative medicine'.

Some 'single-minded' physicians are simply victims of their times, traditions and training. Before the days of evidence-based medicine, when controlled trials were virtually unknown, medical practice was based on what authority figures had said or written. Medical students with inquiring minds, who expressed doubt about particular theories or procedures, encountered hostility among their teachers. From Sinuhe the Egyptian[73] to Arrowsmith the American,[74] students questioning traditional attitudes among their teachers are referred to accumulated clinical experience.

> I asked my teacher [about the evidence for a particular statement]. He merely looked at me as if I were half-witted and said 'It is so written.' But this was no answer.[73]

When Martin Arrowsmith[74] questions the use of ichthyol in the treatment of erysipelas, the professor of materia medica reprimands him in more modern terminology, but the message is the same:

> 'How do they know? Why, my critical young friend, because thousands of physicians have used it for years and found their patients getting better, and that's how they know.'[74]

Martin's question whether there have been any controlled trials elicits a response that is heavy with sarcasm.

> 'Probably not – and until some genius like yourself, Arrowsmith, can herd together a few hundred people with exactly identical cases of erysipelas, it probably never will be tried. Meanwhile, I trust that you other gentlemen, who perhaps lack Mr Arrowsmith's profound scientific attainments and the power to use such handy technical terms as 'control' will, merely on my feeble advice, continue to use ichthyol.'[74]

The modern medical student is no longer encouraged to use ichthyol or discouraged from asking searching questions, but empirical medical training, especially procedural training of interns by residents, remains didactic to this day.

A rigid examination system used to reinforce the attitudes and prejudices acquired by the students during their medical training. Indeed, Molière suggests that the entire system of medical student assessment is designed for only one purpose: the perpetuation of the errors of the medical faculty. In *Le Malade Imaginaire*[75] a chorus of learned physicians appears on stage, singing away in barbarous Latin while they examine a student who is about to graduate. One of the examiners mentions a hypothetical case:

> Last night patientus unus (a patient)
> Chanced to fall in meas manus (into my hands)
> Habet grandem fievram (he had a high temperature)
> Grandum dolores capitis (a severe headache)
> Et grandum malum (and great pain) in his side.

In addition, this poor patient could barely breathe. How would you proceed? asks the examiner. The candidate has been well trained. He prescribes an enema, a venesection and a purge. That's all very well, sings a second examiner, but what if this perverse character should refuse to respond ('non vult se curire'). The candidate gives the 'right' answer. He prescribes further enemas, further bleeding and further purges. The entire Court of Examiners now breaks into a rousing chorus congratulating the young man on his excellent responses and informing him that he is worthy to join their ranks.[75]

If doctors find it difficult to abandon useless, obsolete and dangerous practices acquired from their teachers during their training, it becomes virtually impossible for them to discard theories and therapeutic systems introduced or propagated by themselves. When Pliny[76] fulminates against the physician who introduced the fashion of immersing patients in cold baths and who employed this 'treatment' for all sorts of diseases, he implies that this cold-water torturer is acting from base motives. Pliny does not seem to realize that this doctor who has 'ancient senators . . . chilling and quaking . . . in these baths'[76] more likely regarded himself as an innovative pioneer than a dishonest charlatan.

Dr Sangrado in *Gil Blas*,[77] who bleeds all his patients mercilessly and fills them 'to the tongue' with water, is vaguely aware that his ministrations may do more harm than good, but finds it impossible to change his style because, he admits, 'I have published a book in which I have extolled the use of frequent bleeding and aqueous draughts'.[77]

Dr Hauberger, the Chief of Surgery at the Charité Hospital has, in his younger days, described an operation for trigeminal neuralgia.[78] The 'Hauberger' procedure is, for many years considered standard treatment though newer, more complicated and more effective methods have now been introduced. The chief, of course, persists in using 'his' old method and any of his assistants who dare to mention (let alone employ) the new operation risk instant dismissal.[78] An innocent female medical student asks one of the residents why, if the results of the new operation are better, the chief does not change over.

> 'Because my dear girl,' said . . . [the resident] with a laugh, 'it isn't easy to give up any technique you're used to. When it's become the classical treatment which is found in all the textbooks – well it would be almost like someone asking you to kill your own son and adopt the child next door.'[78]

Detached amusement or intense anger?

In the doctor–patient–author–reader quadrilateral, the doctor's single-minded foibles are generally kept confidential between authors and readers, and contemplated with tolerant disapproval rather than burning anger. Chaucer's remark about the physician who 'knew the cause of every maladie'[79] (no doubt humors and planets) is possibly sarcastic but not angry. Five hundred years later, Dr Thomas Lisse, Professor of Bacteriology,[80] who is convinced that 'a microbe of madness will be discovered in the not very distant future',[80] is treated as an inoffensive eccentric. The company doctor in Conrad's *Heart of Darkness*[81] has some hare-brained hypothesis, which makes him 'measure the crania of those going out there (to the Congo) in the interest of science'.[81] He has no idea how to handle his data and is classified as a 'harmless fool'.

Ellis' Dr Bruneau,[82] a sanatorium doctor in the French Alps, who labors under a preconceived idea about the heredity of tuberculosis, accepts and rejects information according to whether or not it fits in with his theory.

> 'We will begin our acquaintance by learning a few particulars about you. Your parents are both living?' 'Dead.' 'Ah voilà,' said he, with the satisfaction of a man who has just located the missing piece in a jigsaw puzzle. Sensing a misunderstanding, Paul added quickly: 'They died in a car accident when I was two years old.' 'A car accident . . . then they were not ill?' 'No, they were perfectly healthy.' 'Then which member of your family had tuberculosis?' 'None, I am the first.' 'That, monsieur,' said

Dr Bruneau, waving his pen at Paul, 'you do not know. Many are ill and never know it. I have a theory . . .'[82]

The curious beliefs of Graham Greene's Dr Crombie are of a more exotic nature. Crombie, 'a strictly honest man' (and talented train spotter) holds the view that masturbation and 'sexual congress' cause cancer,[83] and, in his role as school doctor, he propagates this opinion among the students. 'Almost one hundred per cent who die of cancer have practiced sex.' These bogus 'statistics' are challenged by one of his students:

> 'But maiden ladies,' I objected, 'they die of cancer too.' 'The definition of maiden in common use,' Doctor Crombie replied, . . . 'is an unbroken hymen. A lady may have had prolonged sexual relations with herself or another without injuring the maidenhead.' . . . 'But the young don't often die of cancer, do they?' 'They can lay the foundation with their excesses.' . . . 'And the saints,' I said, 'did none of them die of cancer?' 'I know very little about saints. I would hazard a guess that the percentage of such deaths in their case was a small one.'[83]

Dr Crombie's outlandish theories cause him to lose his school appointment but, essentially, he seems an inoffensive man, who, apart from missing an authentic case of gonorrhea in a school student, does little harm.

Margaret Drabble describes a variation on the medical one-track-mind theme – the doctor with reserve hypotheses to be used in cases where the principal pet theory is manifestly not applicable.[84] Rosamund Stacey's obstetrician predicts that her baby will be exceptionally small, whereas it actually weighs 'six and a half pounds'. During a postnatal visit, Rosamund's gynecologist tries to explain his incorrect forecast: it must have been her firm abdominal muscles that caused the false impression.

> He turned to me and smiled and said, 'Were you by any chance a professional dancer?' . . . 'Good heavens, no,' I said, 'nothing like that.' 'You must have some athletic pursuits,' he said. 'No, none at all,' I said . . . 'Then you must be just made that way,' he said and smiled and passed on.

Rosamund, the scholarly and sophisticated possessor of the six and a half pound baby and the firm abdominal musculature, 'glowed with satisfaction' at this asinine remark.[84]

Indulgent amusement may even be extended to physicians who use detrimental treatment methods as the result of their old-fashioned or new-fangled theories. Conan Doyle's Dr James Winter,[85] who has fallen *Behind the Times* in his appreciation of medical advances, regards the stethoscope as a 'new-fangled French toy', while the thought of bacteria causing diseases 'set him chuckling for a long time' . . . His favorite joke in the sick room was to say 'Shut the door or the germs will be getting in'.[85] Despite his old-fashioned prejudices and archaic medications, Dr Winter, who 'served out senna and calomel to all the countryside',[85] is still consulted by numerous patients, including some younger doctors. Indeed, Conan Doyle represents him as an ideal physician (*see* p. 90). Similarly, Dr Richard

Gaunt, another old-fashioned English general practitioner 'partial to antiquated remedies', is not resented for his traditional approach.[86]

When surgeons become involved, 'harmless theories' develop into decisive actions that are applied indiscriminately and, once in a while, inappropriately. Bernard Shaw's Dr Cutler Walpole,[87] a leading London surgeon, labors under the delusion that most diseases are due to bacteria and that these unwelcome guests can be made to depart if the 'nuciform sac' is removed, a treatment of which old Sir Patrick Cullen disapproves.[87] 'People pay him five hundred guineas to cut it out. They might as well get their hair cut for all the difference it makes, but I suppose they feel important after it. You can't go out to dinner now without your neighbor bragging to you of some useless operation.'[87] Walpole offers a 'nuciformectomy' to one of his colleagues (who declines) but uses the operation most effectively in an opera singer who is having voice troubles.[87] Here is Walpole being greeted and congratulated on his therapeutic success by his colleague, Sir Ralph Bloomfield Bonnington (BB):

BB:	Walpole, the absent-minded beggar, eh?
Walpole:	What does that mean?
BB:	Have you forgotten that lovely opera singer I sent you to have that growth taken off her vocal cord?
Walpole (springing to his feet):	Great heavens man, you don't mean to say you sent her for a throat operation?
BB (archly):	Aha! Haha! Aha! (trilling like a lark as he shakes his finger at Walpole).
	You removed her nuciform sac. Well, well. Force of habit! Force of habit!
	Never mind. Ne-e-e-ver mind. She got back her voice after it and thinks you are the greatest surgeon alive and so you are, so you are, so you are![87]

Bonnington, who teases his surgical colleague, suffers from the 'one-track-mind' syndrome himself. He uses extraordinary means to 'stimulates the phagocytes' of his artist/patient whose consumption becomes truly galloping as a result. Also in *The Doctor's Dilemma* is Dr Blenkinsop, who tells all his patients to eat a pound of ripe greengages each day half an hour before lunch.[88] On a different 'track' but equally ignorant of any scientific principles, Thomas Mann's Dr Friedrich Grabow[89] prescribes a diet consisting of 'a little pigeon, a little French bread' regardless of whether the patient is a young boy suffering from some acute gastrointestinal disturbance, a middle-aged merchant with a transient ischemic attack of the brain or an old woman dying from carcinoma of the colon.[90]

Truman Capote's unnamed Wichita orthopedic surgeon,[91] whose therapeutic recommendations are cited without comment, constitutes yet another example of the single treatment doctor. Bonnie Clutter, a chronic depressive, has been suffering for more than twenty years from 'an inexplicable despondency – seizures of grief that sent her wandering from room to room in a hand-wringing daze'.[91] There have been several trips into hospital, but during her last admission a young orthopedist provides a new diagnosis.

> Returning from two weeks of treatment at the Wesley Medical Center in Wichita, her customary place of retirement, Mrs Clutter had brought scarcely credible tidings to tell her husband; with joy she informed him that the source of her misery, so medical opinion had at last decreed, was not in her head but in her spine – it was physical – a matter of misplaced vertebrae. Of course, she must undergo an operation and afterwards – well, she would be her old self again.[92]

The young surgeon does not have the opportunity to confirm or refute his hypothesis that a laminectomy will cure Mrs Clutter's depression, because the entire family is murdered *In Cold Blood*,[91] a few days after Bonnie's return.

Even fatal outcomes as the result of the one-track mind are treated with remarkable lenience in the first half of the twentieth century. Clinical details are sparse in Capek's *Giddiness*,[93] which contains a most succinct and witty summary of psychoanalytic theory. Mr Gierke, a wealthy industrialist, is so disabled by his persistent vertigo that he can barely get out of his chair. Various specialists have failed to diagnose the cause of Mr Gierke's problems, so Dr Hugo Spitz, the Freudian psycho-analyst, is called in.

> Spitz based his method on the treatment of . . . repressions . . . His argument was that everybody in their subconsciousness has all sorts of awful ideas or memories or cravings, . . . generally . . . scandalous, . . . that he represses, because he's afraid of them, . . . that . . . these repressed ideas . . . cause nervous disturbances . . . and when a doctor who knows his job . . . drags this repression into the light of day, the patient gets relieved and all is right again.[93]

Dr Spitz decides (on very flimsy evidence) that Mr Gierke has murdered his first wife, that he now contemplates killing his second wife and that his giddiness is due to his inability to decide whether or not to go ahead with his nefarious plan. Gierke is stunned by the doctor's 'revelations', his giddiness disappears for a few moments and he accompanies the doctor to the door of his apartment. Within seconds of Spitz's departure, Gierke falls down a stairwell and dies. 'Suicide', concludes the doctor, while the reader, who has been suspicious of the psychiatrist and his hypotheses all along, decides that an accidental fall (brought on by giddiness) is much more likely.[93] In either case the outcome of the doctor's psycho-analytic efforts can hardly be called successful.

The therapeutic tactics of Dr George Bull, the earthy, irascible and unprofessional physician in Cozzens' *The Last Adam*,[94] are less subtle but equally disastrous. The list of Bull's patients who receive instructions to take castor oil include a boy with acute abdominal pain,[95] a young man who believes he has picked up a sexually transmitted disease from one of the town wenches,[96] a middle-aged man with a fever[97] and sixteen-year-old Molly Ordway, who, the doctor suspects, reports sick because she does not feel like going to school. 'I gave her a dose of castor oil', the doctor gleefully informs his hunting friends, 'so she'd have something to do at home'.[97] Several of the recipients have typhoid fever and die, possibly as the result of Bull's 'treatment'.[98]

Francis Brett Young's Dr Jacob Medhurst[99] does not actually mention castor oil but his therapeutic efforts are obviously aimed in the same direction (*see* p. 80).

Medhurst considers any form of treatment futile, unless it produces immediate and spectacularly unpleasant results, particularly in the gastrointestinal tract. Medhurst's standard prescription consists of

> a bottle of physic that tastes and smells like the devil . . . A mixture . . . that would take the roof off a crocodile's mouth and shift an elephant.[99]

Dr Wills Bolling's therapeutic repertoire is equally monotonous, but at least the record gets changed periodically.[100] When his son and practice partner loses thirty pounds in weight because of persistent vomiting, the doctor inappropriately diagnoses amebiasis. 'That year everything was ameba, another year it was endometritis, and between you and me he took out just about every uterus in Feliciana Parish.'[100]

Writers who have themselves suffered under doctors with a 'one-track mind' are unlikely to look on the perpetrators as inoffensive screwballs. Sophocles expresses some anger towards the 'leech who mumbles charms over ills that need the knife'.[101] In modern terms, this physician should have referred his patient to a surgeon rather than continue to reassure him.

AA Milne's dormouse[102] displays just a hint of irritation with his meddlesome doctor. The creature has been quite happy with his traditional color-scheme ('geraniums red and delphiniums blue') but his physician has other ideas; according to him, a switch to yellow is required.

> The doctor stood frowning and shaking his head
> And he took up his shiny silk hat as he said:
> 'What the patient requires is a change,' and he went
> To see some chrysanthemum people in Kent.[102]

Charms For an Easy Life[103] by Kaye Gibbons displays a strong anti-medical bias. The heroine of the story, self-taught Charlie Kate Birch, with her herbal medicines, her charms and her superstitions, constantly shows that she is a more competent healer than 'proper' doctors, one of whom shows signs of the one-track-mind syndrome. Charlie Kate believes Mareen, the old black maid, has 'intestinal paralysis' and asks a licensed doctor, who lives in 'a neighborhood of grand houses and fine lawns', to admit Mareen to hospital. The MD demurs. 'The only thing that goes wrong below an old colored woman's waist is fibroids. That and too much grease.'[103] Mareen proceeds to die at home, attended by Charlie Kate who then blackmails the 'useless' doctor into an early retirement, even though there is little evidence that hospitalization would have made any difference to the course of the disease.[103]

While single-minded, meddlesome doctors are found in all branches of the profession, the species seems over-represented among ear, nose and throat surgeons. In addition to John Updike's Dr Pennypacker and his pathetic attempts to cleanse his patients' ears and sinuses[64] (*see* p. 208), interventionist ENT doctors are described by Sinclair Lewis,[104] Marcel Proust[105] and Jean Stafford.[106] Dr Roscoe Geake in *Arrowsmith*,[104] whose 'earnest feeling regarding the nasal septum was that it never hurt any patient to have part of it removed',[104] snips out bits of tissue instead of informing his patients that very few people come to harm from a deviated nasal septum. Geake's subsequent departure from the university, and his 'elevation' to the position of vice-president of a medical furniture company, imply that his useless operations are based on pecuniary motives. On the other hand, Proust's ENT surgeon,[105] who suffers from misapprehensions very similar to those of Roscoe Geake, comes across as a fool rather than a knave. During her final illness, when a number of physicians examine (or offer to examine) Marcel's grandmother, an unnamed nose specialist is summoned because the old lady is 'coughing and sneezing a great deal'. As the grandmother refuses point-blank to let herself be examined by this character, the rest of the family

> defer to the desire that he expressed to inspect each of our noses in turn though there was nothing the matter with any of them . . . According to him, however, there was; everything whether headache or colic, heart disease or diabetes was a disease of the nose. . . . To each of us he said: 'I should like to have another look at that nozzle. Don't put it off too long. I'll soon clear it for you with a hot needle.' We asked ourselves. 'Clear it of what?'[105]

Jean Stafford's 'nose bigot'[106] fancies himself not only as a surgeon but also as a psychologist.

> Like many of the medical profession, even those whose specialty was centered on the organ of the basest sense, he interested himself in the psychology of his patients; in several instances, for example, he had found that severe attacks of sinusitis were coincident with emotional crises.[106]

This bumbling fool, with his dreadful bedside manner (*see* p. 75), obviously knows nothing about psychology. Moreover, throughout the lengthy nose-packing procedure the reader is left wondering what on earth this man is doing up 'Pansy's' nose and what benefits (if any) she is likely to derive from his exertions.[106]

Charlotte Gilman's *The Yellow Wallpaper*[107] is the story of a depressive woman writer suffering from chronic fatigue who has to put up with the weird therapeutic notions of her physician-husband. He prescribes 'phosphates', rest and isolation, and decrees that she is 'absolutely forbidden to work'. The patient expresses the view that 'congenial work with excitement and change, would do me good', while John, the authoritarian husband, will not listen to any of his wife's proposals. His 'rest cure' makes her a virtual prisoner in an upstairs room with barred windows and the symbolic 'yellow wallpaper' where, in addition to her fatigue, she develops delusions and hallucinations.*

Some decades after the publication of Charlotte Gilman's book, Sir William Bradshaw, the wealthy and fashionable psychiatrist in Virginia Woolf's *Mrs Dalloway*,[110] still knows of only one treatment for delusional patients.

> When a man comes into your room and says he is Christ (a common delusion) and has a message, as they mostly have, and threatens, as they

---

* Charlotte Gilman, who had herself been subjected to 'rest cure' treatment, was of the opinion that her 'alienist' actually changed his approach after reading *The Yellow Wallpaper*.[108]

often do, to kill himself, you . . . order rest in bed, rest in solitude . . . rest without friends, without books, without messages, six months' rest.[109]

Mrs Dalloway's attitude towards this prominent doctor is one of loathing and contempt.

Even Dr Cottard,[110] Proust's great diagnostician (*see* p. 112), evidently has several diagnostic and therapeutic bees in his bonnet. He infuriates Marcel's family when they tell him that the grandmother (who dies soon afterwards in renal failure) has been taken ill. 'You're sure it's not what they call a diplomatic illness?' – an obviously inappropriate diagnosis in a previously well woman in her seventies. Cottard then goes on to another (equally inappropriate) knee jerk response – he prescribes a milk diet.[110]

Norine Blake in Mary McCarthy's *The Group*[111] has to endure the outdated sexual prejudices of an old-fashioned neurologist, recommended by her mother. Norine's husband is impotent but refuses to seek medical advice, so she goes.

> He asked me whether I wanted to have children. When I said no, I didn't, he practically booted me out of the office. He told me I should consider myself lucky that my husband didn't want intercourse. Sex wasn't necessary for a woman, he said.[111]

Another firm believer in ancient doctrines is to be found in *The Fortunes of Richard Mahony*.[112] Dr Mahony, who himself holds a medical degree, is dismayed to discover, on the night of his wife's confinement, that he has no real confidence in Dr Rogers, her obstetrician.

> Rogers belonged to an old school. His method was to sit by and let nature take its course . . . His old fogyism showed up unmistakably in a short but heated argument they had on the subject of chloroform. He cited such heavy objections to the use of the new anesthetic in maternity cases as Mahony had never expected to hear again: the therapeutic value of pain; the moral danger the patient ran in yielding up her will . . . and the impious folly of interfering with the action of creative law. It had only remained for him to quote Genesis and the talking serpent.[112]

Glasser provides a more recent setting for the one-track-mind syndrome. The physicians in *Ward 402*[113] use renal transplants whenever feasible, while units in other hospitals and other cities prefer chronic dialysis. Robert Berquam, the angry father of one of the children, accuses the doctors of making the patients fit in with their own preferences, prejudices and schedules, rather than adapting the treatment to suit the patients. Here Berquam, a medical technologist, is overheard talking to the father of a child with renal failure. The boy has rejected his second transplanted kidney and members of Dr Kadden's team are talking about a third transplant.[113]

> 'I bet nobody's mentioned home dialysis to you, have they? It's not because they don't know about it. It's because the experts in home dialysis aren't here, they're up in Boston. They're pushing their own thing down here and you pay the price. The patients always have to pay the price. Kadden's thing is recipient typing and transplantation, not dialysis.

If you were in Boston, they'd be talking dialysis, not transplantation. Each specialist pushes his own thing, tears down the other guys ideas while he minimizes the risks and complications of his own. The patient be damned.'[113]

Berquam's outburst, like some of his other statements, contains an element (a small element) of truth. At a time when new techniques are being pioneered, a physician will naturally recommend a treatment that has been tried and established in his own unit.

What causes the medical 'one-track-mind' syndrome?

Regular physicians, unlike 'alternative' practitioners, steer clear of simplistic theories that attribute all of mankind's ailments to a single organ. They denounce the use of particular treatments for all illnesses. Why then should any 'proper' physicians fall into the trap of adopting an approach, which they condemn in charlatans?

Fictional works do not provide an answer to this question but there are a few hints. Deeply entrenched medical misconceptions may simply represent, in individual physicians, an exaggeration of what entire classes or entire generations of students have learnt or mislearnt from their teachers. An enthusiast with an uncritical attitude may have absorbed one message particularly well. He has been conditioned into believing that appearance A is equivalent to disease B and that treatment C must be administered. In the sixteenth and seventeenth centuries, when the urine container was the equivalent of the contemporary stethoscope in terms of the doctor's badge of office, 'urine casting' was mandatory for all serious disorders,[114] despite its subjectivity and notorious unreliability.[115] During the nineteenth and twentieth centuries, diagnostic and prognostic doctrines were based on physical signs such as carotid murmurs, marks on the finger nails and the patient's complexion, which are almost as untrustworthy as the urine sediment. When Tamburlaine's physician declares

I view'd your urine and the hypostasis, thick and obscure doth make your danger great[116]

he is using his 'clinical experience' in much the same way as Lucas Marsh in *Not as a Stranger*,[117] who concludes, by looking at a patient's face, that

her complexion and conjunctivae had the muddiness of chronic gastritis.

Both deductions are highly suspect. 'There's no more credit to be given to th' face than to a sicke man's urine.'[115]

The entire profession may suddenly become afflicted with the one-track-mind syndrome. Lemming-like, all physicians suddenly change direction and adopt theories and practices previously unheard of and subsequently found to be false. In the island of the *Morticoles*,[44] where all human ailments are due to the recently discovered microorganisms, 'the new theories [have] become dogmas and articles of faith, which one cannot contradict without being taken for a fool or a heretic'.[118]* Much of Gawande's *Complications*[70] is taken up with the introduction of innovative surgical techniques, though it would be foolish to assume that, in the long term, the new will invariably prove better than the old.

In addition, the exigencies of their profession make it imperative for doctors to act or seem to act decisively on some occasions. Marcel Proust,[119] using a military analogy, points out that a practicing physician, like a commanding officer under battle conditions, has to make life-and-death decisions on the basis of incomplete data.

> During these brief moments in which [Dr Cottard] deliberated, in which the relative dangers of one and another course of treatment fought it out between them in his mind until he arrived at a decision, this man who was so insignificant and so commonplace, had something of the greatness of a general who, vulgar in all things else, moves us by his decisiveness.[119]

It is no wonder that this decisiveness, once acquired, gets in the way of rational decision making, gives rise to an unvarying treatment strategy and may finally lead to a disaster.

Summary

Doctors by their training and their attitudes are better qualified to intervene in human disorders than other would-be healers. Most 'treatments' consist of relatively simple measures, which provide satisfaction to doctors and patients alike. Spectacular therapeutic successes are largely confined to light fiction, while treatment failures are attributed to clumsiness, inexperience and choice of the wrong treatment. Multiple works of fiction refer to the doctor's 'one-track mind' which may be treated with tolerant amusement or with a sense of outrage.

References

1 Kipling R (1910) A Doctor of Medicine. In: Kipling R (1960) *Rewards and Fairies*. Macmillan, London, pp. 253–76.

2 Sterne L (1759–67) *The Life and Opinions of Tristram Shandy, Gentleman*, Work JA (ed.). Odyssey Press, New York, 1940, p. 168.

3 Galen (2nd century AD) The Affections and Errors of the Soul. In: *Galen, Selected Works*. Translated by Singer PN. Oxford University Press, Oxford, 1997, p. 108.

---

* Most of the events described in *Les Morticoles* are malicious inventions or gross exaggerations but the book contains a few pertinent remarks and observations.

4 Mauriac F (1925) *The Desert of Love*. Translated by Hopkins G. Eyre and Spottiswoode, London, 1949, p. 50.

5 Crichton M (Jeffery Hudson, pseudonym) (1968) *A Case of Need*. Signet, New York, 1969, p. 90.

6 Ellis AE (1958) *The Rack*. Penguin, London, 1988, pp. 140–1.

7 Shaw GB (1906) The Doctor's Dilemma. In: *The Bodley Head Bernard Shaw's Collected Plays With Their Prefaces*, vol. 3. Max Reinhardt The Bodley Head, London, 1971, pp. 230–1.

8 Plato (4th century BC) The Republic. Translated by Jowett B. In: Buchanan S (ed.) (1979) *The Portable Plato*. Penguin, Harmondsworth, pp. 396–7.

9 Bellaman H (1940) *Kings Row*. Dymocks, Sydney, 1945, pp. 254–5.

10 Russell R (1985) *While You're Here, Doctor*. Souvenir Press, London, p. 225.

11 Ibid., p. 66.

12 Bernières L de (1994) *Captain Corelli's Mandolin*. Vintage, London, 1998.

13 Ashton H (1930) *Doctor Serocold*. Penguin, London, 1936.

14 Busch F (1984) Rise and Fall. In: Busch F. *Too Late American Boyhood Blues*. David R Godine, Boston, p. 41.

15 Green G (1956) *The Last Angry Man*. Charles Scribner's Sons, New York, p. 368.

16 Bellaman H and Bellaman K (1948) *Parris Mitchell of Kings Row*. Simon and Schuster, New York, p. 60.

17 Goldsworthy P (1992) *Honk If You Are Jesus*. Angus and Robertson, Sydney, pp. 48–9.

18 James H (1881) *Washington Square*. Bantam Books, New York, 1959, pp. 1–5.

19 Pym B (1980) *A Few Green Leaves*. EP Dutton, New York, p. 13.

20 Angell M (2000) The pharmaceutical industry – to whom is it accountable? *N Engl J Med*. **342**: 1902–4.

21 Busch F (1979) *Rounds*. Farrar Straus and Giroux, New York, pp. 80–1.

22 Rinehart MR (1935) *The Doctor*. Farrar and Rinehart, New York, pp. 12–14.

23 Ibid., p. 408.

24 Green G, op. cit., p. 35

25 Last JM (1967) Quality of general practice. *Med J Aust*. **1**: 780–4.

26 Hoffman ETA (1818) Rath Krespel. In: Bleiler EF (ed.) (1967) *The Best Tales of Hoffman*. Translated by Bealby JT. Dover Publications, New York, p. 232.

27 Dumas A (1848) *The Lady of the Camellias*. Translated by Gosse E. Alan Sutton, Gloucester, UK, 1986, p . 198.

28 Bashford HH (1911) *The Corner of Harley Street: being some familiar correspondence of Peter Harding MD*. Constable, London, 1913, pp. 66–70.

29 Ibid., p. 78.

30 Dawson WJ (1900) John Carson's Wife. In: *The Doctor Speaks*. Grant Richards, London, pp. 133–47.

31 Bennett A (1908) *The Old Wives' Tale*. Hodder and Stoughton, London, 1964, pp. 461–3.

32 Ibid., p. 453.

33 Ibid., pp. 465–6.

34 Ibid., p. 489.

35 Brand M (Frederick Faust) (1941) *Young Dr Kildare*. Ian Henry, Hornchurch, UK, 1977.

36 Turow J (1989) *Playing Doctor*. Oxford University Press, New York, p. 13.

37 Seifert E (1969) *Bachelor Doctor*. Collins, London, 1971, p. 68.

38 Douglas LC (1929) *Magnificent Obsession*. George Allen and Unwin, London, 1944, pp. 38–47.

39 Ibid., pp. 187–221.

40 Ibid., pp. 296–304.

41 Williams T (1948) Summer and Smoke. In: *The Theatre of Tennessee Williams*, vol. 2. New Directions, New York, 1971, p. 142.

42 Shem S (Bergman S) (1978) *The House of God*. Richard Marek, New York.

43 Dooling R (1991) *Critical Care*. William Morrow, New York.

44 Daudet LA (1894) *Les Morticoles*. Fasquelle, Paris, 1956, pp. 142–6.

45 Marquis DRP (1939) Country Doctor. In: Marquis DRP. *The Best of Don Marquis*, Garden City Books, Garden City, New York, pp. 444–63.

46 Cronin AJ (1937) *The Citadel*. Gollancz, London, p. 56.

47 Martin du Gard R (1922–9) *The Thibaults*. Translated by Gilbert S. John Lane The Bodley Head, London, 1939, pp. 323–37.

48 Ibid., p. 576.

49 Warren RP (1946) *All the King's Men*. Modern Library, New York, 1953.

50 Ibid., pp. 399–405.

51 Lightman A (2000) *The Diagnosis*. Pantheon Books, New York, p. 272.

52 Ibid., p. 368.

53 Yglesias H (1972) *How She Died*. Heinemann, London, 1973, p. 14.

54 Proust M (1913–22) *Remembrance of Things Past*, vol. 1. Translated by Scott-Moncrieff CK and Kilmartin T. Penguin, Harmondsworth, 1985, pp. 536–7.

55 Brieux E (1902) Damaged Goods. Translated by Pollock J. In: *Three Plays by Brieux*. Brentanos, New York, 1911, pp. 185–254.

56 Bennett A (1923) *Riceyman Steps*. Cassell, London, 1947, pp. 213–20.

57 Ibid., pp. 264–71.

58 Ibid., p. 308.

59 Kingsley C (1857) *Two Years Ago*. Macmillan and Co., London, 1884, pp. 303–4.

60 Cronin AJ, op. cit., pp. 140–9.

61 Mitchell SW (1885) *In War Time*. The Century Company, New York, 1913, p. 14.

62 Wolfe T (1939) *The Web and the Rock*. Heinemann, London, 1969, pp. 624–8.

63 Hemingway E (1933) God Rest You Merry, Gentlemen. In: *The Complete Short Stories of Ernest Hemingway*. Scribner Paperback Edition, Simon and Schuster, New York, 1998, pp. 298–301.

64 Updike J (1963) The Persistence of Desire. In: Updike J. *Pigeon Feathers and Other Stories*, Andre Deutsch, London, pp. 12–26.

65 Buzacott M (1987) *Charivari*. Picador, Sydney, pp. 200–6.

66 Guibert H (1990) *To the Friend who did not Save my Life*. Translated by Coverdale L. Quartet Books, London, 1991, pp. 38–9.

67 Flaubert G (1857) *Madame Bovary*. Translated by Steegmuller F. Modern Library, New York, 1982, pp. 201–5.

68 Hemingway E (1929) *A Farewell to Arms*. Jonathan Cape, London, p. 349.

69 Cronin AJ, op. cit., pp. 376–80.

70 Gawande A (2002) *Complications: a surgeon's notes on an imperfect science*. Profile Books, London, 2003.

71 Beckett S (1934) A Case in a Thousand. In: Gontarski SE (ed.) (1995) *Samuel Beckett: the complete short prose 1929–1989*. Grove Press, New York, pp. 18–24.

72 Alexander H (2000) *Solemn Oath*. Bethany House, Minneapolis, MN, pp. 149–57.

73 Waltari M (1945) *The Egyptian*. Translated by Walford N. Panther Books, London, 1960, pp. 34–9.

74 Lewis S (1924) *Arrowsmith*. Signet Books, New York, 1961, p. 42.

75 Molière JBP (1673) The Hypochondriack. Translated by Baker H and Miller J. In: *Molière's Comedies*, vol. 2. Dent, London, 1961, pp. 469–71.

76 Pliny the Elder (Gaius Plinius Secundus) (1st century AD) *Natural History*, Book 29. Translated by Holland P. Southern Illinois University Press, 1962, pp. 294–7.

77 Le Sage AR (1715) *The Adventures of Gil Blas Santillana*, vol. 1. Translated by Smollett T. World's Classics, Oxford University Press, London, 1907, pp. 100–15.

78 Soubiran A (1947) *The Doctors*. Translated by Coburn O. WH Allen, London, 1954, pp. 222–3.

79 Chaucer G (approx. 1390) Canterbury Tales. In: Fisher JH (ed.) (1977) *The Complete Poetry and Prose of Geoffrey Chaucer*. Holt, Rinehart and Winston, New York, pp. 17–18.

80 Maartens M (1906) *The Healers*, Constable. London, p. 82.

81 Conrad J (1902) *Heart of Darkness*. Penguin, London, 1988, pp. 37–8.

82 Ellis AE, op. cit., p. 30.

83 Greene G (1965) Doctor Crombie. In: Greene G (1972) *Collected Stories*. The Bodley Head and William Heinemann, London, pp. 128–35.

84 Drabble M (1965) *The Millstone*. Weidenfeld and Nicolson, London, p. 127.

85 Doyle AC (1894) Behind the Times. In: Doyle AC (1934) *Round The Red Lamp*. John Murray, London, pp. 1–8.

86 Ashton H, op. cit., p. 10.

87 Shaw GB, op. cit., pp. 335–40.

88 Ibid., p. 346.

89 Mann T (1902) *Buddenbrooks*. Translated by Lowe-Porter HT. Penguin, Harmondsworth, 1957, pp. 28–9.

90 Ibid., p. 54.

91 Capote T (1966) *In Cold Blood: a true account of a multiple murder and its consequences*. Random House, New York, p. 29.

92 Ibid., p. 7.

93 Capek K (1929) Giddiness. In: Capek K (1967) *Tales From Two Pockets*. Translated by Selver P. Allen and Unwin, London, pp. 177–83.

94 Cozzens JG (1933) *The Last Adam*. Harcourt Brace and Company, New York.

95 Ibid., p. 23.

96 Ibid., pp. 164–6.

97 Ibid., pp. 150–2.

98 Ibid., p. 249.

99 Young FB (1938) *Dr Bradley Remembers*. Heinemann, London, pp. 242–5.

100 Percy W (1961) *The Moviegoer*. Noonday Press, New York, 1977, p. 152.

101 Sophocles (approx. 460 BC) *Ajax*. Translated by Storr F. Loeb's Classical Library, Heinemann, London, 1961, p. 51.

102 Milne AA (1924) The Dormouse and the Doctor. In: Milne AA (1977) *When We Were Very Young*. Methuen, London, pp. 66–7.

103 Gibbons K (1993) *Charms For an Easy Life*. Abacus, London, 1994, pp. 85–8.

104 Lewis S, op. cit. pp. 82–5.

105 Proust M, op. cit., vol. 2, p. 335.

106 Stafford J (1953) *The Interior Castle*. Harcourt Brace and Company, New York, p. 206.

107 Gilman CP (1892) *The Yellow Wallpaper*, Bauer DM (ed.). Bedford Books, Boston, 1998, pp. 41–59.

108 Gilman CP (1935) *The Living of Charlotte Gilman: an autobiography*. University of Wisconsin Press, Madison, 1990, pp. 118–21.

109 Woolf V (1925) *Mrs Dalloway*. Zodiac Press, London, 1947, p. 110.

110 Proust M, op. cit., vol. 2, p. 308.

111 McCarthy M (1954) *The Group*. Signet, New York, 1964, p. 139.

112 Richardson HH (1917–29) *The Fortunes of Richard Mahony*. Penguin, London, 1990, p. 138.

113 Glasser RJ (1973) *Ward 402*. Garnstone Press, London, 1974, p. 145.

114 Silvette H (1967) *The Doctor on the Stage*. University of Tennessee Press, Knoxville, TN, pp. 7–35.

115 Webster J (1623) The Duchess of Malfi. In: Brown JR (ed.) (1976) *The Revels Plays*. Manchester University Press, Manchester, UK, Act I, Scene 1, p. 22.

116 Marlowe C (1590) Tamburlaine Part II. In: Marlowe, C. (1947) *Plays*. Dent, London, Act V, Scene 3, p. 115.

117 Thompson M (1955) *Not as a Stranger*. Michael Joseph, London, p. 335.

118 Daudet LA, op. cit., p. 153.

119 Proust M, op. cit., vol. 2, p. 333.

CHAPTER 7

The 'correct' degree of detachment

A certain measure of insensitivity is not only an advantage but a positive necessity in the exercise of a calm judgment . . . Keen sensibility is doubtless a virtue of high order . . . but for the practitioner in his working-day world, a callousness which thinks only of the good to be effected . . . is the preferable quality.[1]

Most criticisms aimed at physicians entail departures from accepted standards of medical behavior. By contrast, censures of doctors for their emotional detachment from the suffering patient go to the core of medical practice. The degree of aloofness recommended by Osler[1] has been criticized[2] but the question concerning the 'correct' balance between involvement and detachment,[3] which has philosophical implications, will obviously remain unanswered.

The extent to which physicians let themselves become personally caught up in their patients' anguish has captured the imagination of many writers, some of them antedating Osler. Fictional accounts provide examples of doctors who stray too far in one or the other direction, with ensuing therapeutic failures and additional disasters. Over-involvement with their patients' problems produces feelings of self-recrimination and impotence or leads doctors to unwarranted interference in matters that should not concern them. Too much distancing produces less varied but equally detrimental results. In particular, the patient may develop a sense of alienation, which makes any meaningful doctor–patient relationship impossible.

Too detached

The three physicians in Balzac's *The Wild Ass's Skin*,[4] who politely interrogate and examine Raphael de Valentin, behave correctly, they do not hurt the patient and they do not crack jokes at his expense. Unlike other multi-physician consultations described by Balzac[5] (*see* p. 190) this particular examination can certainly not be described as a farce but neither is it a success.

The invalid sought to guess their thoughts, putting a construction on every movement they made . . . All Valentin's observation could discover no trace of a feeling for his troubles in any of the three [senior] doctors. The three received every answer in silence, scanned him unconcernedly and interrogated him unsympathetically. Politeness did not conceal their indifference . . . After spending about half an hour over taking in some sort the measure of the patient much as a tailor measures a young man for a coat . . . the authorities uttered several commonplaces and even talked of politics. Then they decided to go into Raphael's study to exchange their ideas and frame their verdict. 'May I not be present during the discussion, gentlemen?' Valentin had asked them but Brisset and Maugredie* protested against this and, in spite of their patient's entreaties, declined altogether to deliberate in his presence.[4]

The physicians remain cold and detached throughout the examination, they fail to establish a diagnosis, so that the exercise provides neither scientific nor emotional benefits to the patient.

The two army doctors in Weir Mitchell's *In War Time*[7] also display a somewhat uncaring attitude during a tragic deathbed scene. Captain Charles Gray of the Confederate Army, who has been wounded and taken prisoner at Gettysburg, is now dying of septicemia in a Philadelphia hospital. His only child, a motherless girl of fifteen, has somehow managed to visit him just before his death but she arrives too late and he no longer recognizes her.[7] When the two doctors come out of the dying man's room, they talk briefly of the orphaned girl's future but soon go on to other topics. They discuss the possibility of writing a paper on rapidly progressive pyemia: 'We have plenty of material'. They speak of 'Jones in Number Five', who, in their opinion, should be sent back to the front. 'He seems to me a malingerer and a poor actor at that.'[7] Weir Mitchell, himself a physician, gives the impression of feeling some kind of collective guilt at the apparently callous attitude of the two doctors and tries to apologize for them:

> The sense of defeat which waits for the physician as he leaves the room of the dying [is] a keener discomfort than the unthinking public can imagine.[8]

However, as the story illustrates, the 'discomfort' is of very short duration; the subsequent conversation involves the dying man only as a statistic, while 'Jones in Number Five' will be punished for not wanting to finish up the same way as Captain Gray. In Mitchell's military doctors the feeling of 'sympathetic detachment' evidently involves more detachment than sympathy.

Dr Edred Fitzpiers, the flawed medical hero of *The Woodlanders*,[9] who is totally detached, does not even have the excuse of Weir Mitchell's doctors who are dealing with multiple battle casualties and whose dying patient is, after all, an enemy soldier.[7,8] Fitzpiers is a thoroughgoing snob to whom poor patients are 'cases' and who is barely able to recall the relevant clinical details from one visit to the next.[9]

> Fitzpiers entered the sick chamber as a doctor is wont to do on such occasions and pre-eminently when the room is that of a humble cottager; looking round towards the patient with a preoccupied gaze which so plainly reveals that he has well-nigh forgotten all about the case and the

---

* Balzac's fictional characters are believed to be based on authentic physicians practicing at the time.[6]

circumstances since he dismissed them from his mind at his last exit from the same apartment.[9]

An extreme form of 'detachment' is provided by Ellison's 'infallible' robots,[10] whose total disinterest makes them positively dangerous. These appliances perform delicate surgical operations more skillfully than any human, but their designers are unable to build in a bedside manner, which they find 'too nebulous a concept'. The robots lack human emotions such as anger, terror and pity and they need neither fame nor thanks. 'All they needed was their power pack and an occasional oiling.' These deficiencies make the robots unable to give encouragement and reassurance to a bilateral amputee who loses his 'will to live'. A patient from the slums, who suffers from tetanus, makes his woman promise, 'before he started twitching', that she will not take him to the robots in the hospital. 'We'd rather die than go to them. We won't have no truck with them things.'[10]

Too involved

If Balzac's senior physicians,[4] Weir Mitchell's army doctors[7,8] and the supercilious Fitzpiers[9] are perceived as too aloof, other medical characters err in the opposite direction. The fourth doctor who accompanies the three physicians during the consultation in *The Wild Ass's Skin*[4] is young and has 'not yet learned to keep back the . . . tears that obscure a man's clear vision'.[4] This man, a personal friend of the patient, is emotionally too involved to make any intellectual contributions.

Another of Balzac's physicians, Dr Martener in *Pierrette*,[11] discovers soon after commencing medical practice that he lacks the ruthlessness and the aloofness required for a major city hospital appointment. He decides on a career change and becomes a general practitioner in a country town.

> [Martener] had begun by practicing in Paris; but the insensibility to suffering which the terrifying number of patients and the multiplicity of serious cases inevitably impart to the physician, had stricken with dismay his kindly heart . . . So he returned to Provins to marry and settle down and to minister almost with affection to the ailments of a population which he could look upon as one large family.[11]

An unkindly academic might describe Martener's move from Paris to Provins as a 'cop-out' but Balzac certainly does not view it that way.

Strindberg's Dr Ostermark[12] typifies the physician who associates himself too closely with his patients' emotional crises. Ostermark, a vacillating and not very intelligent country doctor, becomes entangled in a bitter domestic fight, which ends in the death of his patient ('The Captain') and 'victory' for Laura, the Captain's stupid but cunning wife. When Ostermark first attempts to call on the Captain, he is hijacked by Laura, who warns him about her husband's mental instability. The doctor makes a token attempt to exercise his own judgement: 'My dear lady, I am honored by your confidence, but as a physician I must observe and examine before giving an opinion'.[12] Having delivered himself of this platitude, he goes on to show that he has already abandoned his independent assessment in favor of Laura's misinformation. He asks: 'Has the Captain shown any symptoms of instability, any lack of will power? . . . Is he dogmatic?' and Laura provides the 'right' answers. When the Captain ultimately appears, he is obviously short-tempered and not particularly polite,[13] but he does not display any signs of insanity. Despite his doubts, Ostermark is irrevocably committed to Laura. He conspires with her to be in the house late at night[14] and when physical violence erupts he procures a straitjacket.[15] Strindberg repeatedly compares Laura to Omphale,[16] the mythological mistress of Hercules who dresses up in his lion's skin and plays with his club, while the strong man has to sit at the spinning wheel and perform other 'female' tasks. Laura and the doctor undergo much the same role reversal. She makes the diagnosis and provides a management plan, while he becomes the menial who carries out her wishes.

Likewise, Dr Richard Diver, the brilliant, tragic hero of *Tender is the Night*,[17] becomes too entangled in his patients' affairs despite his considerable psychiatric talents. The main plot of Scott Fitzgerald's masterpiece relates to Nicole Warren, Diver's beautiful, rich, schizophrenic patient, who becomes his wife, and goes on to destroy him (*see* Book II, Chapter 1). However, his inability to remain aloof from his patients is not confined to Nicole. The woman with 'nervous eczema'[18] and intractable pain evokes such intense pity and love in Richard, that he becomes incapable of discussing her rationally.

> In the awful majesty of her pain, he went out to her unreservedly, almost sexually. He wanted to gather her up in his arms . . . and cherish even her mistakes, so deeply were they part of her.[18]

When this 'scabbed anonymous woman-artist' reaches the final phase of her illness, Richard remains with her for the last three nights of her life,[19] while after her death he refuses to discuss the diagnosis* with his less talented but more detached practice partner.

Dr Samuel Abelman, the hero of Gerald Green's *The Last Angry Man*,[20] whose background and training are quite different from those of Richard Diver, nevertheless suffers from and is ultimately destroyed by the same disability: a severe lack of aloofness. Abelman, a sixty-eight-year-old, irascible Jewish family physician, who practices in what is now a New York City slum, has been in the same neighborhood for forty-odd years. He is consumed by anger against 'fancy specialists', professors and rival general practitioners, all of whom, he believes, are conspiring to steal his remaining patients. He rages against former patients who have let themselves be seduced away,[21] and he is frustrated by the blacks in the area, who wake him up at night, make all sorts of demands but do not appreciate him[22] and are unable to pay.[23] Abelman is more than a paranoid old fool who has failed to move with the times. He enjoys practicing what he believes to be 'true' old-fashioned medicine,[24] without regard to money or diplomatic subtleties. Even in his old age Dr Abelman still visits the medical library[25] and takes an interest in complex clinical problems. Indeed, just before his death, he correctly diagnoses a glioma of the right hemisphere[26] in a black teenage delinquent, from whom he receives no pay, gratitude or

---

* 'Congenital syphilis'[19] may fit in with the general 'Sins of the Fathers' theme of the book. From a medical point of view, disseminated lupus is much more likely, though there are other possibilities.

respect. However, throughout his long medical career Dr Abelman never acquires or sympathizes with the concept of professional detachment. The 'last angry man' is also the 'last honest man' who never learns to dissemble. He treats his patients as if they were members of his own family, loving and protecting them, worrying over them and, when necessary, reprimanding them and even becoming angry at them.[27]

This is how Dr Abelman lectures one miserable couple, who are evidently suffering from a 'folie à deux':

> 'There's not a goddam thing wrong with either of you, medically . . . What do you want from me? . . . If I give you a diet you won't follow it, and if I give you medicine you'll call up after the first dose and complain you're still sick. Go home, love each other, get interested in your kids, get a hobby. You're not sick.'[27]

The patients respond in kind, and act as if

> Sam was their father. The kind of father you talk back to and you love sometimes and you hate other times.[28]

Lengthy disputations and ghastly 'family scenes' ensue. Abelman cannot quite understand why neither his enemy, young Dr Baumgart,[25] nor his friend and classmate, Doctor Max Vogel,[27] have such problems. They never lose their tempers and they never have to deal with angry patients.[29] Vogel gives Abelman a lecture on how to cultivate an atmosphere of aloofness. 'The worst thing you can do', declares Dr Vogel, . . . '[is to make] friends out of patients'.[30] He wears a white coat (*see* p. 72), he hires an Irish nurse 'who wiggles her ass on schedule', he installs flashing red lights and he will not allow his patients to call him by his first name.[30] To Abelman all this is empty flummery, designed to impress and deceive the public, but he has sufficient insight to realize that his 'neat, cool and aloof' colleagues in their white coats present themselves as models of professional competence[25] while he regards himself as a father figure and complains about the ingratitude of his 'children'.[23]

Contrasts between two extremes

Chekhov, a physician-author, provides examples of both types of errors – too much and too little involvement. Dr Eugene Lvov in *Ivanov*,[31] a recent medical graduate, knows all about truthfulness and decency but he lacks tact and he is evidently unfamiliar with the concept of professional objectivity. Like the behavior of Dr Ostermark[12] (*see* p. 175), Lvov's meddlesome eagerness to 'straighten the crooked' benefits no one, but hastens the death of one patient[32] and causes the suicide of another.[33] Dr Lvov has under his care Anna/Sarah Ivanov who is dying of tuberculosis. He advises a change of climate and absolute rest but Anna gets neither; a stay in the Crimea is too expensive, while the strained relations between her and her husband, Nicholas Ivanov, make a restful existence impossible. Instead of carrying on professionally under these difficult but not unique circumstances,

Lvov assumes the role of Anna's advocate and troubadour. He lectures Nicholas on a daily basis, accusing him of having married Anna for her money and, when that is not forthcoming, trying to get rid of her so that he can marry another unsuspecting young maiden.[34] The doctor asks Anna (uselessly and unprofessionally) how she ever came to marry Nicholas who, despite his faults, is basically a generous man.

> 'Tell me . . . how you, a decent, intelligent woman with a nature almost angelic, have let yourself be taken in so blatantly? . . . What have you in common with that callous, insensitive' . . .[32]

He leaves the sentence unfinished but his meaning is obvious. Lvov personally escorts Anna to a neighboring property where she faints after witnessing signs of her husband's infidelity.[32] When, a year after Anna's death, Nicholas is about to marry again, the doctor turns up at the house of the new bride, publicly calls Nicholas an 'unmitigated swine' in order to 'open the eyes' of the young girl, and Nicholas responds by killing himself.[33] The 'provincials' thoroughly disapprove of this interfering 'do-gooder' and treat him with contempt. Lebedev, an old drunkard, sarcastically addresses Lvov as 'medical genius'. Shabelsky, another stage buffoon, calls him 'reverend high priest of science'.[35] Behind his back the doctor is called a 'shallow, narrow-minded medico. . . . Puts himself on a high moral pedestal and abuses everyone who doesn't squawk like him'.

By contrast, another of Chekhov's physicians, also called Eugene, is so well trained in detachment that he has become almost totally insensitive to his patients' sorrows. Dr Eugene Dorn in *The Seagull*[36] has under his care an impoverished retired public servant (Peter Sorin) who walks with a cane and who feels that life has passed him by. Dorn does not even put on a show of compassion.

> 'To go to your doctor when you're sixty and complain that you didn't enjoy yourself as a young man . . . that's just silly.'[36]

Two years later, Peter Sorin, by now in a wheelchair, still wants 'a bit of life'.[37] He complains that he is not receiving any medication. Once again, Dr Dorn is quite brutal. "What would you like?' he asks Sorin, 'Valerian drops? Soda? Quinine?' The message, which may not be entirely clear to Sorin, implies that no medication is going to make the slightest difference to his condition. Dorn expresses himself more explicitly a few minutes later when he informs Sorin 'All life must end'.[37]

William Faulkner's *The Wild Palms*[38] contains descriptions of four medical men displaying different degrees of detachment though Faulkner does not use this term. The unnamed forty-eight-year-old landlord-physician, intellectually, emotionally and physically sterile, is unlikely even to understand the concept.

> [He] had graduated nearer the foot of the class than the head[39] . . . married the wife his father had picked out for him and within four years owned the house which his father had built and assumed the practice which his father had created, losing nothing from it and adding nothing to it.[39]

This doctor sleeps in a 'stale bed', he eats stale food and he practices stale medicine.[40] On the one occasion when we see him called upon to treat a patient, to help a woman bleeding to death after a bungled abortion, he becomes moralistic, produces a gun and calls the police.[41] The notions of 'love', 'lust', 'tolerance' and 'compassion' mean nothing to this mediocrity. The 'bright wild passion had somehow passed him up when he had been young enough'.[41]

The second physician in *The Wild Palms* is Dr Henry Wilbourne, the principal male character. Wilbourne, twenty years younger than his medical landlord, is well on the way to becoming equally sterile. He has led a monastic existence throughout his training period and is still a virgin at twenty-seven,[42] when he is virtually hijacked by Charlotte Rittenmeyer,[42] a wild, impulsive woman whose husband has failed to satisfy her emotionally and sexually. Wilbourne leaves his hospital position and ceases functioning as a doctor from that moment. He is interviewed for a number of other posts but despite his 'degree from a good medical school and his twenty months' internship in a hospital which was known',[43] the interviews go badly.[43] 'Always after the first three or four minutes something began to happen.' Whether quiet or aggressive,[44] Wilbourne manages to convince his interviewers on each occasion that he is unsuitable for medical work. Faulkner does not reveal what is said at these interviews but the reader wonders whether Wilbourne's poverty and his unconventional lifestyle have enhanced his compassion for the more unfortunate members of society. He earns a little money writing stories for pulp magazines but a lot of his time is spent sitting on park benches 'among the bums'.[43] He performs two abortions, the second on Charlotte, who dies as the result of the procedure, and he finishes in the State Penitentiary[45] (*see also* Book IV).

In contrast to these medical eunuchs, Faulkner introduces a third physician, a virile 'real' doctor and an embodiment of competence and aloofness. Dr Richardson's surgical skills are legendary,[46] though he fails to save Charlotte. He asks a few crisp questions, recognizes that Wilbourne holds a medical degree, but remains 'perfectly impersonal' throughout.[47]

> 'How do you account for it? Instruments not clean?' 'They were clean.' 'You think so.' 'I know it.' 'Your first attempt?' 'No. Second.' 'One other come off? But you wouldn't know.' 'Yes, I know. It did.' 'Then how do you account for this failure?'[47]

Wilbourne has no answer to this question but asks Dr Richardson in a half-hearted way whether he can see Charlotte once more. 'Why? She wouldn't know you.'[46] Richardson continues his emotional non-involvement and asks the police officer to take Wilbourne away.[46] The deputy sheriff, despite his 'sadist's eyes' and 'air . . . of . . . formally pre-absolved brutality',[48] is more compassionate than Dr Richardson, and allows Wilbourne to stay in the hospital until Charlotte dies.

The fourth doctor in *The Wild Palms*, the 'mild man' on the Mississippi steamboat,[49] is shown as a true physician. He is shrewd and yet compassionate, tough but willing (and able) to help his convict-patient. He provides medical treatment, he offers financial assistance (which is declined[49]) and after a moment of doubt ('I don't know how far out of bounds I am on this occasion') he persuades the captain to put the convict and his party ashore. This doctor is no naive 'do-gooder'. He evaluates every one of the convict's statements ('it's like he's watching the way my hair grows on my head'[49]) but for a brief moment the two achieve an ideal doctor–patient relationship.

Simenon[50] contrasts the behavior patterns of two doctors, caring for the same patient. René Maugras, a prominent newspaper editor, who has sustained a massive stroke with profound aphasia and right hemiparesis is being treated by Professor Pierre Besson d'Argoulet, a personal friend,[51] and Professor Audoire, a neurologist, who remains totally detached. Neither of the physicians achieves a satisfactory relationship with René. Besson, who sees the patient soon after the onset of the devastating symptoms, uses all the tricks at his disposal to reassure his paralyzed and speechless patient-friend:

> 'There is nothing seriously wrong with you, René. That's confirmed by all the tests . . . It'll probably be a few days before you can speak . . . You trust me don't you? . . . I promise you that in your case it's merely a temporary aphasia. . . . You don't believe me. You think I'm trying to reassure you with claptrap.'[51]

Besson's bedside voice (*see* p. 73), the clichés he considers appropriate to the occasion and his hearty, professional optimism all fail to impress Maugras.

> Why these circumlocutions, this painstaking speech? He was being treated like a child or rather like a very sick man, which indeed he was . . . The doctor . . . presumably . . . spoke in that convincing voice to all of his patients who were seriously ill. . . . It . . . struck him as odd that this distinguished person, a Commander of the Legion of Honor . . . was now sitting at his bedside and wasting time in futile explanations.[51]

On another occasion Besson's attempts to restore his friend's confidence not only fail to convince but actually cause him to become angry. The doctor, 'elegant and self-possessed', has been talking to Maugras' wife,[52] who worries because her husband refuses to see her.

> 'I reassured her . . . I explained that for the first week you'd have your ups and downs.'

Maugras resents these prognostications.

> They were at it again! They knew, day by day, what his mental state as well as his physical state must be. Why didn't they write it down beforehand on the chart at the foot of the bed at which Besson merely cast a casual glance . . . 'Let's get down to business old fellow' . . . Besson uttered this remark with the bogus joviality of some boulevard comedian and Maugras looked at him . . . discovering that the great man, with all his medals, was after all merely a grotesque figure.[52]

Besson tries desperately to strike the right note so as to improve his friend's negative attitude:

> 'With some patients we have to cheat, because they are incapable of understanding. That's not the case with you.'[53]

He goes on to present details of the natural history of the illness. He provides the results of René's blood sugar and serum cholesterol estimations.[53] Rapport is not established because Maugras is unimpressed by what he considers a theatrical performance, even though the doctor seems sincerely concerned. 'Actors too feel genuine emotion as they say their parts.'[54] There is an additional factor: the two former friends, Besson the physician and Maugras the patient, no longer cherish the same values. Maugras, threatened by death or permanent disability, has ceased to care for worldly success. 'He had crossed an invisible barrier and now found himself in a different universe' whereas Dr Besson lives in the familiar world and speaks its language of exaggeration and deceit.[54]

Maugras' second physician, Professor Audoire,[55] remains aloof throughout Maugras' illness. While Besson's garrulous messages fail to reach their target, Audoire, the neurologist, makes no attempt to send any messages whatever.

> He seemed to be avoiding Maugras' eyes and the latter suddenly wondered if this was out of gaucherie or shyness. . . . Dealing with sickness he was on his own ground. Dealing with a sick man he felt less at his ease and avoided contact.[55]

After the neurological examination, Audoire asks the patient to say a few words.

> Maugras was seized with panic . . . Hesitantly he opened his mouth. 'Aaaa . . . ' He could not recognize his own voice. 'Don't be afraid . . . Say something, whatever you like . . . ' The first word that occurred to him was Monsieur. 'Mon . . . ' Audoire nodded encouragingly to him. The word came out almost normally. 'Monsieur . . . ' 'You see! . . . You'll have to practice even if it's discouraging to begin with . . . ' For no apparent reason . . . Maugras had [suddenly] become hostile. How could he explain to them that they were disturbing him, that he had resigned himself, that he did not want their encouragements, that what had happened to him was bound to happen, that he accepted it . . . And since that was the case what was the good of making him ridiculous in his own eyes by forcing him to bleat: 'Mon-sieur.' All they had succeeded in doing . . . was making him want to cry.[55]

The next day, when Maugras shows signs of aspiration pneumonia, and a tracheal suction procedure is performed, Dr Audoire not only frightens his patient, but also makes him feel totally dehumanized. Maugras is given no preparatory explanations and no anesthetic.[56]

> He was at their mercy. He had no defense against them . . . They understood one another without saying a word . . . There was a conspiratorial world about him to which they all belonged. . . . They were holding him still like a dog at the vet . . . 'Open your mouth' . . . He wanted to signal to them that he was choking, that he couldn't bear it any longer

but the procedure continues for fifteen minutes

> the most unpleasant he had ever experienced . . . He had felt like an
> animal and he realized that he had behaved like one . . . If he could have
> bitten them he would have done so.[56]

Initially resentful of both doctors, Maugras comes to recognize, during the recovery
phase, that the 'division of responsibility' between an involved and an aloof doctor is
logical and achieves a balanced effect.[57] The reader of *The Patient* is less convinced
and wonders whether a close friend like Besson can ever provide efficient medical
care for a serious illness, and whether a little less aloofness on the part of the
neurology professor might have spared Maugras at least some of his anguish.

Susan Cheever, in *Doctors and Women*,[58] describes another pair of doctors, one
aloof and efficient, the other emotionally involved with his patients and disorga-
nized. The careers and work habits of the two men, who both work at the
'Parkinson Hospital and Cancer Center', differ sharply. Dr Peter Mallory, the
Chief of Surgery, who doles out sympathy in measured amounts, retains sufficient
spare time to perform research and conduct his administrative duties. Dr Macklin
Riley, the oncologist, who is full of self-doubts, suffers with his patients and blames
his own deficiencies every time one of them deteriorates. He spends so much time on
the wards that he becomes incapable of performing any meaningful research, and
comes very close to dismissal.

Mallory's strategy of giving the patients the impression that he has 'all day to
chat', while spending no more than three minutes at each bedside,[59] succeeds almost
all the time.

> Mallory walked in and sat down on the empty chair next to the bed. He
> tried to give the impression that he was at leisure to talk about anything
> and everything. 'Well Mrs Rosen, how are you doing today?' he said.
> 'I'm scared.' (Mrs Rosen is due for surgery the next day) . . . 'Wait I have
> a list of questions for you.' 'Terrific.' Inwardly Mallory cursed. These
> written lists of questions took too much time. First the patient had to find
> the list – Mrs Rosen was right now groping helplessly in the drawer of
> her night table. Then they had to decipher each question, squinting to
> read their own illegible handwriting. It went faster if Mallory took the
> list from them and read it himself but often they wouldn't relinquish it.
> Sometimes the questions had already been answered by the resident – or
> they were so . . . irrelevant that Mallory could see they were just a way of
> talking out fear, of maintaining closer contact with him.[59]

Mrs Rosen who has evidently lost her little list is allowed only one question: 'Was it
all right for her to drink?' Obviously, to a woman who is in hospital for the removal
of an abdominal tumor this sort of question can only be an opening gambit.
Dr Mallory, who wants to be on his way to the next patient and his research
laboratory, decides that the question requires a 'straight' answer. He tells Mrs
Rosen: 'There's no reason why you shouldn't have a glass of wine', and stands up as
an indication that the interview is over.[59]

Mallory uses the same tactics on his clinic patients who come from all over the
USA. In order to save time, he does not ask names and other personal details but

simply looks at the next chart and begins by asking cheerfully: 'How are you doing, Mr Doe?' Occasionally, when the nurses have provided the wrong chart, the schedule is disrupted and an uncomfortable silence ensues while the correct chart is obtained.[60] Most of the time, Mallory is in control.

> 'Now, what else can we do for you?' he always said at the end of the exam as if he had time to attend to the patient's every need . . . His manner was sympathetic and positive. He talked only about what could be done not about what couldn't. . . . Mallory didn't talk about survival. Instead . . . he said . . . 'In my opinion this would be a case for [regional] perfusion. . . . We may have to think about losing the leg but we may not . . . I'm not changing the percentages but I think there are things we can do here.'

The daughter of a patient with a pancreatic carcinoma asks:

> Should we encourage him to eat? He's so thin.' . . . 'Encourage him to eat, but don't be upset if he can't.' Patients often asked Mallory about diet and bowel movements when they meant to ask questions about life and death. His answers were always about diet and bowel movements.[60]

Dr Macklin Riley, the oncologist, who lacks Mallory's cheerful optimism and decisiveness, is not adept either at emotional detachment or at rationing his time. He does not try to distract his patients with trivialities when they want to talk to him about life and death, but such conversations drain him emotionally and burn up his time. When a ten-year-old boy who knows he is dying of leukemia presents Riley with his most precious possession – a baseball cap – as a parting gesture, the doctor is moved to tears.[61] He manages to control himself but it is the dying child that has to remind him of his 'real' duties: 'Listen . . . it's nice of you to come down and see me but don't you have other things to do around here?'[61] During the lengthy consultation with Dorothy Clay, who is dying from breast cancer with hepatic metastases, Dr Riley hides behind his surgical colleagues: '*They've* decided not to do another operation',[62] while Dorothy, who does not hide her chemotherapy-induced baldness under a turban, is much more direct. 'Are you sending me home to die?' she asks bluntly.[62] Dr Mallory would either not have given Dorothy the opportunity to ask this sort of question or would have answered 'Of course not'. Dr Riley, on the other hand, fiddles with his pen and gives half-answers. 'It's true that the operations haven't been as successful as we had hoped . . . we're still not sure about the effects of the various drugs . . . and compared with some of my other patients you are actually doing very well.' Mrs Clay does not let up. She asks whether she ought to take out an expensive insurance policy in case she dies before the New Year. Riley, after first trying to withhold this information, finally capitulates and tells Mrs Clay to reinsure her property. She accepts her death sentence calmly and continues to consult him during the brief remainder of her life.[62] At this internationally renowned academic institution, Riley's inability to 'detach' is seen as a liability. He comes close to getting dismissed and, naturally, it is Mallory who will make the final decision whether or not Riley will have to go.[63] (He is allowed to stay.)

A recent addition to the theme of 'too much or too little detachment' is to be found in Goldsworthy's *Three Dog Night*.[64] Felix, the patient, is a marginalized and angry surgeon, who acquires hepatitis C through a needle-stick incident. He has now developed a hepatoma with pleural metastases, and his prognosis is measured in months. Felix' connections with his former classmates are not based on official doctor–patient relationships, but offers of help come from two colleagues, characteristically belonging to specialties with opposite traditions of detachment. Frank Boyd, a self-satisfied, successful surgeon with a loose tongue, a braying laugh and groping hands, offers to display his political powers by providing some scraps of work like administrative duties or the performance of endoscopies. Felix, uninterested in Frank's charity, replies 'You disgust me'.[65] Martin Blackman, a psychiatrist and former friend of Felix, is more tactful when he asks what he can do to make the remainder of the sick doctor's life less unhappy. Half as a joke, Felix inquires whether he might spend a night with Martin's wife, Lucy.[66] At this point, instead of sending a semi-humorous but clear 'nothing doing' message, Martin and Lucy, also a psychiatrist, remain 'undetached' from their patient. Out of compassion and a mixture of other motives, Lucy leaves her husband for the dying man, follows him literally into the wilderness, with Martin in pursuit. The two psychiatrists nurse Felix through his final few days but their marriage is irretrievably damaged by this episode.

Just right

Several novels, old and recent, describe doctors with exactly the right degree of detachment. Charlotte Bronte's Lucy Snow, the heroine of *Villette*,[67] describes the annoying antics of a delinquent teenage student (Désirée) who has 'declared herself ill'. Lucy, a boarding-school teacher, is full of admiration for the doctor whose 'correct' behavior is followed by the 'patient's' complete recovery.

> That possessed child had a genius for simulation, and captivated by the attentions and indulgences of a sick room, she came to the conclusion that an illness would perfectly accommodate her tastes and took to her bed accordingly.[67]

Despite Lucy's conviction that Désirée is malingering, the girl's mother decides to treat the symptoms seriously. Enter Dr John Graham Bretton,[67] who, to Lucy's surprise, shows no signs of irritation with the dreadful girl, and avoids any sort of behavior that might lead to a confrontation. The doctor

> consented tacitly to adopt madam's tactics and . . . to play his part in the farce . . . I wondered that Doctor John did not tire of the business. [He] wrote harmless prescriptions [and] Désirée [was] suddenly cured of her ailments.[67]

Howells' Dr Rufus Mulbridge[68] also displays the 'right' mixture of concern and detachment. Unlike Charlotte Bronte's teenager, who complains of 'non-organic' symptoms, Dr Mulbridge's patient suffers from a 'real' illness – pulmonary tuberculosis. She deteriorates under the treatment of Dr Grace Breen, who is quite unable to be dispassionate and engages in much self-recrimination. At the patient's request she calls in a male doctor who provides a lesson in good professional behavior.

> He was perfectly kind without being at any moment unprofitably sympathetic. He knew when to listen and when not to listen, to learn everything from the quivering bundle of nerves before him without seeming to have learnt anything alarming.[68]

Dr Stephen Maturin, Captain Jack Aubrey's friend, confidant and physician,[69] provides yet another example of 'correct' professional detachment. Maturin remains quite unperturbed when he discovers that the captain has sought help from 'alternative' practitioners. When the captain mentions that he has been to see a Mr Martin who has 'singular powers, . . . [who has] performed some wonderful cures, . . . [and has] rubbed Aubrey's spine with a certain oil',[69] Maturin refrains from giving his friend a lecture concerning quacks and their secret remedies. He 'had seen too many quite well educated people run after men with singular powers' and simply goes on to provide a dose of orthodox medicine. He bleeds the Captain and gives him an enema.[69]

Richardson's Dr Mahony[70] remains aloof even when a patient's husband confesses his murderous intentions. Mahony, who before his mental and physical deterioration (*see* Book II, Chapter 8) has the makings of a talented obstetrician, is summoned on a stormy night to attend to Matt Doyle's wife who has gone into premature labor. After being literally dragged through a flooded creek, Mahony arrives, soaking wet, at Doyle's cottage where he performs a 'skillful procedure under the worst possible conditions'. The next day, a grateful Matt Doyle confesses to Mahony:

> 'I don't mind telling you now, I'd me shooting-iron here . . . and if you'd refused – you was the third mind you – I'd have drilled you where you stood.'

Mahony bears Doyle no malice.

> 'Much good that would have done your wife, you fathead.'[64]

Summary

As long as suffering people come to physicians asking for help, doctors will have to ask themselves how hard they should try to participate in their patients' physical and emotional distress. Fictional literature does not and cannot answer this question, which is clearly one of degree, but it can provide instances of the pendulum swinging too far in one or the other direction.

References

1   Osler W (1889) *Aequanimitas*. HK Lewis, London, 1920, p. 5.

2   Spiro H (1992) What is empathy and can it be taught? *Ann Int Med.* **116**: 843–6.

3 Kim J (2001) Emotional detachment and involvement of physicians in literature. *The Pharos of Alpha Omega Alpha*, vol. 64, Spring, pp. 32–8.

4 Balzac H de (1831) *The Wild Ass's Skin*. Translated by Marriage E. Dent, London, 1960, pp. 199–201.

5 Balzac H de (1847) *Cousin Pons*. Translated by Hunt HJ. Penguin, Harmondsworth, 1968, p. 117.

6 Poynter FNL (1968) Doctors in the human comedy. *JAMA*. **204**: 105–8.

7 Mitchell SW (1885) *In War Time*. The Century Company, New York, 1913, p. 57.

8 Ibid., pp. 60–1.

9 Hardy T (1886–7) *The Woodlanders*. Oxford University Press, Oxford, 1988, pp. 77–8.

10 Ellison H (1957) Wanted in Surgery. In: Ellison H (1979) *The Fantasies of Harlan Ellison*. Gregg Press, Boston, MA, pp. 120–52.

11 Balzac H de (1840) *Pierrette*. Translated by Ives GB. George Barrie and Sons, Philadelphia, PA, 1897, pp. 215–16.

12 Strindberg A (1887) The Father. In: Strindberg A (1962) *Twelve Plays*. Translated by Sprigge E. Constable, London, p. 20.

13 Ibid., p. 22.

14 Ibid., p. 31.

15 Ibid., p. 48.

16 Ibid., p. 56.

17 Fitzgerald FS (1934) *Tender is the Night*. Penguin, Harmondsworth, 1998.

18 Ibid., pp. 202–4.

19 Ibid., pp. 262–3.

20 Green G (1956) *The Last Angry Man*. Charles Scribner's Sons, New York.

21 Ibid., p. 308.

22 Ibid., p. 384.

23 Ibid., pp. 2–9.

24 Ibid., p. 368.

25 Ibid., p. 423–4.

26 Ibid., p. 349.

27 Ibid., p. 322.

28 Ibid., p. 344.

29 Ibid., p. 152.

30 Ibid., p. 188.

31 Chekhov AP (1887–9) Ivanov. In: *The Oxford Chekhov*, vol. 2. Translated by Hingley R. Oxford University Press, London, 1967, p. 174.

32 Ibid., p. 191.

33 Ibid., pp. 226–7.

34 Ibid., pp. 207–8.

35 Ibid., p. 200.

36 Chekhov AP (1896) The Seagull. In: *The Oxford Chekhov*, vol. 2. Translated by Hingley R. Oxford University Press, London, 1967, p. 250.

37 Ibid., pp. 270–1.

38 Faulkner W (1939) *The Wild Palms*. Random House, New York.

39 Ibid., p. 4.
40 Ibid., pp. 12–14.
41 Ibid., pp. 279–89.
42 Ibid., pp. 40–4.
43 Ibid., pp. 84–5.
44 Ibid., p. 219.
45 Ibid., p. 321.
46 Ibid., pp. 298–301.
47 Ibid., p. 297.
48 Ibid., p. 293.
49 Ibid., pp. 241–9.
50 Simenon G (1963) *The Patient*. Translated by Stewart J. Hamish Hamilton, London, 1963.
51 Ibid., pp. 1–13.
52 Ibid., pp. 54–5.
53 Ibid., pp. 56–9.
54 Ibid., p. 66.
55 Ibid., pp. 34–6.
56 Ibid., pp. 90–3.
57 Ibid., p. 178.
58 Cheever S (1987) *Doctors and Women*. Methuen, London, 1988.
59 Ibid., pp. 43–5.
60 Ibid., pp. 182–7.
61 Ibid., p. 190.
62 Ibid., pp. 210–13.
63 Ibid., p. 229.
64 Goldsworthy P (2003) *Three Dog Night*. Penguin, Australia.
65 Ibid., pp. 82–4.
66 Ibid., p. 135.
67 Bronte C (1853) *Villette*. Penguin, Harmondsworth, 1983, pp. 161–5.
68 Howells WD (1881) *Dr Breen's Practice*. James Osgood, Boston, MA, p. 107.
69 O'Brian P (1992) *The Truelove*. WW Norton, New York, pp. 15–35.
70 Richardson HH (1917–29) *The Fortunes of Richard Mahony*. Penguin, London, 1990, p. 205.

CHAPTER 8

'It's all a cruel hoax'

Doctors are . . . pigs, everybody knows that[1]

Resentment against individual doctors on account of their greed (Chapter 1), their poor communication skills (Chapters 3 and 5) or their lack of therapeutic success (Chapter 6) may culminate in the patients' conclusion that the entire practice of medicine is a cruel trick. Unlike relatively harmless swindlers like dishonest salesmen or lawyers, physicians, so this concept runs, not only defraud their unsuspecting clients but actually cause them physical harm. In literature, this notion may surface in one-line remarks or in lengthy diatribes. It may even comprise the theme of entire novels.

Irrational hatred of the entire system

Ancient and modern authors like Pliny,[2] Montaigne[3] and Thomas Bernhard[4] express frustration with or contempt for all members of the medical profession and their useless endeavors. The degree of resentment varies from gentle irony to blazing hatred, depending, presumably, on the writer's own contacts with doctors and the outcome of particular illnesses. Lucian of Samosata[5] does not provide the clinical background of the woman who detests all physicians:

> Towards everyone else she is very civil and gentle . . . but if she sees any physician . . . she is . . . exasperated against him.

However, his sarcastic comment that this irrational dislike of the medical profession 'constitutes proof that her condition is bad and incurable'[6] suggests that he considers the lady's 'exasperation' not at all unreasonable.

According to this assessment of the medical cosmos, all clinical activities are futile and all practicing doctors are either fools or scoundrels. The physical examination, a meaningless ritualistic hocus-pocus, contributes no information, but continues to be performed for traditional and theatrical indications. Summoned to see a dying patient Céline's Dr Bardamu

> listened to his heartbeat just to be doing something, [to produce] the few gestures people expect under those circumstances.[7]

Medical consultations, particularly consultations involving multiple doctors simultaneously, are dramatic shows, put on for the gratification of the patients or their families but most unlikely to produce any medical benefits.

> As they took leave of one another on the threshold of the main entrance, they were letting science and truth out of the bag and chatting together as doctors do, once the farce of a consultation is over.[8]

Treatment is an elaborate torture, designed to make the patient miserable. Dryden's 'nauseous draft'[9] enriches the doctor, does nothing for the patients other than make them want to vomit, and is considerably less effective than a healthy lifestyle, which is available to everyone free of charge.

Chekhov's Count Shebalsky,[10] an elderly stage buffoon, sums up this point of view with the standard denunciation of the medical profession, whose members are uniformly deceitful and incompetent:

> Doctors are like lawyers, only lawyers just rob you while doctors rob you and murder you as well. . . . I've paid out twenty thousand odd in doctors' bills in my time and never met a doctor yet who didn't strike me as a licensed swindler.[10]

Curiously, the dying patient's sense of frustration against an individual doctor or against the medical profession in general,

> the furious hatred that must seize a man condemned when he compare(s) himself with the doctor, sane and healthy, who ha[s] the inestimable privilege of life,[11]

does not seem to extend to non-elite health professionals. The doctor is the most prominent and the most privileged of the healers and the easiest target for rational and irrational resentment. Buzacott's delinquent Lisa Pembroke,[12] ex-stripper and angry terminal cancer patient who has been receiving chemotherapy against her wishes, writes this in her diary a few days before her death:

> The nurses, they're great. It's the doctors I hate. They should shoot every one of the doctors and give their pay to the nurses. Give the money to the people who work for it, not the people whose parents paid their way through medical school.[12]

Bad experiences

A general dislike of physicians may have its origin in a particular illness, which fails to respond to the doctor's therapeutic endeavors. Samuel Richardson's Belton, on his deathbed, curses physicians for their diagnostic and therapeutic incompetence and blames their medications for his decline.[13] He exempts surgeons from his denunciations but few other angry patients make such fine distinctions.

Sick and depressed patients, whose careers (and lives) are coming to an end, cannot help comparing themselves with their 'plump and healthy'[14] doctors, some of them at the height of their professional careers. When the 'afflicted mortal'[15] suffering from a fatal or incurable disease asks himself 'Why me? . . . Why not that stinker Smith? Why not that louse Jones?'[15] his next question might well be 'Why not this foolish and arrogant doctor?' Instead of remaining focused on an individual physician, the patient's and the family's anger may be extended towards the entire medical profession.

Eugene O'Neill's homosexual Charles Marsden initially keeps his dislike of doctors to himself[16] (*see* p. 104) but after his mother's death, he becomes openly hostile towards all the 'useless' members of the medical profession, who, by definition, are unable to cure incurable disorders.

> You were right, Doctor Darrell. It was cancer . . . But the doctor you sent me to and the others he called in could do nothing for her – absolutely nothing. I might just as well have imported some witch doctors from the Solomon Islands! They at least would have diverted her in her last hours with their singing and dancing, but your specialists were a total loss! . . . I think you doctors are a pack of Goddamned ignorant liars and hypocrites![17]

The hatred of the medical profession expressed by Heller's Bob Slocum[18] clearly stems from the inability of a variety of doctors to diagnose and treat his mentally handicapped child. The Slocums have remained together, despite his infidelities and despite her drinking habits, for the sake of their children, particularly their youngest son, Derek, a severely retarded boy.[18] Multiple physicians offer conflicting opinions, leaving the parents confused at first, and then, when they finally get the picture, seething with rage.

> By now my wife and I have had our fill – are sick and glutted to the teeth – of psychologists, psychiatrists, neurologists, neurosurgeons . . . with their inability to help and their lofty patronizing platitudes that we are not to blame, ought not to let ourselves feel guilty and have nothing to be ashamed of. An outsider wouldn't believe the number of conflicting opinions the different doctors gave us . . . 'The prognosis is good'. . . . 'The prognosis is bad.' 'It wouldn't be possible to offer a prognosis at this time.' . . . 'You are making too much of it.' . . . 'He will never speak.' . . . We hate them all, the ones who were wrong and the ones who were right.[18]

'Josephine', the central character in Jenefer Shute's *Life Size*,[19] also suffers from a disease not readily amenable to treatment – anorexia nervosa. Naturally, this woman who detests herself, her parents and her sexual partners, can't stand her doctors.

Dislike of specific medical traits

Some of the general dislike for physicians stems from an aversion to what are essentially parts of medical behavior. These traits, exaggerated and distorted, become a source of anger towards the physician as a person and, by extension, towards all members of the profession. The necessity to inflict occasional discomfort is attributed to sadism; decisiveness is equated with arrogance, while the limitations of medical knowledge turn all doctors into ignorant poltroons.

Cruelty

Daudet's *Les Morticoles*,[20] a polemical anti-Utopian story, consists of a bitter attack on medical practice and almost all members of the medical profession. The doctors who control the island of the 'Morticoles' (= the deadly charlatans) for their own benefit are interested only in their own intellectual gratification while the patients are tyrannized, tortured and experimented upon. Unlike Molière's ignorant but essentially good-natured buffoons, the physicians in *Les Morticoles* are knowledgeable but vicious and sadistic.* Felix Canelon, a shipwrecked sailor on the island, is told contemptuously by one of the interns:

> Did you really believe, you idiot (espèce de sauvage) that we practice medicine to cure the patients? You are quite wrong (Erreur grave!). All we want is to find things out (Constater).[22]

Most of Daudet's exaggerations are quite outrageous but his resentment at the doctors' lack of respect for the body of a recently deceased young woman seems based on a real episode. 'Suzanne', who occupies bed number 20 in the female ward, dies after a brief illness despite attempts at resuscitation.

> At that moment there occurred a most unseemly racket. [Two doctors] followed by their students, burst into the room talking at the top of their voices. . . . [One of them] called out triumphantly 'I was right. . . . Acute tuberculosis . . . [Let's see] if there was any edema, that'll settle the point.' The two lost no time in removing the covers. There was no edema. . . . They departed leaving the body uncovered.[22]

Martin du Gard, unlike Leon Daudet, is not a 'doctor-basher'. On the contrary, his Dr Antoine Thibault is one of the great medical heroes in twentieth-century literature.[23,24] Yet, when Martin du Gard speaks of

> the callousness common to doctors for whom the sufferings of others count only as so much experience or profit or professional advantage; men to whose fortunes death and pain are frequent ministers,[25]

he is merely restating Pliny's complaint made almost two thousand years earlier: 'They learn their skill by endangering our lives'.[2] Translated into common parlance this means: 'We (the patients) are suffering while they (the doctors) are furthering their careers'. Kenneth Fearing's Helen Russell, a gentle, non-aggressive woman,

---

* It has been suggested[21] that much of the hostility against the medical profession expressed in *Les Morticoles* stems from the author's unsuccessful attempts to study medicine.

harbors no hostility towards doctors or anyone else. However, even she wonders, as she waits outside the chest clinic in a charity hospital, how the doctor, as he arrives,

> can walk . . . between the benches crowded with patients, . . . how can he act so casually, as though this were just an ordinary visit and another day.[26]

Sylvia Plath,[27] who had good reasons to be dissatisfied with her physicians, implies that some of them received their training at Auschwitz.

> So, so Herr Doktor.
> So, Herr Enemy.
> I am your opus,
> I am your valuable
> The pure gold baby
>
> That melts to a shriek.
> I turn and burn.
> Do not think I underestimate
> Your great concern.[27]

Arrogance

In a brief anti-medical outburst in *The Brothers Karamazov*,[28] Dostoyevsky castigates doctors collectively for another perceived failing – their conceit (*see also* p. 25). Unlike Chekhov, who was himself trained as a physician, and who put his 'licensed swindler'[10] remark into the mouth of a stage clown (*see* p. 190), Dostoyevsky expresses his opposition to doctors through Nikolai ('Kolya') Krasotkin, a precocious thirteen-year-old grammar school student who comes across as the sort of boy the author would have chosen for his own son. Kolya is a prankster who knows 'when to stop', a courageous fighter, a talented dog-trainer, a capable baby-sitter, a voracious reader and a budding philosopher with evident leadership qualities. This likeable youngster declares that all doctors are rogues, 'a dirty lot, generally speaking and, of course, individually',[28] with Dostoyevsky providing an illustration to substantiate this opinion a few pages further on. At the house of a classmate who has terminal tuberculosis, Kolya overhears a famous Moscow specialist informing the boy's father, as a parting gesture, that the climate in Sicily might be beneficial. The patient's parents are desperately poor so that this piece of advice serves no purpose other than to make them feel helpless and guilty. Kolya promptly and openly expresses his contempt for this pompous physician 'who looked . . . as though . . . he were . . . afraid of dirtying himself'.[29] 'Don't worry doc,' he called out, 'my dog won't bite you'. . . . 'Good bye, doc, we shall meet in Syracuse.' When the Moscow doctor flies into a rage at this impertinent behavior, Kolya threatens to set his dog on him, and while the boy is dissuaded from carrying out his threat,[29] Dostoyevsky implies that this arrogant and useless physician (and most of his colleagues) thoroughly deserve a dog bite on the leg if not more proximally.*

---

* In *The Brothers Karamazov* there is also an account of a 'dear old' doctor,[30] but from a medical point of view he is as useless as the arrogant Moscow specialist.[31]

Anne Sexton,[32,33] whose illness was a little less severe than that of Sylvia Plath, applies more restraint, and her doctors are not portrayed as concentration camp supervisors. However, she fulminates against the power doctors wield (or think they wield) and the arrogance generated by this power.

No reason to be afraid, my almost mighty doctor reasons.[32]

Sexton sees the doctors' overconfidence as a deadly menace.

> The doctors should fear arrogance
> More than cardiac arrests.
> If they are too proud
> And some are
> Then they leave home on horseback
> But God returns them on foot.[33]

Sexton's dislike for medical pride is evidently more compelling than her concern for the patient, who is also likely to come to grief when the doctor falls off his horse.

Simone de Beauvoir's resentment against all the members of the medical team taking care of her mother[34] is based on very similar considerations. The doctors are healthy, well groomed and knowledgeable, whereas her mother is sick, disheveled and lacks formal education. They make the decisions while the old lady has to take what is dished out to her.

> 'Dr J, Professor B, Dr T: Neat, trim, shining, well-groomed, bending over this ill-kempt, rather wild looking old woman from an immense height: Great men; bigwigs. I recognized that piddling self-importance: It was that of the judges on the bench when they have a man whose life is at stake before them.'[34]

Simone, who is not particularly fond of her mother, is nevertheless outraged by the physicians' patronizing attitude towards her mother's work, which is considered a kind of purposeless play, while their work, by implication, is focused and serious.

> What right had B to say to me 'She will be able to potter around again?' I objected to his scale of values.[34]

Ignorance

Ignorant doctors come in two categories. On the one hand are simple characters, like Chekhov's Dr Ivan Chebutykin,[35] who has forgotten all he learnt in medical school and has not opened a textbook since he graduated. This kind of ignorance constitutes a menace but is easy to recognize. Thomas Hardy[36] hints, in one devastating sentence, that a second type of medical ignorance may be found in doctors who are very much up to date with diagnosis and treatment, and who may even possess the much-vaunted 'Sherlock Holmesian' powers of observation

> That quick glittering empirical eye, sharp for the surface of things if for nothing underneath.[36]

This second kind of ignoramus may practice 'correct' medicine but fails because of a lack of depth and insight.

Venice Harpenden in Arlen's *The Green Hat*[37] shares Thomas Hardy's view that doctors, despite their questioning and probing, lack the capacity to penetrate the core of their patients' problems. Venice is an early exponent of the dangerous notion, widely held among contemporary feminists, that there is nothing a doctor, especially a male doctor, can tell a woman about her body that she does not know herself. Convinced that she is sterile, Venice nonetheless stubbornly refuses to see a doctor. 'I can't have a baby . . . I just feel that I can't, in my bones I feel it.' The suggestion that she ought to seek medical advice is not well received (*see also* p. 105). How can a doctor, after 'poking about', tell her anything she does not already know?[37] There is no visit to a fertility specialist. Venice dies in an automobile crash at an early age and without issue.

Virginia Woolf's Clarissa Dalloway[38] resents Sir William Bradshaw, the prominent London psychiatrist and, by implication, psychiatrists in general, for the same reason; they poke around inside their patients' minds, but fail to provide relief. Bradshaw is thoroughly professional. He 'never hurried his patients . . . he gave (them) three-quarters of an hour' and he even asks at the end 'if Mrs Warren Smith was quite sure she had no more questions'. Mrs Dalloway, no doubt speaking for Virginia Woolf, finds this professionalism offensive while the psychiatric interview itself is an act of indecency[39] (*see* p. 109).

To James Tate,[40] the disease, the doctor and the treatment are all part of the same purposeless process, though the doctor, simple clown that he is, does not quite comprehend this line of reasoning.

> Dr Bitterroot right away
> diagnosed a rotten cancerous bitterroot
> and reached for his bitterroot which he stabbed
> into her bitterroot up the bitterroot canal.[40]

Raymond Chandler, who seems to dislike most doctors, is particularly sarcastic about 'omniscient' characters. Here is his assessment of this medical stereotype as expressed by Philip Marlowe.[41]

> Dr Zugsmith will see you now, Mrs Whoosis. [The receptionist] would hold the door open with a little smile and Mrs Whoosis would go past her and Dr Zugsmith would be sitting behind his desk as professional as hell with his white coat and his stethoscope hanging around his neck. A case file would be in front of him and his note pad and prescription pad would be neatly squared off. There was nothing that Dr Zugsmith didn't know. You couldn't fool him. He had it all at his fingertips. When he looked at a patient he had the answers to all the questions he was going to ask just as a matter of form.[41]

In *The Long Good-Bye*[42] Chandler refers to a medical practitioner as

Some jerk in a white coat with a stethoscope hanging around his neck, and while this particular remark relates to a doctor in a television commercial, Chandler's medical characters generally fit this description.[43]

Tillie Olsen[44] describes yet another clever/ignorant doctor who is summed up in the remark 'Doctors are bills and foolishness'. The patient in this instance is Eva, who migrated to the USA early in the twentieth century and who has gradually become isolated because of her deafness, her visual impairment, her grinding poverty and her stunted intellectual development. Eva resents her cheerful, gregarious husband, who first tries to persuade her to enter a retirement village, and subsequently hauls her around the country to visit friends and relatives, when all she wants is to stay home and use her remaining energy in keeping the place tidy. Various doctors advise Eva 'correctly' from the medical point of view but inappropriately in her particular case.

> 'What did the doctor say?' 'A real fatherly lecture. Sixty-nine is young these days. Go out, enjoy life, find interests. Get a new hearing aid; this one is antiquated. Old age is sickness only if one makes it so.'[44]

Eva's physical disintegration and the indignities associated with her final illness make her reject her husband's suggestions, while the doctor's glib advice to 'find interests' is as useless to her as his dietary recommendations.[44]

Thomas Bernhard detests everything about doctors, who are either totally ineffective or possessed by delusions of grandeur or both.[4] In any case 'they can only harm the patient'. Bernhard, who tends to exaggerate, repeats over and over that doctors are ignorant and impotent but, at the same time, arrogant and self-serving. They are unable to communicate with the patients, who are rebuffed because of the medical profession's 'overweening self-importance [and] its . . . perverted need to impress'.[45] Bernhard suspects that both his grandfather and his mother died because of their doctors' ignorance but provides insufficient details in support of his accusations.[46]

Three anti-medical novels

In addition to *Les Morticoles*,[20] a polemical nineteenth-century satire against the medical 'establishment' of the time, three major twentieth-century works,[47–49] from three countries, have as their principal theme the unsatisfactory and harmful nature of medical activities in the face of disorders that do not respond to treatment. These works are discussed in some detail.

'Doctor' John Tremont in William Wharton's *Dad*,[47] who entertains medical ambitions during his teens[50] but goes on to acquire a PhD in psychology instead, is resentful of medical doctors for a variety of reasons. Dr Santana, his father's urologist, is 'reading X-rays' while Tremont tries to tell him about Dad's cancerophobia. The old man has transitional cell carcinoma of the bladder and despite John's pleading, Santana insists on telling 'Dad' the truth[51] (*see also* pp 133–4).

The relationship between John Tremont and his father's internist (Dr Ethridge) is strained almost from the moment of their first contact.[52] Dr Ethridge does not like taking telephone calls from patients' family members who complain about his urological colleague.

'Mr Tremont, these are decisions we doctors make. If your father uses our hospital facilities you must trust our judgment in these matters.' Then he goes into a harangue on the theme 'we know best'. I listen till he winds down.[52]

A second telephone encounter is equally unrewarding.[53]

After the usual runaround, I'm put through. I tell Ethridge Dad's home with me on Dr Santana's suggestion. I get a very cold response; he's still on his high horse playing 'boss man'. 'Dr Ethridge, I don't know why it is but my father keeps crying. He's been crying the whole day; he won't eat and is not responding.' There is a slight delay. 'Does he seem depressed?' I guess that's a logical question but it sounds stupid. No, Doctor, he's not depressed he's only crying. 'I would say he is, Doctor. He seems terribly depressed.' 'Well, it sounds as if we should try some Elavil*; that will bring him around. These kinds of severe depressions are not unusual with older people after surgery.'[53]

Tremont finds the last remark, with its double negative, particularly annoying. Dr Ethridge implies that 'Dad's' behavior is not unique, that other patients have experienced this sequence of events and that antidepressant drugs may resolve the setback. The suggestion that his father is one of a series of cases infuriates Tremont. 'He's talking as if we're discussing a puppy with a case of worms.' There is worse to come. The drug causes adverse reactions, including hypertension and tachycardia.

I call the hospital and fight my way through to Ethridge. I tell him what's happening and what I've done so far. 'Mr Tremont, who took your father's blood pressure?' 'I did, Dr Ethridge.' 'What do think you are, a doctor, Mr Tremont?'[53]

Tremont is incensed by his inability to reach Doctor Ethridge at a moment's notice, he is outraged by the doctors' apparent detachment and he deeply resents their real or perceived authority.† Most importantly, he believes that his father's anguish elicits only mild professional interest from the hospital's medical staff. Dr Ethridge's rudeness and incompetence obviously exacerbate the situation but the anti-physician sentiments of this PhD antedate 'Dad's' deterioration.

Ellis' semi-autobiographical *The Rack*[48] is a formidable indictment of the entire medical profession whose members are unable to cure Paul Davenport's pulmonary tuberculosis, to give him meaningful information or even to let him die in peace. With one exception (*see* pp 40–1) the doctors in *The Rack* are authoritarian, incompetent or dishonest. Dr Vernet, who initially laughs at rather than answers Paul's questions, gradually becomes frustrated by Paul's failure to improve or deteriorate. After Paul is discovered in bed with a female patient, Vernet adopts the silent ostracism treatment as a kind of punishment. He now conveys the

---

* *See* footnote p. 124.
† Tremont exempts two non-authoritarian 'hippy'-type doctors from his censures. One is dressed in 'tight pants',[54] the other wears a full black beard.[55]

impression that he has lost interest in Paul's case and that no kind of intervention will make the slightest difference to the outcome.[56]

> Dr Vernet sat down at his desk and, to show that the interview was at an end, he started to sort some papers. Paul put on his jacket. 'It's over six months since I've had an X-ray plate,' he said. Dr Vernet did not look up. 'And you haven't examined me since I left Les Alpes.' 'No?' 'Nor have I had a blood or sputum test.' 'Tiens!' 'And you have expressed no opinion as to my condition.' 'I told you last autumn you could return to England.' 'Yes – and nothing since.' Dr Vernet gave no indication of having heard the remark. Paul hesitated a moment, then said: 'I think that after all you would prefer me to go to another doctor.' Dr Vernet put down the papers, which he had been sorting. 'Monsieur Davenant' he said, his whole voice dangerously controlled, 'you can do what you like and you can go where you like. If you want another doctor, tell me and I will hand over your dossier. Until then, have the courtesy not to examine me respecting my methods.'[56]

The other physicians in *The Rack* are no better. The pessimistic and somewhat venal Dr Bruneau, whose career has been destroyed by tuberculosis, feels obliged to give his patients a poor prognosis.[57] David Bean, the medical student who has lost two brothers from tuberculosis, also oozes pessimism.[58] Dr Florent, who cannot find a job when the sanatorium closes,[59] is too junior, too ignorant and too ineffectual to give much comfort to Paul despite his pathetic attempts at being friendly.[60] Dr Bertin,[61] 'a notoriously dubious character . . . a drunkard and a drug addict', does not actually appear, leaving the reader to wonder why Dr Vernet would recommend this particular colleague to Paul. Is it meant as a hint that Paul's case is hopeless and that he might as well put himself in the hands of an impostor?

Dr Roussel, apparently 'brisk, sympathetic . . . courteous and optimistic' promises [Paul] that he will be cured by the beginning of the summer and fit to get married.[62] Roussel's Pollyanna attitude evaporates when his 'creosote' treatment produces a number of complications. When he discovers that Paul can no longer pay for his stay in hospital, he declares 'the treatment has served its purpose; it is time for it to be stopped'.[62] Even the kind and generous Dr Dubois displays an initial 'coldness',[61] due to a letter from one of Paul's previous medical attendants. The contents of this letter are not disclosed but it presumably describes Paul as a 'difficult' patient. Professor Klauss, the famous Swiss specialist, 'an enormous man, bald, bearded and frock-coated', constitutes Paul Davenant's last court of appeal.[63] Klauss, courteous and analytical with only one lapse into sarcasm (*see* p. 83) and one glance at his watch (*see also* p. 60), summarizes the various treatment options. The realistic choices, neither of them satisfactory, lie between doing nothing and, after two and a half years of complications resulting from the first pneumothorax, inducing a second pneumothorax.[63]

The book ends with Paul recapitulating his entire treatment as a prolonged torture with himself stretched on 'the rack'.[63] Everything has failed in his case except for the doctors' 'success' in preventing him from taking an overdose of barbiturates. Unfortunately Paul suffers from a disease which is largely uninfluenced by any treatment modality available at the time. Generous or rapacious, kindly or sarcastic, none of his physicians are able to help, and the final outcome would presumably have been much the same if the unspeakable Dr Bertin[61] had been in charge.

Malègue, in *Augustin, ou, Le maître est là*,[49] is more subtle in his condemnation of medical behavior in the face of mortal illnesses, but the message is the same. The doctor is as useless and as annoying as the blowfly which drones round the sickbed and which Augustin, the principal character, is longing to kill.[64] ('L'envie de la tuer démangeait Augustin.') Malègue's book, which is not available in English, is cited extensively because it describes multiple encounters between patients and doctors, all of them, to a greater or lesser extent, unsatisfactory.

The young physician, who diagnoses tuberculous meningitis in a one-year-old boy,[65] behaves 'correctly' at all times, but Augustin Méridier, the child's uncle and only male relative, finds him irritating almost from the moment he first sets foot inside the house.

> The doctor asked bits of questions sandwiched between long periods of silence in order to disguise his uncertainty and his fear of the unknown.[64] (Le docteur . . . enchâssait des bouts de question dans ces morceaux de silence où se dissimulent les incertitudes et le pressentiment de l'inconnu.)

Augustin, a university professor, knows nothing about medicine but senses that the doctor is fumbling in the dark and concealing his ignorance behind an assortment of gestures designed to increase his credibility. When the doctor finally inspects the child's mouth and decides that the problem is due to 'teething troubles' his former lack of confidence is replaced by a new-found certainty. He reassures the family with a resounding 'Oui'

> not one of those drawn out soft 'ouis' that hide all sorts of fears in a never ending vowel. This was a definitive 'Yes', a 'Yes' that closed off all escape routes. You don't go on, after such a 'Yes.'[64] (Pas de ces Oui traînés et mous, où toutes les craintes peuvent se terrer dans une voyelle qui n'en finit pas. Un Oui définitif qui barre toutes les routes. On ne passe plus après un tel Oui.)

The doctor's initial opinion that the child's symptoms are due to teething troubles[64] ('il est en pleine crise dentaire') is perfectly reasonable in the light of medical beliefs current at the time, though a less resounding 'Yes' would have been more appropriate. Sadly, two weeks later[66] it becomes obvious that the infant is seriously ill and the doctor is summoned once more. Again his behavior is pretentious and outlandish. When he is told about the baby's projectile vomiting he remarks 'Like a fountain', and draws a parabola in the air.[66] (Son geste dessine la parabole.) There is a bizarre role reversal between the adult physician with his childish antics and the semi-conscious child who seems to possess the secret of meditating quietly.

For a little while, the doctor seems to play with the child and its toys. He lifts its legs, he tries to raise its head off the pillow and gradually the reader and Augustin come to realize that there is some method behind these apparent stupidities. While handling the little boy's teething ring and talking in exasperating baby language[66] (une exasperante imitation du parler enfantin – *see* p. 76) the doctor comes to the conclusion that the child has a fatal illness. He is not at all concerned about the fact that he had not performed a lumbar puncture sooner. 'You don't do lumbar punctures every time a baby vomits.'[66] ('On ne fait pas de ponction pour un seul vomissement.')

When the doctor tells Augustin that the child's prognosis (in 1932) would have been just as hopeless if the diagnosis had been made one or two weeks earlier, he is technically correct. His statement, that if the child indeed has tuberculous meningitis, consultations with even the most senior colleagues would be quite pointless,[66] is also true. ('S'il l'a, il est parfaitement vain d'appeler le Président de l'Académie de Médecine ou qui que se soit au monde.') What the reader finds disturbing is the apparent heartlessness of these remarks; the young doctor seems cheerful and comfortable with the inexorable progression of the child's illness.

The little boy is handled gently, the lumbar puncture is accomplished without difficulty[67] and the dreadful diagnosis is confirmed.[68] A senior consultant arrives from Clermont, one hundred kilometers away, charges an enormous fee (*see also* p. 27) and confirms that no one can do anything for the child other than prevent unnecessary suffering.[68] The local doctor visits each day, he tries to distract the family members with small talk and he does his best to reassure them that the baby is not in any pain.[69] After the child's death, which is described in minute detail,[70] he strongly and wrongly advises the mother not to tell *her* mother (who is on *her* deathbed) about the tragedy.

Despite all this medical 'correctness' Augustin's resentment against the doctor is never far from the surface. He is irritated by this young upstart ('arriviste') and his pride in having made the right diagnosis.[66] The prescription forms, which show the doctor's surgery hours, his telephone number and the fact that he was once an intern in one of the Lyon teaching hospitals, are obviously considered vulgar. The new, illegally parked[66] automobile is mentioned without comment, though it is hinted that this latest symbol of the doctor's 'success' is somehow connected to his ability to use platitudes like 'we are both men'. Augustin, who is still an agnostic at the time, expresses the view that the old priest with his hocus-pocus and his cruel remarks is better at handling death than the doctor.[69]

When Augustin himself starts coughing up blood, his own encounters with the medical profession are equally unsatisfactory. The family doctor is friendly enough with his practiced smile,[71] which Augustin has already experienced during his little nephew's fatal illness. Initially, the doctor is somewhat reluctant to come up with a diagnosis. 'What is it you've got? Oh, a little lung problem. We'll talk about it again in a few days time when you're better. You don't mind waiting that long?'[71] A few days later when Augustin is well enough to ask for the unvarnished truth he is told that he has 'a few little tuberculous spots . . . that's all' ('de petits lésions tuberculeuses . . . voilà tout') and that he will of course get better. 'That's a statistical fact.'[71] The doctor goes on: 'Fifty per cent of all patients get better. When they are cooperative, intelligent, persistent and . . . well off, the rate goes up to eighty per cent. And you needn't complain – you're in the better group. Tuberculosis isn't a democratic illness . . . Democracy doesn't exist in real life.'[71] Angry and frustrated, Augustin wants to protest. 'Not so much against the truth which hadn't fully penetrated' his consciousness but against the messenger. 'Against his artificially cheerful tone of voice, his inappropriate sociological remarks, his obvious desire to talk about something else and his red lips.'[71] ('Moins contre la vérité qui ne le pénétrait pas encore complètement, que ces accessoires plus à sa portée: ce ton faussement léger, cette sociologie déplacée, cet envie trop visible de parler d'autre chose, ces lèvres rouges.')

Augustin asks for a sputum analysis.

> 'I want to be quite certain.' 'The clinical signs are clear enough,' said the
> doctor after a silence that lasted several seconds. 'Of course I can't
> explain those to you.' He turned towards Christine and declared with
> what one might call affable condescension (pitié amicale): 'Naturally,
> we'll do a sputum analysis. Intelligent lay persons always think that
> laboratory results equal certainty and that there is no certainty apart
> from laboratory results. That's the sort of opinion that has been
> propagated by the current popularization of medical topics.'[71]

The sputum test is positive and Augustin goes off to Paris, where he consults one of
the leading chest physicians in the country.[72] This doctor is surrounded by the
trappings of a highly lucrative private practice. There is a valet, a sexy nurse-
receptionist, and an efficient though somewhat brusque radiographer. The corridors
are lined with bound volumes of German and American professional journals.
Between the bookshelves, the walls are decorated with Impressionist and Cubist
paintings.[72] The famous specialist, a full Professor of Medicine at the University of
Paris and a senior physician at one of the major hospitals,[72] seems to have reached
his exalted position on merit rather than by nepotism. He is a versatile scholar
whose erudition and powerful intellect are reflected in his scientific papers. He has
even studied in the United States.[72] So long as he is not contradicted, he manages to
keep his aggressive tendencies well under control.[72] The great man recommends a
two years' stay in a Swiss sanatorium, 'longer if necessary', and he produces a glossy
prospectus advertising a particular establishment. He dictates an appropriate letter,
indicating that Augustin requires an extended leave of absence. 'You should be there
within a week' says the lung specialist.[72]

Despite all these rational instructions, Augustin feels very negative. 'If I don't get
better, what sort of time frame is there before they carry me away?' The doctor
dislikes that question. 'Monsieur Méridier, what you are asking doesn't make sense.
All the medical evidence is in favor of your recovery. I've sent patients [to that
sanatorium] that were a lot worse than you and they got better. You'll get better.'[72]

Augustin is not satisfied. He wants to consider both possibilities, recovery and
death. But his time is up; doorbells are ringing and the valet is ready with the
doctor's overcoat. The fixed smile on the doctor's face does not change. He remains
perfectly polite but one can sense his annoyance with this encroachment on his
time.[72] 'His voice was not totally free of that hint of arrogance which he could never
quite suppress when someone contradicted him.' ('Sa voix ne fut pas tout à fait
exampte de cette hauteur nuancée qu'en face d'une contradiction il n'était jamais
totalement maître de retenir.')

Augustin takes the physician's advice, he enters the recommended sanatorium,
but he fails to improve and dies within a few weeks. His only comfort during that
time comes from an old school friend, now a Jesuit priest, who restores his faith in
God.[73] Malègue does not actually quote the book of Job[74] but he seems to share the
biblical view that being a physician is almost synonymous with being 'worthless' and
that there is only one True Healer.

Summary

An irrational dislike of the entire medical profession, dating from classical times, persists to this day. It stems from a variety of causes including a deep resentment of powerful experts with their semi-secret knowledge, who promise results but fail to deliver.

References

1 Céline LF (1932) *Journey to the End of the Night*. Translated by Manheim R. New Directions, New York, 1983, p. 353.

2 Pliny the Elder (Gaius Plinius Secundus) (1st century AD) *Natural History*, Book 2. Translated by Holland P. Southern Illinois University Press, 1962, pp. 294–7.

3 Montaigne M de (1580–8) *Essays*, vol. 2, Book 3. Translated by Trechmann EJ. Oxford University Press, London, 1927, pp. 564–6.

4 Amm M (1996) Utterances of Discontent: the physician in the œuvre of Thomas Bernhard, Wien. *Klin Wochenschr.* **108**: 478–82.

5 Lucian of Samosata (2nd century AD) Disowned. Translated by Harmon AM. In: *Lucian*, vol. 5. Loeb's Classical Library, Heinemann, London, 1972, pp. 477–525.

6 Ibid., p. 487.

7 Céline LF, op. cit., p. 322.

8 Balzac H de (1847) *Cousin Pons*. Translated by Hunt HJ. Penguin, Harmondsworth, 1968, p. 117.

9 Dryden J (1699) To My Honour'd Kinsman, John Driden, of Chesterton in the County of Huntingdon, Esquire. In: Dearing VA (2000) *The Works of John Dryden*, vol. 7. University of California Press, Berkeley, CA, p. 199.

10 Chekhov AP (1887–9) Ivanov. In: *The Oxford Chekhov*, vol. 2. Translated by Hingley R. Oxford University Press, London, 1967, p. 170.

11 Maugham WS (1919) *The Moon and Sixpence*. Penguin, Harmondsworth, 1953, p. 201.

12 Buzacott M (1987) *Charivari*. Picador, Sydney, pp. 200–6.

13 Richardson S (1747–8) The History of Clarissa Harlowe. In: Stephen L (ed.) (1883) *The Works of Samuel Richardson*. Henry Sotheran, London, vol. 7, p. 378; vol. 8, pp. 111–12.

14 Tolstoy L (1886) The Death of Ivan Ilych. Translated by Maude L and Maude A. In: Simmons EJ (ed.) (1966) *Leo Tolstoy, Short Novels*, vol. 2. Random House, New York, p. 47.

15 Runyon D (1946) Why Me? In: Runyon, D. *Short Takes*. Somerset Books, New York, pp. 364–6.

16 O'Neill E (1928) Strange Interlude. In: O'Neill E (1988) *Complete Plays*, vol. 2. Library of America, New York, p. 660.

17 Ibid., p. 724.

18 Heller J (1974) *Something Happened*. Jonathan Cape, London, pp. 531–2.

19 Shute J (1992) *Life Size*. Houghton Mifflin Company, Boston, MA.

20 Daudet LA (1894) *Les Morticoles*. Fasquelle, Paris, 1956.

21 Salières F (1948) *Écrivains contre médecins*. Denoël, Paris, pp. 31–40.

22 Daudet LA, op. cit., pp. 94–7.

23 Martin du Gard R (1922–9) *The Thibaults*. Translated by Gilbert S. John Lane, The Bodley Head, London, 1939.

24 Martin du Gard R (1936–40) *Summer 1914*. Translated by Gilbert S. John Lane, The Bodley Head, London, 1940.

25 Martin du Gard R, *The Thibaults*, p. 332.

26 Fearing K (1939) *The Hospital*. Ballantine Books, New York, p. 7.

27 Plath S (1965) Lady Lazarus. In: Plath S (1976) *Ariel*. Faber and Faber, London, p. 18.

28 Dostoyevsky F (1880) *The Brothers Karamazov*, vol. 2. Translated by Magarshack D. Penguin, Harmondsworth, 1977, pp. 603–16.

29 Ibid., pp. 655–9.

30 Ibid., pp. 789–95.

31 Ibid., vol. 1, pp. 211–12.

32 Sexton A (1962) The Operation. In: Sexton A. *All My Pretty Ones*. Houghton Mifflin, Boston, MA, p. 13.

33 Sexton A (1975) Doctors. In: Sexton A (1981) *The Complete Poems*. Houghton Mifflin, Boston, MA, pp. 465–6.

34 Beauvoir S de (1964) *A Very Easy Death*. Translated by O'Brian P. Andre Deutsch and Weidenfeld and Nicolson, London, 1966, pp. 21–2.

35 Chekhov AP (1900–1) Three Sisters. Translated by Hingley R. In: *The Oxford Chekhov*, vol. 3. London, 1964, pp. 74–7.

36 Hardy T (1886–7) *The Woodlanders*. Oxford University Press, Oxford, 1988, pp. 77–8.

37 Arlen M (1924) *The Green Hat*. George H. Doran, New York, p. 221.

38 Woolf V (1925) *Mrs Dalloway*. Zodiac Press, London, 1947, pp. 104–13.

39 Ibid., p. 203.

40 Tate J (1976) Who Gets The Bitterroot. In: *Viper Jazz*. Wesleyan University Press, Middletown, CT, p. 43.

41 Chandler R (1949) *The Little Sister*. Houghton Mifflin, Boston, MA, pp. 235–6.

42 Chandler R (1953) *The Long Good-Bye*. Pan, London, 1979, p. 254.

43 Ibid., pp. 134–5.

44 Olsen T (1962) *Tell Me a Riddle*. Virago, London, 1990, pp. 84–5.

45 Bernhard T (1978) Breath – A Decision. In: Bernhard T (1985) *Gathering Evidence*. Translated by McLintock D. Alfred A Knopf, New York, pp. 240–1.

46 Bernhard T (1981) In the Cold. In: Bernhard T (1985) *Gathering Evidence*. Translated by McLintock D. Alfred A Knopf, New York, p. 301.

47 Wharton W (1981) *Dad*. Alfred A Knopf, New York.

48 Ellis AE (1958) *The Rack*. Penguin, London, 1988.

49 Malègue J (1932) *Augustin, ou, Le maître est là*. Spes, Paris, 1935, 2 vols.

50 Wharton W, op. cit., p. 237.

51 Ibid., pp. 102–19.

52 Ibid., pp. 129–30.

53 Ibid., pp. 159–62.
54 Ibid., p. 63.
55 Ibid., p. 249.
56 Ellis AE, op. cit., pp. 242–3.
57 Ibid., pp. 97–8.
58 Ibid., pp. 35–6.
59 Ibid., p. 264.
60 Ibid., p. 154.
61 Ibid., pp. 259–60.
62 Ibid., pp. 349–51.
63 Ibid., pp. 352–7.
64 Malègue J, op. cit., vol. 2, pp. 117–19.
65 Ibid., p. 20.
66 Ibid., pp. 213–20.
67 Ibid., p. 230.
68 Ibid., pp. 277–83.
69 Ibid., pp. 323–9.
70 Ibid., pp. 341–51.
71 Ibid., pp. 380–5.
72 Ibid., pp. 415–22.
73 Ibid., p. 489.
74 The Bible (7th–4th century BC) Revised Standard Version. Oxford University Press, New York, 1977, Job, 13: 4.

CHAPTER 9

The ward round

The purpose of rounds; favorable portrayals

In the real world, formal ward rounds serve three objectives:

1 A senior staff member assesses the patient's progress and orders appropriate treatment changes.
2 The house staff and students receive clinical instruction at the bedside.
3 The sick individual is provided with information and reassurance.

These aims, which require different attitudes and tactics, are not incompatible,[1] and generations of physicians have learnt clinical medicine on rounds.

In literature, a few writers portray the round for what it can be – a useful and even dramatic teaching exercise with appropriate patient participation. Noah Gordon's *The Physician*[2] contains many anachronisms, improbabilities and supernatural events, but its description of a ward round in Avicenna's Isfahan Hospital gives some indication of how a great physician might have behaved on rounds. The 'prince of physicians' has been told about a camel driver with kidney stones and now wants to question the patient himself.

> 'Amahl,' he said [to the camel driver] 'I am Husayn the physician . . . These (his entourage of eleven other physicians and students) are my friends and would be thine. Where are you from?'[2]

The language is flowery and inconsistent but at least there is an attempt to put a frightened hospital patient at ease.

Cable's *Dr Sevier*,[3] written in 1883 but set in 1856, describes a ward round in a New Orleans charity hospital in relatively factual terms.

> The group stretched out and came along, the doctor first and the young men after . . . pausing, questioning, discoursing, advancing, moving from each clean slender bed to the next, on this side and on that, down and up the long sanded aisles among the poor, sick women. Down at the far end of one aisle was a bed whose occupant lay watching the distant, slowly approaching group with eyes of unspeakable dread.[4]

The patient, the heroine of the story, has, in better times, seen the doctor privately, and now feels mortified by her poverty and her enforced stay in a charitable institution. Dr Sevier recognizes the woman and decides that a formal teaching round would distress her. He dismisses the students and comes back alone.[4]

A moving and unique scene from Sobel's *The Hospital Makers*[5] is quoted in full. Dr Rintman, the famous internist, is able, in the space of a few minutes, to achieve all three aims of the ward round. He refutes a lethal diagnosis, he provides an important message on liver disorders and, despite his patronizing attitude, he makes the patient feel happy and privileged.[6] The setting is a 'Nightingale' ward in a New York teaching hospital in the 1930s before the days of reliable imaging and before the ready availability of biochemical procedures. All the patients are neatly tucked into bed and everything is very quiet as Rintman's observations to his staff and students carry across the entire room. The group reach the bed of a 'seventy-four-year-old white male', who has been admitted because of severe jaundice, due, the house physician informs Rintman, to a pancreatic carcinoma.[6] Rintman reaches a different conclusion. After performing a theatrical rectal examination,

> [he] sat on the edge of the bed and took one of the old man's hands between his own. 'I must disagree with you, my friend,' he said firmly. 'I am sure you don't have cancer.' 'Well, you're the great Dr Rintman,' the old man said. Rintman laughed. 'This time I must agree with you.' The old man laughed too. 'That's why you are the great Dr Rintman, you know when to agree and to disagree.' Now everyone laughed. Rintman slid up toward the head of the bed. 'What are you taking for your cough?' he asked like a fellow conspirator . . . 'You're sure you won't scold me?' Rintman patted his hand. 'Of course not. I only scold doctors.' The old man opened up the drawer of his bedside table and took out an unlabeled bottle half full of a clear colorless liquid. Rintman pulled out the cork and smelled it. 'This isn't cough medicine. This is cleaning fluid' . . . Rintman stood up and tapped him on the chest. 'Do you know why you are sick, why you have yellow jaundice . . . It's because of this.' He pointed to the bottle . . . 'Let's make an exchange. You give me the bottle and I'll give you . . . your life.' . . . [Dr Rintman] turned to the doctors who were now clustering around the bed . . . 'I like this colorful old man. He has courage, imagination and a sense of humor. He's stolen a little of the divine fire and, like Prometheus, he's having trouble with his liver.' . . . He handed the House Physician the bottle of cleaning fluid. 'There's your cancer of the pancreas,' he said, and walked away, slowly. To everyone's consternation, the old man climbed out of bed and put on his bathrobe. Rintman stopped and turned around when he heard the shuffling steps. The old man was trying to catch up with him. Everyone waited, quietly. 'Thank you, Doctor, thank you,' said the old man standing very straight. 'It is you who have stolen the divine fire.' The great internist bowed and walked briskly to the door. That was one thing about Rintman, everyone agreed. He knew when to bring down the curtain. As he crossed the threshold of the silent room, it was as if he were being ushered out by thunderous applause.[6]

Bad teaching

The 'happy-clappy' atmosphere described by Sobel in this memorable passage[6] is rarely found in literature. On the contrary, rounds are generally perceived as relatively ineffective teaching exercises. At best, they amount to mini-lectures as a swarm of white-coated individuals moves from bed to bed, and the instructor, using the patients as 'teaching material', delivers himself of words of wisdom at each station ('shifting dullness'). The recipients of this distilled knowledge, whether respectful students scribbling in their notebooks,[7] or skeptical residents longing to escape so they can attend to their other duties, are treated to a smorgasbord of truisms, half-truths and untruths. At worst, the instructor uses the 'education-by-insult'[8] approach, with the pivotal message that the trainee or the student is an absolute idiot. 'Didn't you people learn anatomy a year or two ago or is that no longer on the curriculum?'[9]

Dr Watson Kreck* of the Paradiso Veterans Administration Hospital[10] who is making rounds with his new resident, Dr Redshield, demonstrates both techniques. First, Redshield is regaled with one of his preceptor's favorite mantras: 'Remember Redshield, the longer a man lives the less he's going to live. No matter what he's got.'[11] Then comes the 'boot camp' method.

> Kreck threw a piercing look at Redshield. 'Now then Redshield. What's the first thing you think of . . . when you see a red tattoo?' 'I don't know.' 'Syphilis, Redshield. When you see a red tattoo, think of syphilis . . . Hasn't anyone ever taught you that?'[11]

A recipe for the humiliation of patients

From the patient's point of view, rounds, especially teaching rounds, are disasters. The doctor's bedside manner during these futile exercises is cruel or indifferent, with only occasional attempts (mostly unsuccessful) to communicate with the patient. Rounds even provide occasions for mirth at the expense of the sick.

Ken Harrison, the quadriplegic in *Whose Life Is It Anyway*,[12] resents the relative ranks of the chief physician who descends 'like Zeus from Olympus with his nymphs and swains',[12] and that of the patient who is treated as an object to be viewed and discussed. Simenon's René Maugras,[13] a journalist, attends Professor Besson's ward rounds as a spectator and is appalled by the degradation of the patients, despite Besson's good-nature:

> Wasn't it a cruel sport? An unfeeling hand lifted up the sheet and disclosed a feverish body, malformations, bedsores, while the professor in his lecture-room voice, uttered his comments and the students took notes . . . Each of [the patients] waited his turn, listening eagerly, trying to understand the doctor's comments, which might just as well have been made in Latin. And yet Besson was a humane man. He knew most of his

---

* Several of Schneiderman's characters bear 'catchy' names of medical pioneers like 'Henderson', 'Hasselbalch' and 'Klippelfeil' with or without slight variations from the original.[10]

patients by name and would address them familiarly. 'Well, here's my old friend who's going to ask me a lot of questions again.' Sometimes he would give them a pat on the cheek or on the shoulder, particularly if he knew that the bed would probably be empty or have another occupant, at his next visit.[13]

Patients find themselves particularly frustrated and humiliated when the doctors abruptly cease talking to them so as to resume teaching the students and residents. Staff members ask questions but then proceed to talk to each other rather than listen to the replies. Marjorie Kellogg in *Tell Me That You Love Me, Junie Moon*[14] provides a typical case:

A large group of doctors, nurses, medical students and usually a visiting dignitary or two went from bed to bed to discuss the patients' progress or decline . . . 'How are you feeling?' A tall older man always began this way after the resident had recited the facts. 'I feel better, doctor.' 'That's good.' 'There's only one thing, doctor.' 'Yes?' But the doctor had turned to the resident. 'By the way, the Schilling test showed what?'[14]

Surgical rounds are worse. The attending surgeon in Frede's *The Interns*[15] (Dr Riccio) does not even make a token effort to talk to the patients, the house staff or the students.

Rounds had been swift – an almost cursory stop by each of the six beds in each of the six rooms, that comprised, along with three semiprivate rooms, Ward B of Male Surgery. A brief summary by . . . the chief resident at each stop. Usually only a grunt from Riccio. A few times a comment like 'Discharge this man' or 'Who the hell ordered high protein for this patient?' Twice bandages were removed and Dr Riccio looked – and grunted and moved on to the next bed.[15]

Riccio himself is not very impressed with the educational effects of the exercise on the large group of residents, interns and students. 'Some group', he complains to the chief resident after the rest have departed, 'they don't know their ass from their elbow; and they're not interested in finding out . . . Forty-two patients and not one intern asked a question'.[15]

Rounds in hospitals for chronic diseases, like old-fashioned tuberculosis sanatoria, are worse still. The laconic surgeon, who expresses himself in a variety of grunts,[15] at least provides some overall supervision and checks the patients for postoperative complications. In establishments for long-term inmates, where nothing changes from month to month, formal, regular rounds at set times are perceived as meaningless rituals even by the medical participants.[16]

Temperature charts were laid in readiness across the bottom of each bed. Whilst Dr Vernet assessed keenly the implications of the interlaced graphs of temperature, weight and pulse, Dr Bruneau lolled apathetically against the wall, stared out of the window or if a book or magazine lay to hand, seized it so purposefully as to suggest that its perusal constituted the sole reason for his visit.[16]

Paul Davenant and his fellow-patients in *The Rack*[16] have to submit to this degrading charade on a weekly basis in the

> humiliating perspective from which the horizontal view the vertical.[16]

After enduring these visitations for three years, Paul becomes so disenchanted that the idea occurs to him the doctors might as well make rounds in the graveyard, the 'ideal extension of a sanatorium. Here prognosis hugged diagnosis . . . here [lay] the mute graduates of the Alpine academies'.[17]

Also suffering from tuberculosis, Thomas Bernhard, who regards almost all doctors as ignorant fools or megalomaniacs[18] (*see* p. 196), believes that from the patient's point of view the ward round is not only meaningless and degrading but also positively harmful.[19]

> The ward round unfailingly . . . brought an icy chill with it and all it left
> behind . . . were doubts about the art of medicine and its pretensions . . .
> Every day they appeared in front of my bed, a white wall of unconcern

providing no information, let alone reassurance for the intelligent, sick young apprentice who is totally in their power.[19]

Shem provides an instance of actual physical harm ensuing from the outrageous behavior of an attending physician during a ward round. Dr Donowitz, one of the multiple negative role models in *The House of God*,[20] attempts to demonstrate a physical sign for amyloidosis. The diagnosis is inappropriate, the sign (easy bruising) useless and in the process 'Donowitz . . . ripped a big chunk of flesh from the guy's arm'.[20] Dr Donowitz' patient must have been particularly stoical or stupid not to complain, but the 'right' degree of provocation on a ward round, especially a perceived affront, may cause smoldering resentment to burst into an open blaze with the development of a major confrontation.

Two of Noah Gordon's patients in *The Death Committee*[21] reach this point when new investigations or changes in treatment strategies are first mentioned during rounds. Unlike 'Amahl' in one of Gordon's other novels,[2] who is treated with elaborate courtesy (*see* p. 205), Gertrude Soames, a 'colored woman whose red hair came from a cheap bottle',[21] is told 'cheerfully' by the chief resident in front of fourteen other residents and interns that she needs a liver biopsy. ' "There's something wrong with your liver and we won't know how to help you unless we make this test". . . . "I'm not your damn guinea pig" ', says Gertrude[21] and signs herself out of the hospital.[22] Another patient becomes equally angry when he learns during a 'Socratean' conversation between the chief resident and an intern that he needs a femoral arteriogram. 'I can't take that kind of business', he declares.[21]

The ward round in Dooling's *Critical Care*,[23] which takes place in the 1990s, involves, like Dr Rintman's round in the 1930s,[6] the chief of medicine (Dr Richard Hofstader), residents, interns, medical students and, of course, a patient. But here the resemblance ends. The setting is now the intensive care unit at the University Medical Center where machines hiss and whirr and eight desperately ill patients are being kept alive on various types of apparatus. The 'teaching case' on this occasion is a man with Goodpasture's syndrome whose hands are tied to the bed rails and whose 'support system' includes an endotracheal tube, a nasogastric tube, an intravenous line and a urinary catheter. His 'wrists and elbows were bruised and bloody from lab sticks and . . . arterial blood gas sampling'. Throughout the story, this patient is referred to as 'Bed Two'.[23]

The chief's attitude has also changed over six decades. Rintman, despite his glaring faults,[24] is capable of communicating with his patients on a person-to-person basis, while his successor's erudition and administrative skills no longer include the ability to deal with living or dying patients. Indeed, Dooling implies that the prominence of a physician is negatively correlated with his clinical skills. Dr Richard Hofstader

> knew more about internal medicine than any other human being living within five hundred miles . . . He had stopped seeing or touching patients in the traditional office setting years ago. His time was too valuable to be squandered in seeing patients one at a time . . . What the patient said about his pain . . . and the gross examination . . . were matters best left to lower level physicians who could then edit and compress the information into a page or two.[23]

This 'medical visionary' is about to impart his knowledge to his 'clones'. Unfortunately, his capacity to appreciate a patient's anguish is so atrophied that even his other functions during the round – assessment of progress, supervision of treatment and teaching – lose their credibility.[23]

> 'Dr Hofstader . . . spoke in short, succinct, crisply enunciated sentences reviewing the latest vicissitudes in Bed Two's treatment, the persistent complications and system failures attending the imminent demise . . . [He] faced the clone brigade and held forth on the relative virtues of corticosteroids, azathioprine and mercaptopurine . . . Bed Two rattled the bed rails, clawed at his restraints and made a motion [a medical student] recognized as a request for pencil and paper . . . Bed Two scrawled in huge . . . hardly legible letters: 'WATER' . . . Everyone smiled at the medical impossibility of Bed Two's request. Everyone knew that Bed Two could not have any water. Everyone except Bed Two.

The systematic torture continues. Dr Hofstader points out various physical signs and makes all his disciples listen to an 'impressive' pericardial friction rub. The assembly remains quite unmoved by a further scrawl from the patient that reads 'DIE'. Dr Hofstader comments 'The patient's confusional state is probably the result of hypertensive encephalopathy'.[23] An intern who displays his ignorance of renal medicine is let off lightly. Dr Ernst, the only staff member who recognizes the futility of the entire exercise, is roundly berated for having missed the diagnosis. For the patient, there is not a word of comfort or sympathy. We do not even learn his name.[23]

Summary

The formal ward round is perceived unfavorably because the juggling act of assessing, teaching and comforting at the same time is beyond the capacity of most physicians. Moreover, the concept of regular rounds, as it evolved for the patients who occupied the wards of teaching hospitals between 1850 and 1950, is probably inappropriate for very acute and very chronic conditions.

References

1   Lehmann LS, Brancati FL, Chen MC, Roter D and Dobs AS (1997) The effect of bedside case presentations on patients' perceptions of their medical care. *N Engl J Med.* **336**: 1150–5.

2   Gordon N (1986) *The Physician.* Simon and Schuster, New York, p. 306.

3   Cable GW (1885) *Dr Sevier.* James R Osgood and Company, Boston, MA.

4   Ibid., p. 102.

5   Sobel IP (1973) *The Hospital Makers.* Doubleday, Garden City, NY.

6   Ibid., pp. 20–6.

7   Bashford HH (1911) *The Corner of Harley Street: being some familiar correspondence of Peter Harding MD.* Constable, London, 1913, p. 13.

8   Hecht B (1959) Miracle of the Fifteen Murderers. In: *A Treasury of Ben Hecht.* Crown Publishers, New York, p. 191.

9   Roe F (1989) *Doctors and Doctors' Wives.* Constable, London, pp. 35–8.

10 Schneiderman LJ (1972) *Sea Nymphs by the Hour.* Authors Guild Backinprint.Com, Lincoln, NE, 2000.

11 Ibid., pp. 55–8.

12 Clark B (1972) *Whose Life Is It Anyway.* Amber Lane Press, Ashover, UK, 1978, p. 11.

13 Simenon G (1963) *The Patient.* Translated by Stewart, J. Hamish Hamilton, London, 1963, pp. 33–4.

14 Kellogg M (1968) *Tell Me That You Love Me, Junie Moon.* Popular Library, New York, pp. 39–41.

15 Frede R (1960) *The Interns.* Corgi, London, 1965, pp. 32–3.

16 Ellis AE (1958) *The Rack.* Penguin, London, 1988, pp. 99–100.

17 Ibid., p. 230.

18 Amm M (1996) Utterances of Discontent: the physician in the œuvre of Thomas Bernhard, *Wien. Klin Wochenschr.* **108**: 478–82.

19 Bernhard T (1978) Breath – A Decision. In: Bernhard T (1985) *Gathering Evidence.* Translated by McLintock, D. Alfred A Knopf, New York, pp. 240–1.

20 Shem S (1978) *The House of God.* Richard Marek, New York, pp. 43–44.

21 Gordon N (1969) *The Death Committee.* The Book Society, London, 1969, pp. 38–41.

22 Ibid., p. 332.

23 Dooling R (1991) *Critical Care.* William Morrow, New York, pp. 93–104.

24 Sobel IP, op. cit., pp. 11–16.

CHAPTER 10

The physician's social status

> Everyone of our patients whether he is the richest man in the land or the poorest, has everything done for him that we can do. We have no secrets in reserve for the rich.[1]

> His wife's affiliation to the 'best people' brought him a good many of those patients whose symptoms are, if not more interesting in themselves than those of the lower orders, at least more consistently displayed.[2]

The discrepancies between the social and financial positions of the patients and those of the doctors introduce an important feature into the relationship between the parties. Idealistic doctors may delude themselves into believing that all patients, regardless of their social status, receive the same treatment. Most authors of fictional works have no such fantasies. Fictional characters, rich and poor, convey the message that, despite lofty declarations to the contrary, the social standing of the patients and their bank balances strongly influence the quality of their medical care (though not necessarily the ultimate outcome). Elsie Sprickett, the domestic servant in *Riceyman Steps*,[3] does not express this notion openly but she has 'well-implanted in her, the not groundless conviction that doctors were apt to be more summary with the sick poor than with the sick rich'. The greater the divergence between the position of the doctor and that of the patient in the social hierarchy, the more complex the establishment of meaningful interactions. In addition, the relative rank of patients on the perceived power scale determines whether resentment and hostility towards physicians remain latent or erupt into open conflict.

Rich and powerful patients

CP Snow's Katherine Getliffe, 'born scandalously rich',[4] regards a doctor as 'someone whose time you pay for and whose advice you consider rather as you would an electrician's when he brings a new type of bulb'.[4] Naturally, she 'harried her doctors, wanted to know the reasons for their actions and would not be put off by bedside patter'[4] or, presumably, by unpronounceable medical terms which so impressed less privileged women of a previous generation[5] (*see* pp 80 and 111).

Mary Rinehart's hero, Dr Noel Arden,[6] explains that in order to get even close to the Katherine Getliffes of this world, a new general practitioner has to work his way up the domestic ladder.

We usually begin with the servants. After that, if we're good, we get the children. And of course, in due time, and if we're very, very good we get the family. Like trying it on the dog.[6]

Arden does not explain how the doctor's performance is judged in this scenario but, no doubt, part of 'being good' consists of not disagreeing openly with the strongly held prejudices of the mistress of the house. Dr Lydgate of *Middlemarch*,[7] in his more idealistic days, does not want to prove himself to the 'leaders of society'. Medical practice among the rich, says Lydgate, 'is . . . monotonous . . . One has to go through more fuss and listen more deferentially to nonsense'.[7] He prefers to practice among poor and ignorant patients, who ask few questions and express even fewer opinions.

The interaction between a distinguished writer (Sir Lewis Eliot), who has sustained a second detachment of his left retina,[8] and his ophthalmologist (Dr Christopher Mansel) is described in detail in CP Snow's *Strangers and Brothers*.[8,9] The ophthalmologist, a thoroughly competent individual, displays exactly the right mixture of firmness and deference so that the doctor–patient relationship, while a little reminiscent of the eighteenth century (*see* p. 215), remains excellent despite various setbacks. Eliot, who has not been born into the English squirearchy, has nevertheless moved around the 'Corridors of Power' sufficiently to be able to check Mansel's credentials via a tycoon friend and the President of the Royal College of Surgeons.[9] Mansel calls his patient 'Sir', while Eliot calls the doctor by his first name. Here is Dr Mansel examining Sir Lewis with Lady Margaret Eliot looking on..

'Not quite in the same place as before,' he remarked. Then with some irritation he said that there hadn't been any indication or warning the last time he examined me only a month before. 'If we were cleverer at spotting these things in advance . . . Well, we shall have to try and make a better go of it this time.' 'Look Christopher,' I said, 'is it really worth while?' His antennae were quick. 'I know it's an awful bore, sir, I wish we could have saved you that –' 'What do I get in return? It's only vestigial sight at the best. After all that.' Mansel gazed at each of us in turn, collected, strong-willed. 'All I can give you is medical advice. But anyone in my position would tell you the same. I'm afraid you ought to have another operation.' 'It can't give him much sight, though, can it?' Margaret wanted to be on my side. 'This sounds callous but you both know it, as well as I do,' said Mansel. 'A little sight is better than no sight. There is a finite chance that the other eye may go. We're taking every precaution but it might. Myopic eyes are slightly more liable to this condition than normal eyes . . . If the worst did come to the worst and you'd only got left what you had yesterday in the bad eye – well, you could get around, you wouldn't be cut off.' 'I couldn't read.' 'I'm not pretending it would be pleasant. But you could see people you could even look at TV. I assure you, sir, that I've seen patients who would give a lot even for that amount of sight.' Margaret came and sat by me. 'I'm afraid he's right,' she said quietly. 'Would you like to discuss it together?' Mansel asked with firm politeness. 'No,' I said. 'Intellectually you are right. Let's get it over with.' I said it in bad grace and a bad temper but Mansel didn't mind about that. He had, as usual, got his way.[8]

During the operation, which is performed under general anesthesia, Sir Lewis Eliot suffers a cardiac arrest and Dr Mansel performs open cardiac massage. The next day when Sir Lewis becomes aware of what has happened, he expresses transient mistrust and irritation but harmonious relations with Doctor Mansel are soon restored.[8] Throughout his illness, Sir Lewis shows no hint of resentment against Dr Mansel's elegant clothes, his 'English Upper Class' accent or even his lack of therapeutic success.[8] On the contrary, Mansel is praised for his deft fingers, his efficiency and his strong will.[8,9] Snow obviously identifies with his rich and prominent patient and while the ophthalmologist is certainly not a lackey, his status and intellect are clearly inferior to those of Sir Lewis.* One does not harbor resentment against one's inferiors – one abuses them or dismisses them. Also, the relationship might have been less harmonious if, like Ivan Illych[10] (*see* pp 105 and 130), Sir Lewis had suffered from some incurable malignancy rather than a treatable eye condition.

A knowledgeable patient with a strong personality and in a position of power may even succeed in making a doctor alter his plan of management. Inspector Dalgliesh in PD James' *Shroud for a Nightingale*[11] has been hit over the head with a golf club and the gash in his scalp requires sutures. The inspector had interviewed the doctor (Stephen Courtney-Briggs) a few days earlier in connection with a murder, so that the relationship between the two is different from that normally found between a senior surgeon and a member of the police force. The doctor proposes to give the inspector a general or a local anesthetic.

> 'I don't want any anesthetic. I just want it stitched.' Courtney-Briggs explained patiently as if to a child. 'It's a very deep cut and it's got to be sutured. It's going to hurt badly, if you won't accept an anesthetic.' 'I tell you I don't want one. And I don't want a prophylactic injection of penicillin or anti-tetanus. I just want it sutured.' Then Courtney-Briggs spoke, curiously formal. 'If you'd prefer another surgeon . . .' 'No. I just want you to get on with it.' There was a moment's silence. Then the surgeon spoke. 'All-right. I'll be as quick as I can.'[11]

The doctor as lackey

In the days when doctors were content to serve as lackeys to the socially prominent (and some continue to serve in that capacity to the present-day), the squire would bark a brisk order and the doctor would obey as best he could. In the opening lines of Smollett's *Humphry Clinker*,[12] Squire Bramble, who suffers from chronic constipation, writes to his doctor informing him that his current medication is ineffective, and demands a stronger purgative:

> Doctor, the pills are good for nothing . . . I have told you over and over how hard I am to move . . . prithee send me another prescription.[12]

---

* Sir Lewis' anesthetist, who orders fluid restriction in the postoperative period, evidently occupies a lower spot in the medical hierarchy than Mansel, and is considered a fit subject for harassment.[8]

In due course, the new prescription arrives but it is highly unlikely that Bramble's physician would have suggested, at any stage, that there are better ways of dealing with bowel problems.

The irascible and immensely rich Earl in Warren's *Rich and Poor*[13] is dangerously ill. The diagnosis is allegedly 'gout [of the] stomach and bowels' but more likely renal failure or some abdominal malignancy complicated by pulmonary embolism. 'His lordship, . . . [who] had a tolerable knowledge of medicine' has dismissed his physician whose medications, he imagines, are poisoning him. 'He did it on purpose. He had a spite against me.' The new physician wants to continue with the same treatment.

> 'I am afraid, my lord,' said I hesitatingly, 'that I shall find myself compelled to continue the use of the medicine which Dr – prescribed.' 'I'll be – if you do,' replied the Earl, continuing to mutter indistinctly some insulting words about my 'small acquaintance with the pharmacopeia.'[13]

The doctor swallows his pride and ignores the Earl's derogatory remarks.

John Fairthorne, another rich and irascible invalid,[14] is not as sick or as angry as Samuel Warren's Earl, but his relationship with his physician follows a very similar pattern. Fairthorne complains to one of his visitors: 'I am not very strong today . . . If that confounded doctor did not dose me I should be better. I have no faith in his tribe.' After one of Fairthorne's nieces points out to her uncle that he would be most unhappy if the doctor did not attend each day, he declares that he prefers the doctor's conversation to his medications. He then goes on to admit that he wants the medications, too. 'We all believe in drugs, sort of fetich [sic], a survival of the medicine man.' When the doctor finally arrives, Fairthorne introduces him to another visitor as 'my daily nuisance'.[14]

Charles Dickens' Dr Alexandre Manette,[15] who is kidnapped by the aristocratic St Evremonde brothers, has the status of a slave rather than a lackey. 'They were armed. I was not.' The aristocrats need a physician to attend to a peasant girl they have seduced and impregnated, and to the girl's brother who has received a sword-thrust during a subsequent fight. The peasants (who both die) are referred to as 'patients', while the St Evremonde brothers, who are not treated by Dr Manette, are 'clients'.[15] Another of Dickens' doctors, 'Mister Chillip', who attends the birth of *David Copperfield*,[16] does not have to face armed kidnappers, but this 'mildest of little men' is so terrified of the baby's formidable great-aunt that he prefers 'to sit upon the stairs in the dark and strong draught rather than face her stony silence and occasional outbursts by the parlor fire'.[16]

Samuel Pickwick's medical adviser, created by Bernard Shaw rather than Charles Dickens,[17,18] might not have been as timid as Mr Chillip but he would have been equally reluctant to comment adversely on his patient's insobriety.

> Had Mr Pickwick's doctor gone on to forbid Mr Pickwick to drink brandy and water whenever he felt chilly, and assured him that if he were deprived of meat and salt for a whole year he would not only not die but would be none the worse, Mr Pickwick would have fled from his presence as from that of a dangerous madman.[18]

Similarly, Thomas Mann's Doctor Grabow,[19] who is building up a practice among the prosperous merchants of a city in north Germany, has no intention of offending his patients by telling them the truth about their unhealthy lifestyles. He takes good care not to criticize their gluttony and their lack of physical exercise even when early symptoms of vascular disease are already apparent.

> He . . . was not the man to upset the habits of these prosperous, comfortable tradesmen and their families. He would come when he was sent for, prescribe a few days' diet . . . and assure the family that it was nothing serious this time. Young as he was, he had held the head of many an honest burgher who had eaten his last joint of smoked meat and his last stuffed turkey.[19]

On the other hand, Dr Maturin is extraordinarily candid with his superior officer, Captain Aubrey: 'You eat too much, you drink too much, and you do not take enough exercise'.[20] There is no hint that this anachronistic advice provokes any tension between the two men.

The personal physician to a bloodthirsty tyrant has to take particular care with his bedside manner; one wrong gesture may cost the doctor his life, especially when the patient imagines that the sharks circling the sick room are looking for ways and means to gain entrance. Alexei Tolstoy's Dr Jacobi,[21] who treats Czar Ivan the Terrible during his final illness, manages to avoid summary execution by emphasizing that there is some hope. The Czar is paranoid, superstitious and full of premonitions concerning his impending demise. He orders the execution of the soothsayers when they predict his death but he is also deeply suspicious of the doctor who believes Ivan may survive.[21]

> Ivan: Am I doomed to death? Speak thou, I wish to know.
> Jacobi (feeling his pulse): Thou art ill great Czar but death at present does not threaten thee.
> Ivan: Tis false. I soon shall die . . . Thinkst thou that I am blind? . . . Who bribed thee?

The doctor proceeds as if he had not heard the question or the accusation.

> 'Mighty Czar, thy long night vigils have overwrought thy brain.
> Permit me to prepare a draught.'[21]

In a subsequent scene, Jacobi discusses the medical situation with Boris Godunov, one of the Czar's 'advisers', and unwittingly becomes involved in a palace conspiracy.[22]

> The Czar's disease . . . is most complex.
> His suffering is not of the flesh alone;
> His mind is also ill. Accustomed from
> His youth to have all else to give way before
> His own imperial will, he could not bear
> This last humiliation.

Jacobi recommends rest and protection from agitation.

> Godunov: And if – which God forbid, his spirit should be roused to
>   wrath?
> Jacobi: Then we could surely not
>   Answer for the result. The channels
>   That conduct the blood out from the heart and
>   Into the heart* are under such a strain
>   That they may burst if he be agitated.[22]

The subservient status of physicians in Russia continues well into the nineteenth
entury. Pushkin[23] tells of a doctor summoned by a postmaster to diagnose and treat
a sick traveler. The doctor recognizes that the 'patient', an army officer who
subsequently abducts the postmaster's daughter, is perfectly healthy. He suspects
some mischief but keeps silent 'through fear of [the Hussar's] whip'.[23]

Even in the second half of the twentieth century the power structure in Russia still
works against physicians. The communist official who makes a scene in *Cancer
Ward*[24] (*see* p. 55) evidently feels that his position entitles him to bully the doctors.

A late British example of the forceful patient–meek doctor syndrome is described
by Anthea Cohen in *Angel of Vengeance*.[25] The protagonists, Major Abbott and
Dr Stephenson, are discussing Abbott's three-year-old daughter, who has been
admitted to hospital for the third time. On this occasion the child has facial injuries
and a fractured skull, while the two previous admissions were for a broken arm and
a broken leg. In addition, the X-ray films show two healed rib fractures so that
Stephenson, a hospital pediatrician, clearly has to consider child-battering. Abbott,
an aggressive army type, begins the interview.

> 'Mind if I smoke?' . . . He lighted the cigarette before Stephenson had had
> time to reply. . . . 'Want to talk to me about my kid? . . . The wife's
> expecting to have her home tomorrow . . . OK?' Dr Stephenson turned
> away, faced the wall in front of him . . . thinking how to start this
> conversation. 'Yes I did want to see you. It's just the fact that your little
> girl seems to be accident-prone. First the leg, then the arm and now
> this.' . . . 'What are you suggesting?' asked the major.[25]

Doctor Stephenson, an indecisive character who has already lost one round when he
fails to prevent the major lighting a cigarette in a non-smoking area, will not come to
the point. He talks about fragile bones, about accident proneness, behaving all the
time as if he were on the defensive. Finally he mentions his suspicion that the child
may have been hit.

> Abbott jumped to his feet . . . 'Are you suggesting . . . You'd better be
> careful doctor.' 'I'm not suggesting anything . . . It is just that the child
> has received several injuries and we must see to it that these are properly
> explained and accurately diagnosed.' . . . 'Surely you know that one of
> the injuries was sustained in the nursery school playground. Is that

---

* Anachronism. At the time of Ivan's death in 1578, William Harvey was six years old.

> supposed to be something to do with me?' 'You are taking this far too
> personally' . . . Dr Stephenson's voice was placatory . . .

Major Abbott responds by taking his daughter out of the hospital and informing
Dr Stephenson that his services are no longer required. The child is re-admitted some
weeks later, almost battered to death by her alcoholic mother.[25]

Dr Steven Rushton, another diffident, somewhat insecure British doctor[26] who
seems to attract argumentative patients,[27] has made himself even more vulnerable by
choosing to work in a 'one-man practice' in a small English town. A local politician
(Ken Horrocks) becomes particularly obstreperous when, after a consultation with
Dr Rushton, Mrs Horrocks decides to change her lifestyle.[28] Ken phones to enquire
what was said during the session and turns hostile when Rushton reminds him of
doctor–patient confidentiality.

> 'Oh, come now,' he snorted, 'what's that supposed to mean? Sounds as if
> you're hiding behind the party line about medical ethics . . . I *am* married
> to the woman when all's said and done.'[28]

Mr Horrocks becomes more strident as the telephone conversation goes on. He
informs Rushton that he has no time for 'all this female self-fulfillment stuff' and
concludes with a piece of gratuitous advice before he hangs up in the doctor's ear.

> 'May I suggest that in future you [restrict your activities] to sore throats
> and nappy rashes, where any blundering by yourself will at least be
> confined to the unfortunate individual you are treating.'[28]

The lackeys strike back

For the most part, doctors shrug off their powerful patients' outbursts of anger as
signs of illness. Dr Dontsova, the abused oncologist in *Cancer Ward*,[24] displays 'no
trace of the bitterness that naturally comes from a quarrel, for she could see . . . the
fist-sized tumor under . . . [the patient's] jaw. Who could she feel bitter against? The
tumor?'[24]

A few remind their patrons, by subtle or unsubtle means, that they are not
domestic servants. One such episode occurs in Duhamel's *Les Sept Dernières
Plaies*,[29] which is set in a military hospital in 1914. Colonel Piâtre, the star patient
and martinet of the establishment, is recovering from a bullet wound of the left
elbow. He tyrannizes and humiliates his male nurse, and now tries to show
Dr Cauchois where he belongs in the military hierarchy. When Cauchois enters
the Colonel's room he finds his patient immersed in official documents, barely giving
any indication that he has seen the doctor. ' "Your dressing, Colonel." "All right;
just get on with it." ' (' "Votre pansement, mon colonel!" "C'est bon, marchez." ')
The Colonel lets himself be attended as if he were having a haircut and pointedly
pretends to be busy. 'He continued to read his papers and relinquished his left arm
with an indifference that verged on insolence.' ('Il continuait de lire les feuilles et
m'abandonnait son bras gauche avec un désintéressement voisin de l'insolence'.) The
Colonel is duly chastised for his lack of respect for the medical profession. Cauchois

pulls the injured arm out of the plaster cast and examines it with such minute attention to detail that the patient calls out in pain. At first he growls 'Hey, look out'. The examination continues relentlessly. Then comes 'You're hurting me', but Cauchois still goes on with his punitive ministrations. He finally desists when Piâtre complains meekly: ' "You hurt me a bit, doctor". . . . The Colonel was no longer in the barber shop'.[29] (Le colonel n'était plus chez le coiffeur.')

Somerset Maugham's Dr Audlin,[30] in a stronger position in relation to his distinguished patient than a military doctor vis-à-vis an irascible colonel, is able to set the ground rules early in the course of the relationship. Lord Mountdrago, a senior British cabinet minister, is made to understand on Day One that the doctor will treat him exactly the same way as he treats his other patients. Audlin declines to undertake a home visit, despite the offer of a large fee and His Lordship is informed that unless he comes to Dr Audlin's office, the doctor will not see him.[30]

> When Lord Mountdrago was . . . shown in, he did not come forward but stood at the door and insolently looked the doctor up and down. Dr Audlin perceived that he was in a rage . . . 'It seems that it is as difficult to see you as a Prime Minister, Dr Audlin. I am an extremely busy man.' 'Won't you sit down?' said the doctor. His face showed no sign that Lord Mountdrago's speech in any way affected him. Dr Audlin sat in his chair at the desk. Lord Mountdrago still stood and his frown darkened. 'I think I should tell you that I am His Majesty's Secretary for Foreign Affairs,' he said acidly. 'Won't you sit down?' the doctor repeated. Lord Mountdrago made a gesture, which might have suggested that he was about to turn on his heel and stalk out of the room; but if that was his intention he apparently thought better of it. He seated himself. Dr Audlin opened a large book and took up his pen. He wrote without looking at his patient.[30]

Then comes the finishing stroke. The doctor, who is almost certainly aware of the prominent politician's personal details, asks his standard opening question: 'How old are you?'[30]

Dr Adam Stanton in *All the King's Men*[31] is anything but a lackey. Stanton, an idealistic Southern aristocrat, 'son of Governor Stanton, grandson of Judge Peyton Stanton and great-grandson of General Morgan', has nothing but contempt for Governor Willie Stark, a ruthless and unscrupulous demagogue, and for Stark's loathsome associates. The politicians thoroughly reciprocate. They regard Stanton as an idiot savant who 'does not like to play with the rough boys. He is afraid they might dirty his Lord Fauntleroy suit'.[32] Despite this antagonism, Stanton lets himself be persuaded to head up the new Stark medical facility, mainly out of altruistic motives. However, he is not happy in his position as 'court surgeon' or his proximity to the seat of power, and when he discovers that his sister has been sleeping with Stark, he declares that he will not be looked upon as her pimp and kills the governor.[33]

Dr Rushton's revenge against the obstreperous Alfred Groves is considerably less dramatic. Groves, who is forever complaining about the 'system' and Dr Rushton's perceived faults, is constipated after his recent stay in hospital and demands some medicine to move things along. The doctor maliciously prescribes a powerful purgative, which causes Alfred to soil his pants during a car trip.[26]

The doctor as despot; 'doctor's orders'

In the days when medical treatment was opinion- rather than evidence-based, the medical examination, whether gentle or brutal (*see* pp 107–8), was followed by a set of 'doctor's orders', which were delivered with a significant degree of firmness. Molière was obviously unimpressed both by the content and the style of these orders and used a sham doctor to ridicule the process.[34] Sganarelle, the clownish woodcutter who displays a remarkable talent for imitating the behavior of real doctors, has barely been 'anointed' as a member of the medical profession when he shows himself as a master of the bedside manner (*see* p. 72), especially when it comes to issuing decisive commands. The bogus doctor clears his throat, spits on the ground and, pointing to the blob of sputum, barks at the attendants 'Step on that – doctor's orders'. The servants are most impressed by this 'authentic' medical conduct.[34]

Henry Fielding contrasts the flexibility of doctor's orders for the rich with the 'take it or leave it' approach adopted for the poor. Having instructed *Tom Jones'* landlady[35] that the patient's diet is to consist of nothing but water-gruel, the surgeon is quite ready to relax his rigid position in the interest of finance.

> 'Won't you allow him sack-whey?' said the landlady. 'Ay, ay, sack-whey,' cries the doctor, 'if you will, provided it be very small.' 'And a little chicken-broth too?' added she. 'Yes, yes, chicken-broth,' said the doctor, 'is very good.' 'Mayn't I make him some jellies too?' said the landlady. 'Ay, ay,' answered the doctor, 'jellies are very good for wounds, for they promote cohesion.' And, indeed, it was lucky she had not named soop (sic) or high sauces, for the doctor would have complied, rather than have lost the custom of the house.'[35]

The same surgeon reluctantly agrees to defer bleeding Tom who 'persisted obstinately in his refusal'.[35] However, when the doctor discovers that Tom may be poor, he reverts to his usual high-handed approach.

> 'And have I suffered such a fellow as this,' cries the doctor, in a passion, 'to instruct me? Shall I hear my practice insulted by one who will not pay me! I am glad I have made this discovery in time. I will see now whether he will be blooded or no.'[36]

In addition to their firmness, opinion-based doctor's orders are characterized by their considerable detail (*see* p. 148). Doctors give instructions concerning the closure of windows, the kind of fish the patients are to eat for lunch[37] and whether or not they should or should not go out for a drive.[38] One type of soup is preferable to another and fruit may or may not be allowed.[39] Father Knellwood in *Circumstance*, who is recovering from some unidentified illness, complains bitterly that his doctor 'had forbidden work and had laid remorseless orders on him as to diet and times of rest'.[40] The ordinances in this case[38–40] are issued by the decisive Dr Sydney Archer, the medical hero of Weir Mitchell, who was himself trained as a doctor.

During the first half of the twentieth century the status of the doctor reaches its high point. While some rich and influential patients continue to harass their physicians, the power structure has shifted heavily in favor of the doctors. In Europe, general practitioners are no longer members of the 'lumpen-bourgeoisie',[41] they are now able to imitate their more prominent colleagues and impose their values and opinions on their patients. In the USA, where the status of doctors was high at a relatively early stage, a middle-aged, male gynecologist[42] refuses to fit a young woman with a diaphragm because she is not wearing a wedding ring. 'When you're married you come back with a ring and a license. We don't fit unmarried women.' The young woman meekly accepts this refusal, she pays her hefty bill and the matter goes no further.[42]

In the cities, teaching hospitals using poor patients as 'clinical material' were well established and there was little opportunity for such patients to express their dissatisfaction with the physicians who virtually controlled these establishments. Indeed, as Orwell reports in *How the Poor Die*,[43] it was not unusual for a doctor, an intern and a troop of students to ignore 'uninteresting' patients 'day after day [in spite of] imploring cries'. Open confrontations are unlikely to occur under these conditions.

Until relatively recent times (when nurses enlisted the help of patients in their power struggle against doctors), 'difficult' hospital patients were promptly subjugated by the combined forces of the two professions who presented a united front against any form of insubordination. Marilyn French, in *The Women's Room*,[44] provides a confrontational scene involving a patient–nurse–doctor triangle. A woman in labor had let out

> a piercing shriek. A nurse ran in. 'What is it now Mrs Martinelli?' There was irritation and contempt in her voice . . . 'It's time for the spinal,' the woman wailed in the irritating whine of the child, the helpless, the victim known and accepted. 'Tell the doctor to come, it's time.' The nurse was silent; there was a ruffling of a sheet. 'It's not time yet.' The woman's voice rose hysterically. 'It is, it is! I ought to know, I've had five kids. I know when it's coming. It'll be too late, it happened before, it was too late and they couldn't give it to me at all. Tell him, tell the doctor!' The nurse left and after a time a gray-faced man in a rumpled suit entered. He went to Mrs Martinelli's bed. 'Well, what's this I hear about you stirring up a rumpus, Mrs Martinelli? I thought you were a brave girl.' The woman's voice cringed and whimpered 'Oh, Doctor, please give me the spinal. It's time. I know it's time. I've had five kids . . .' 'It's not time yet, Mrs Martinelli. Quiet down now and don't bother the nurses. Don't worry. Trust me. Everything will be fine!'[44]

(Mrs Martinelli's baby arrives, without the benefit of an epidural anesthetic, a few minutes later.)

In military institutions doctors decide not only whether a man is sick and what treatment he is to receive but also whether a recalcitrant conscript is 'well enough to go to the front'.[45] The Good Soldier Svejk in World War I, reluctant to 'fertilize the vast fields' of the Fatherland with his blood, pretends to be half-witted.[46] He is craftily and obsequiously respectful to the senior army doctors who address him as 'you swine' and who have the authority (and use it) to subject him to a variety of tortures.[46]

In World War II Sergeant Alfonso Columbato in Wharton's *Birdy*[47] takes good care not to express his resentment against the 'doctor-major' openly.

> I ask what's the matter with Birdy but he's sly and manages not to answer. Suddenly he gets to be the major talking to the sergeant . . . All doctors in the army ought to be privates.[47]

For the time being Major Weiss is considerably more powerful than Alfonso, who salutes at opportune and inopportune moments, provides misinformation about his friend Birdy, and laughs loud and long at Weiss' weak jokes.[48] In Vietnam, Dr Lenhardt, who 'believes in the War and the sacrifice and the need for making a stand and dying for it . . . [sends] troopers back to the paddies with thirteen-inch thoracotomy scars'.[49]

Even in the 1970s the chronic inmates of the neurology ward in the Paradiso Veterans Administration Hospital continue the military tradition of expressing disapproval of their doctor's activities by guile and passive resistance rather than by open rebellion.[50] These old warriors do not appreciate tests or treatment. They know they will not improve and they want to be left alone 'in the cozy atmosphere of the ward' which is a second home to them. The last thing they want is a young doctor anxious to 'fight disease'. When they suspect that their new resident, like his meddlesome predecessors, will insist on performing useless and unpleasant tests they prepare to show their displeasure by coughing, vomiting and other gestures that might 'scare him away'. Bernstein, the doyen of the establishment, realizes that young Dr Redshield has one saving grace – he is lazy. In the environment of the Paradiso VA Hospital laziness is a virtue rather than a vice.

> Rather than bothering with those annoying complicated tests the new doctor would eat all his meals and linger over coffee . . . Rather than fluttering, tense and angry, over every dying patient as though each symptom were an insult, each fever a slap of the glove across the face which could be settled only by a flashy show of cold steel and frightful bloodshed . . . [this doctor] would yield mercifully.[50]

Only George Washington Carver, the foul-mouthed, angry, long-term malingerer exhibits signs of mutinous conduct. Carver, younger than the other veterans, becomes aggressive within a few seconds of meeting Dr Redshield. During the initial interview he asks the questions, sneers at the doctor and remarks:

> 'You're full of shit, Doc.' The words jolted him. Doctors spoke that way – among themselves. And even lay people in their own circles, were entitled to the expression. What bothered him was its miscegenation . . . It bothered him to be put down this way by a non-doctor.[51]

The patients revolt; ethnic minorities

The ignorant and superstitious poor look upon the doctor as a benign or malicious miracle worker, depending on the outcome of a particular illness. This suspicious mistrust was in evidence in the eighteenth century when physicians acted as purveyors of cheap and harmful medications and it persists to this day among members of cultural or linguistic minorities especially when they are admitted to state-of-the-art hospitals.

The sullen hostility of the 'lower orders' occasionally turns into violence with doctors as the target of 'peasant revolts' or individual acts of 'insubordination'. Gil Blas,[52] the physician's apprentice, and his master, Dr Sangrado, have to put up with the rage of bereaved relatives. 'Those afflicted people whose reproaches we were obliged to undergo were sometimes very brutal in their grief and called us ignorant assassins. My master who was used to such accidents heard them without the least emotion.'[52]

Dr Edward Hope in Martineau's *Deerbrook*[53] also has to face angry villagers and an eruption of physical violence. In his case, the anger of the 'masses' is not entirely spontaneous but surfaces as the result of agitation by the doctor's political enemies who almost drive him out of town when he refuses to vote for the squire's candidate in a parliamentary election.

> He stopped to speak to one man of eighty-three who was sitting in the sun at his door but he could get no answer out of him, nothing but growls about the doctor being a pretty doctor not to have mended his patient's eye-sight yet. Not a bit better could he see now than he could a year ago with all the doctoring he had had; and now the gentleman would not try anything more. A pretty doctor indeed! But it would not be long before there would be another who would cure poor people's eyes as if they were rich. And poor people's eyes were as precious to them as rich people's.[54]

Hope ultimately wins back the confidence of the villagers but not before his surgery has been ransacked and all the windows of his residence smashed.[54]

The modern equivalent of this syndrome is described by Hellerstein in *Children of the Valley*.[55] A poor immigrant couple, who speak only Spanish, are not in the least grateful for the medical care provided for their mentally and physically handicapped child at the University Hospital. On the contrary, they suspect the resident staff of 'experimenting on their baby', they refuse permission for any tests and they take the infant home against medical advice. We do not hear about broken clinic appointments but there are statistical data from real life indicating that marginalized patients are likely to express their discontent with the system by simply not turning up for scheduled visits.[56–58]

In Hellerstein's *The Battle for the Dead*,[59] the overt and unremitting mistrust of the Chiapas family for their gringo physicians, which is reciprocated with mild contempt on the part of the resident staff, makes any meaningful rapport between the parties virtually impossible. Old Simon Chiapas has lived in Brooklyn for fifty years but he is still unable to converse in English so that his wife, 'a short gaudy Puerto Rican with hennaed hair', has to translate for him. The two of them cannot accept that Simon's disease is undiagnosed and they suspect the doctors of suppressing information. Every blood test becomes a confrontation. Chiapas 'screams like a baby' while his wife declares: 'The tests hurt him so much. And what do you find? Nothing'. The family members watch the intern's every move during Simon's final hours and they become 'hysterical with grief' when the old man dies. Permission for autopsy is refused.

> 'No doctor, he suffered enough already . . . I ain't going to let you cut him up, understand? You tortured him long enough when he was alive, understand? . . . You been lying to me all along, now you make more lies to me. I ain't signing nothing.'[59]

Patients from ethnic minorities, even those without linguistic problems, may feel sufficiently alienated to become openly hostile when they believe they are being treated insensitively or incorrectly. Sidney Sheldon's Mr Sparolini[60] is more integrated into mainstream American society than Hellerstein's Mr Chiapas[59] and he does not suffer from any serious illness. Nevertheless, he feels aggrieved by his treatment and he puts on an act of rebellion against what he sees as the 'authorities'. Seventy-year-old Sparolini has a young wife who decides, after her sixth child, to talk the 'horny old goat' into a vasectomy, which is performed on an inpatient basis. A day later, the patient regrets his decision and confronts the medical staff.

> As soon as Dr Hutton approached the bed, the patient yelled: 'Gonzo! I'm going to sue you, you dirty son of a bitch.' 'Now, Mr Sparolini . . .' Don't Mr Sparolini me! You turned me into a fucking eunuch!' . . . 'Mr Sparolini, you agreed to have the vasectomy, and . . .' 'It was my wife's idea. Damn bitch! Just wait till I get home.' They left him muttering to himself.[60]

A confrontational scene in the emergency ward of the *House of God*[61] involves a tactless and useless intern, a black woman with abdominal pain and her black boyfriend, who does not attempt to contain his anger. The physical examination and the relevant tests are negative and she is told that no treatment is indicated.

> She accepted that and began to put on her clothes, but her boyfriend did not and said, 'Hey, wait a minute, man. You mean to tell me you're not going to do anything for her? Nothing?' 'I can't find anything I can treat.' 'Listen dude, my woman is in pain, real pain and I want you to give her something for it.'[61]

Instead of prescribing some mild analgesic, Dr Roy Basch refuses to give the black woman any medication. 'I don't want to mask what's going on.' Tempers rise and there would have been a punch-up if the nurses had not called security who 'stood around until the couple left'.[61]

The twenty-first century code of behavior: rules and exceptions

As the social, financial and educational positions of patients in developed countries begin to approach those of the physicians, the current code of behavior gradually evolves. Office and even clinic appointments are kept in the majority of instances.[56]

The patient arrives on time, suitably attired, possibly accompanied by a spouse or a grown-up daughter, but not by a tribe of undisciplined children.[62] The doctor's questions, his physical examination and the tests that he arranges are anticipated and accepted. Unlike the 'lower orders' of the nineteenth century,[2] who tended to ramble, the 'better' patients give consistent and coherent accounts of their symptoms. So long as the doctor provides appropriate explanations, his opinion is not challenged openly.

Knowledgeable patients (and patients who consider themselves knowledgeable) become the norm, so that in addition to his other contractual obligations, the doctor now has to avoid curt, evasive or dogmatic answers, which are likely to lead to arguments rather than silent resentment. Piercy's docile patient (*see* p. 222) who meekly pays the doctor's bill for a 'consultation' after being refused contraceptive advice[42] is now likely to be represented by a self-assertive young woman with a cell phone, a water bottle (which she uses during the interview), a navel ring and similar accoutrements. Such a person is unlikely to accept 'you come back with a ring and a license'[42] and unless the doctor tempers his advice to suit the times she is likely to walk out on him. The pregnant patient who declares that she does not want an episiotomy now elicits the grudging response 'You seem to know all the answers',[63] rather than 'That's for me to decide'.

As their part of the contract, physicians do not pursue their patients into the street to see whether their prescriptions are being taken to the pharmacy and whether their therapeutic recommendations have or have not been accepted. A doctor who advises a fellow invitee at a party about his eating or drinking habits is not only in a considerably weaker position than if he were to proffer the same advice in his office; he is provoking an open mutiny. When Doctor Webster Civet, one of the guests of the *Great Gatsby*,[64] tries to tell Miss Baedeker, a drunken, hysterical fellow-guest, to reduce her alcohol intake, her response is entirely predictable.

> 'Speak for yourself,' cried Miss Baedeker violently, 'your hand shakes. I wouldn't let you operate on me.'[64]

Rosenbaum[65] describes a physician who

> if he encountered one of his patients smoking, . . . would pull the offending cigarette from the patient's mouth and snuff it out. In a restaurant, if he saw a patient of his eating forbidden food he would publicly berate the poor soul and demand that the waitress remove the offending dishes.'[65]

Unless this doctor uses a 'double standard' and confines his inappropriate enforcement tactics to women and physical weaklings, he is likely to be beaten up as a reward for his therapeutic efforts.

'Lunatics', inebriates, minors

Several groups of patients, in addition to members of ethnic minorities,[55,59-61] do not feel themselves bound by these conventions and do not bother to suppress their resentment. The propensity of delirious patients to become aggressive towards their physicians has been known since classical times.[66] Psychotics, by virtue of their disease, are almost expected to cause disruption of appointment schedules, to frustrate the doctor's therapeutic efforts and, if the spirit so moves them, to turn violent. Doctor Baryton in *Journey to the End of the Night*,[67] who visits the wealthy patients in his asylum each day and charges large fees (*see* p. 25), is forcibly made aware that in this establishment the resentful patients do not always conceal their sentiments. On the contrary, from time to time, they receive him with a couple of clouts across the face. Likewise, Hellerstein's 'Ambrose', currently incarcerated in a prison for the criminally insane on a charge of rape, is physically and emotionally quite capable of throttling his physicians and gives every indication that he is about to assault them.[68]

Shem tells of an intern's unsuccessful attempt to examine a demented old woman who had been transferred from the 'Massada Nursing Home' to *The House of God*.[69]

> Potts did what the text books said to do: Introduced himself saying 'Hello Mrs Goober, I'm Dr Potts. I'll be taking care of you.' Upping her volume, Ina screamed, 'Go avay, go avay, go avay.' Potts next tried to engage her, using the other textbook method, grasping her right hand. Quick as lightning Ina struck him a southpaw blow with her purse knocking him back against the counter.[69]

Young Dr Potts, a gentleman from South Carolina, is mortified by Ina's lack of appreciation for his subtle clinical approach.

Drunks constitute another group who may forget the parts they are meant to play in the 'doctor–patient relationship' and, instead, resort to verbal abuse and physical violence. Morton Thompson[70] is obviously on the side of Dr Runkleman (MD, Creighton, 1889) who is threatened by an aggressive drunken patient with a broken ankle.

> Dr Runkleman turned the foot slightly. 'Hey!' the man shouted. 'Hey! Goddamn you!' 'Yes,' said Dr Runkleman, 'I think it's broken. We'll have an X ray.' . . . Dr Runkleman pressed the man's knee. 'Does it hurt here?' The man's face contorted in pain. 'You son-of-a-bitch –' he drew back a heavy forearm – 'you do that again, you bastard, I'll smash your face in.' . . . Dr Runkleman looked up coldly. 'You just try it!' he said.[70]

Runkleman, who has apparently participated in similar encounters in the past, 'punishes' the patient by withholding narcotics – 'little pain won't hurt him' – and by making the patient hobble to the ambulance without assistance – 'he's very strong, this fellow, let him help himself'.[70]

Children are also likely to regard the doctor as part of the disease rather than as a healer and may express themselves vigorously on the subject. In a much-quoted passage in *The Use of Force*,[71] William Carlos Williams describes a confrontation between a physician and Mathilda Olson. Mathilda is a schoolgirl, young enough to sit on her father's knees but old enough to knock off the physician's spectacles while he is trying to examine her throat. Mathilda is forcibly held down and is found to suffer from diphtheria.[71]

In Dr Bardamu's case[72] strong opposition comes from a sickly two-year-old boy who lives with his grandparents and his unmarried mother. The recently graduated doctor, who combines inexperience with cynicism, has not yet learnt how to restrain himself in the face of such a hostile reception and uses this inopportune moment to relieve himself of his pent-up frustrations.

> The child lying swaddled on his back in the middle of the table, let me palpate him. To begin with, I pressed the wall of his abdomen, ever so carefully and slowly, from the navel to the testicles, and then still very gravely I auscultated him . . . Then the child had enough of my exploring fingers and began to yell as children can do at that age, incredibly. . . . What screams! . . . I was at the end of my rope . . . 'Hey,' I said to this little bellower, 'don't be in such a hurry, you little fool . . . You'll have plenty of time for bellowing. Never fear, you little idiot, there'll be time to spare . . . There'll be enough misery to melt your eyes and your head and everything else if you don't watch out.' 'What are you saying, doctor?' the grandmother asked with a start. I repeated simply: 'There will be plenty!' [The child's mother promptly becomes hysterical.] 'Mama he's mad.' She bellowed so hard she almost choked. 'The doctor's gone mad! Mama, take my baby away from him!' . . . They snatched the baby out of my hands as if they were rescuing him from the flames. The grandfather who had been so deferential only a short while ago, unhooked an enormous mahogany barometer from the wall, it was as big as a club . . . and he pursued me at a distance to the door, which he slammed violently behind me.[72]

Embellished reports of the incident circulate throughout the neighborhood and Dr Bardamu's practice does not flourish.[72]

Delany's precocious, traumatized, suicidal nine-year-old 'mind-reader'[73] has no inhibitions about informing her psychiatrist of her contempt. 'Your thoughts, they're just as clumsy and imprecise as the others. How can you . . . help people who are afraid and confused . . . ? I don't want to stumble around in all your insecurities and fears.'

Adolescents who are taken to the doctor by their parents because of trouble with the authorities may also lack docility. Such 'patients' have no clinical problems but it is hoped the physician will be able to provide a medical label as well as an excuse (or at least an explanation) for the teenager's 'deviant' behavior and/or lack of achievement. Alternatively the parents may bring along a fifteen-year-old because of what they regard as abnormalities of height, weight or pubertal development. The perceived problems ostensibly do not bother the 'children', who have no desire to discuss them in this context and who express their contempt for the entire exercise clearly though non-verbally. Weir Mitchell, himself a physician, tells the story of 'Sarah Grace', an 'impassive and sallow'[74] teenager who suffers from bulimia and who is advised 'to eat less and walk more'.[74] Mrs Grace makes up for her daughter's reticence by volubly airing her own views concerning the etiology of the girl's condition.[75]

One of the best examples of an encounter between a physician and a recalcitrant teenager is to be found in Levenkron's *The Best Little Girl in the World*.[76] Neither Francesca ('Kessa') Dietrich, a fifteen-year-old school student with anorexia nervosa, nor her domineering father are at all enthusiastic about seeing Dr Alexander Smith, a fashionable Park Avenue psychiatrist. Harold Dietrich finds the very idea of telephoning a psychiatrist repulsive. Psychiatrists treat 'crazy people' and here he is calling a psychiatrist 'to treat his own daughter'. The doctor answers in a

> calm, flat voice . . . Emotion was lacking, even feigned emotion. 'I can see you and your wife and daughter on Thursday at one.' 'An evening appointment would be more convenient.' 'I don't have evening appointments Mr Dietrich.' There was no arrogance in the voice, only the same matter of fact flatness. Harold thought of Francesca and subdued his anger.[76]

On the following Thursday Harold Dietrich, Grace Dietrich and Francesca are shown into Dr Smith's office.

> There were two chairs in front of the huge mahogany desk, both considerably smaller than the high-backed one behind it. Dr Smith drew up a third for Francesca and the interview began. 'How old are you Francesca?' Dr Smith asked, pencil poised above a yellow legal pad. Kessa said nothing. 'Fifteen,' Grace replied. 'And what seems to be the problem?' Still no sound from Kessa. 'The problem is,' Harold said impatiently, 'that she won't eat. Exactly what I told you on the phone.' 'Is that true Francesca?' Kessa sat small and sullen in the big chair, her eyes riveted on the floor. 'I think I'll have a word alone with Francesca,' Dr Smith said to her parents.[76]

Rapport is not established and after six visits Francesca ceases to attend (*see* p. 45).

Criminals and semi-criminals; the 'class struggle' in the doctor's office; physical violence

The 'undeserving' poor generally regard doctors as 'gentry' and keep away unless they are desperately ill or in need of a medical certificate. Under those circumstances, open class-warfare is avoided, though the doctor may complain about having to treat dirty, smelly and ignorant patients. Relations become more complicated when a child belonging to a 'lumpenproletariat' family becomes ill. The drunken, semi-criminal father who is incapable of affection for his infant, resents the doctor's visits, his orders and his medications all of which he regards as alien pretentiousness. The child's mother may lack the educational background to make a good nurse but she wants her baby to recover and is prepared to put up with the doctor's harassment. Dr Jonathan Godwin's patient is the infant son of Reuben Daines, a violent, murderous Australian ex-convict.[77]

> Godwin, going into the Daines' hut winced at the squalor of it: the slab
> walls lined with smoked and stained sail cloth; the earth floor compacted
> with wood ash . . . 'Good day to you Mrs Daines. How's the baby?' 'He
> seems much the same, sir. Not better, nor worse. It's the coughing that
> keeps him weak.' 'Have you been giving him his linctus?' 'Yes sir.' The
> whining voice told him she was lying. . . . She stood cringing and
> wringing her hands. 'I'm doing everything you said sir . . . But he don't
> seem to like the stuff and Daines says it won't do the kid no good if he
> can't bide it.' He went to the cradle and stood looking down into it,
> frowning at the filth, knowing there was next to no hope for the child
> because the slatternly mother and her surly, mean-spirited husband
> expected it to die and would not believe that any medicine could save
> it.[78]

Reuben Daines, the vicious father, is so suspicious that he believes Dr Godwin only
makes home visits so as to spy on him.

> 'It's going to die ain't it? And Godwin knows it. He's only keeping it alive
> so's he can come here spying. Better for all of us if it was dead already.'[79]

'Bobo', the repulsive pimp in Remarque's *Arch of Triumph*[80] who represents the
French 'nasty type', provokes a violent encounter with the doctor of one of his
'protegées'. Dr Ravic has performed an emergency hysterectomy on Lucienne
Martinet who developed septicemia after a bungled abortion. As a cost-saving
measure he has discharged Lucienne from the hospital somewhat prematurely and is
now visiting her at home.

> Lucienne . . . was not alone. A fellow of about twenty-five slouched on a
> chair. He wore a cyclist's cap and was smoking a home made cigarette,
> which stuck to his upper lip when he talked. He remained sitting as Ravic
> entered. 'How are you, Lucienne?' Ravic asked without taking any notice
> of him, 'You're wise to stay in bed.' 'She should have been up long ago,'
> the boy declared. 'There's no longer anything wrong with her.' . . . Ravic
> turned around and looked at him. 'Leave us alone,' he said. 'What?' 'Get
> out. Out of the room, I'm going to examine Lucienne.' The boy burst out
> laughing. 'You can do that just as well with me here . . . And why
> examine? You were here only the day before yesterday. That costs for an
> extra visit, eh?' 'Brother,' Ravic said calmly, 'you don't look as if you
> would pay it . . . And now, get out.' . . . The boy grinned and sprawled his
> legs comfortably. He wore tapered patent leather shoes and violet socks.
> 'Please, Bobo,' Lucienne said. 'I'm sure it will only take a moment.' Bobo
> did not pay any attention to her. He stared at Ravic . . . [and] . . . said, 'If
> you think you can bleed us for hospital bills, operations and all that –
> nothing doing! We didn't ask to have her sent to the hospital – not to
> mention the operation . . . You ought to be glad we don't ask for
> compensation! For an unauthorized operation.[80]

The scene ends in a brief scuffle. Bobo makes a clumsy attempt to garrote the doctor,
but Ravic, by far the stronger of the two, has no difficulty pushing the pimp out of

the room and locking the door behind him. Bobo evidently decides to decamp and is nowhere to be seen when the doctor emerges.[80]

The terms 'class-struggle', 'confrontation' and 'litigation' do not occur in Deeping's *Sorrell and Son*[81] but these problems clearly worry Dr Maurice Pentreath, a family doctor in 'Millchester', who has been treating a young girl for a broken wrist. The child's father, Pentreath's chauffeur, has made no overt threats as yet, but he has emitted a few hints that he considers Dr Pentreath's treatment inappropriate. Pentreath, 'a nervous fumbler' and procrastinator, does not want to lose face by formally obtaining a second opinion from a senior colleague, and, instead, tries to arrange a 'chance encounter' between the little girl and his old medical school friend, Christopher (Kit) Sorrell, now a prominent London surgeon.[81] Pentreath takes the affair so seriously that he makes a pre-emptive trip to London to arrange the consultation with Sorrell. Warwick Deeping, who tells this story in considerable detail, had graduated in medicine.[82]

Henpecked Pentreath is a sorry figure of a doctor. His knowledge of medicine is minimal and his ability to make logical decisions is non-existent. In front of Sorrell he cringes and whines.

> 'I can't make up my mind.' 'Whether there was a fracture?' 'Oh yes, there was a fracture. I had it X-rayed. But whether I –' 'Didn't you have it X-rayed again?' 'No.' 'My dear old chap, why not?' 'Simply – because I was afraid – afraid of what I might see.' He gave Christopher a mute and deprecating look.[81]

Sorrell decides to accept Pentreath's invitation to spend a weekend as Pentreath's house guest. On his arrival, he is met at the train station by the mistrustful chauffeur. If Pentreath is perceived as a somewhat contemptible character, the chauffeur who has the temerity to question a doctor's judgement is seen as a poisonous species of vermin.

> The fellow at the wheel was a rodent, a nasty, acute little man with . . . bright, insolent, treacherous little eyes. Sorrell was determined to speak to this villain just long enough to ensure that he would bother Pentreath no further.[81]

At the appointed time, Sorrell strolls into Pentreath's office, pretending to be looking for a medical journal and 'happening' to see the chauffeur, his daughter and Pentreath, he approaches the group.

> 'Anything interesting?' . . . 'A Colles. Care to have a look? We're rather proud of our pet fracture, aren't we, Gladys?' The little girl simpered and her father made a scraping sound with his feet, a sound of potential protest.

Sorrell is satisfied with the result. There is indeed a mild deformity, but wrist and finger movements are normal. Pentreath had done a reasonable job.

> He patted the girl's wrist. 'Very nice – very nice.' Instinct warned him that the father was about to say something and he did say something in a

little acid, threatening voice. 'What's that lump there?' 'That? Bone, my friend.' 'There wasn't no lump like it before.' 'Exactly, said Kit, 'and now you are wiser.' 'I don't know what you gentlemen think but it looks all wrong to me.'

The conversation continues a little longer with Sorrell talking about the healing process in bone and about plumbers' joints but in essence informing the chauffeur that he regards him as an ignorant lout. Pentreath is full of gratitude when he accompanies Sorrell to the railway station the next day. The two doctors walk up and down the Millchester platform.

'Nothing more to suggest about that case?' Christopher stood watching the engine of the incoming train. 'No,' he said slowly. 'Nothing. But at the next convenient opportunity I should sack your chauffeur.'[81]

Francis Brett Young's Dr Jonathan Dakers[83] and AJ Cronin's Dr Andrew Manson[84] both refuse to write medical certificates for trade unionists, who are perceived as 'socialist agitators' and malingerers. Young's patient

a plausible and fluent malingerer . . . with symptoms that simulated sciatica, [was] craftily polite to Jonathan. Until his turn came he had been boasting loudly to the other patients about his racing pigeons and whippets. In Jonathan's presence he was mild as milk; a decent down-right fellow, disappointed at being unfit for work.[83]

Cronin's patient

was a great lump of a man, rolling in fat who smelt strongly of beer and looked as if he'd never done a day's work in his life. 'Certificate' he said without minding his manners. 'What for?' Andrew asked. 'Stagmus.' Even from a cursory inspection he felt that Chenkin had no nystagmus.[84]

A shouting match results in each case, but there is no physical violence.[83,84] The writers, both of them physicians, are clearly in sympathy with the honest, hard-working doctors who protect society from lazy and corrupt unionists. These undeserving characters, unable to speak the 'King's English', are nevertheless sufficiently cunning to defraud their employers.

Simenon is more subtle in handling a description of a dishonest demand for a medical certificate.[85] Dr Bergelon has assisted at an obstetric disaster during the night – mother and child both died – but the doctor is now back in his office, seeing the usual assortment of patients.

'What's the trouble, Madame Barmat?' 'It's about a medical certificate for my husband. He couldn't get out of bed this morning . . . He still has those dreadful stomach pains.' This was a lie. Her husband had nothing at all the matter with him, but he had decided to repaint the whole of the inside of his house while continuing to draw his wages. Only yesterday he would have refused,[85] but the catastrophic events of the night have made him less inclined to identify with the 'establishment'. Monsieur Barmat is recommended for leave of absence on medical grounds.[85]

On the other hand Reade's opera singer, who is thinking of canceling her contract, has no doubt she will be able to obtain an appropriate medical certificate. She is well aware 'how readily a doctor's certificate can be had to say or swear that the great creature cannot sing or act without peril to life'.[86]

Actual physical fights between non-psychotic, non-criminal, sober adults and their physicians are particularly rare, and only one such brawl was found.[87] Robert ('Herb') Berquam, the 'rebellious' father of a dying child in Glasser's *Ward 402*, who assaults the intern and resident of his dying child, is not intrinsically a nasty character. Berquam, a senior medical technologist who is knowledgeable but lacks power and status, initially decides to let Mary, his leukemic daughter, 'die in peace' without submitting her to chemotherapy protocols. He is now incensed against the doctors at the University Hospital who talked him out of his original decision, especially when, after a very brief remission, Mary develops meningitis, generalized purpura and a cardiac arrest. During a dramatic night she is resuscitated but she remains unconscious and when the parents arrive early the next morning they are dismayed by her sudden deterioration.[87] Despite his wife's plea for calm, Berquam loses his temper with the intern who is telling the story.

> He seized [his wife's] hand and dragged her over to the bed. 'Look at your child. See what they've done to her.' He pulled back the sheet. 'Go on, look at her.' . . . I grabbed the sheet from his hand. 'What the hell . . .' 'Shut up,' he hissed through clenched teeth. His wife was sobbing now . . . 'Berquam,' I said, 'I want you out of here. Just get the hell out of here. Now.' 'Why you arrogant young –' . . . I got my arm up but his fist skidded off my forearm and caught me on the side of the jaw.[87]

The fighting becomes more intense when the resident enters the room and tries to separate the combatants. He subsequently requires sutures and the father of another child, who tries to help Berquam, sustains a broken nose. The fight might have been avoided if someone had succeeded in notifying the Berquams of Mary's cardiac arrest before they left for the hospital. The symbolic seizure of the sheet should obviously not have resulted in a counter-seizure and in a territorial conflict between an angry father and an exhausted intern.[87]

Summary

Despite declarations to the contrary, the doctor–patient relationship is strongly influenced by the relative social positions of the parties. Physicians attending rich and powerful patients develop a degree of subservience, which only some manage to overcome. The poor and marginalized raise 'antibodies' in their physicians. Members of various subgroups do not feel bound by the usual obligations governing the doctor–patient relationship. In developed countries the medical code of behavior works best as a contractual arrangement between equals.

References

1 Brieux E (1902) Damaged Goods. In: *Three Plays by Brieux*. Translated by Pollock J. Brentanos, New York, 1911, pp. 185–254.

2 James H (1881) *Washington Square*. Bantam Books, New York, 1959, p. 125.

3 Bennett A (1923) *Riceyman Steps*. Cassell, London, 1947, pp. 271–81.

4 Snow CP (1958) The Conscience of the Rich. In: Snow CP (1972) *Strangers and Brothers*, vol. 1. Charles Scribner's Sons, New York, p. 720.

5 Young FB (1938) *Dr Bradley Remembers*. Heinemann, London, pp. 242–5.

6 Rinehart MR (1935) *The Doctor*. Farrar and Rinehart, New York, p. 41.

7 Eliot G (1871–2) *Middlemarch*. Penguin, London, 1988, p. 327.

8 Snow CP (1970) Last Things. In: Snow CP (1972) *Strangers and Brothers*, vol. 3. Charles Scribner's Sons, New York, pp. 731–53.

9 Snow CP (1968) The Sleep of Reason. In: Snow CP (1972) *Strangers and Brothers*, vol. 3. Charles Scribner's Sons, New York, pp. 388–417.

10 Tolstoy L (1886) The Death of Ivan Ilych. In: Simmons EJ (ed.) (1966) *Leo Tolstoy, Short Novels*. Translated by Maude L and Maude A. Random House, New York, p. 47.

11 James PD (1971) *Shroud for a Nightingale*. Sphere Books, London, 1988, pp. 277–8.

12 Smollett T (1771) *The Expedition of Humphry Clinker*. Knapp LM (ed.) (1971) Oxford University Press, London, p. 5.

13 Warren S (1832) Rich and Poor. In: Warren S. *Diary of a Late Physician*, vol. 2. Blackwood, Edinburgh, pp. 223–43.

14 Mitchell SW (1901) *Circumstance*. Century Company, New York, 1902, pp. 126–31.

15 Dickens C (1859) *A Tale of Two Cities*. Oxford University Press, London, 1988, pp. 394–406.

16 Dickens C (1849–50) *David Copperfield*. Signet Books, New York, 1962, pp. 21–4.

17 Dickens C (1837) *The Pickwick Papers*. Signet Classics, New American Library, New York, 1964.

18 Shaw GB (1906) The Doctor's Dilemma. In: *The Bodley Head Bernard Shaw, Collected Plays with their Prefaces*, vol. 3. Max Reinhardt, The Bodley Head, London, 1971, pp. 295–6.

19 Mann T (1901) *Buddenbrooks*. Translated by Lowe-Porter HT. Penguin, Harmondsworth, 1957, p. 29.

20 O'Brian P (1992) *The Truelove*. WW Norton, New York, pp. 15–35.

21 Tolstoy AK (1865) The Death of Ivan the Terrible. In: Noyes GR (ed.) (1961) *Masterpieces of the Russian Drama*. Translated by Noyes GR. Dover Publications, New York, 1961, vol. 2, Act IV, Scene II, p. 514.

22 Ibid., Act V, Scene I, pp. 533–4.

23 Pushkin AS (1830) The Postmaster. In: Yarmolinsky A (ed.) (1936) *The Poems, Prose and Plays of Alexander Pushkin*. Translated by Keane T. Modern Library, New York, p. 523.

24 Solzhenitsyn A (1968) *Cancer Ward*. Translated by Bethell N and Burg D. Bodley Head, London, 1970, pp. 57–8.

25 Cohen A (1982) *Angel of Vengeance*. Quartet Crime, London, pp. 85–9.

26 Russell R (1985) *While You're Here, Doctor*. Souvenir Press, London.

27 Ibid., pp. 8–11.

28 Ibid., pp. 202–5.

29 Duhamel G (1928) *Les Sept Dernières Plaies*. Mercure de France, Paris, pp. 25–31.

30 Maugham WS (1940) Lord Mountdrago. In: Maugham WS (1975) *Collected Short Stories*, vol. II. Pan Books, London, pp. 268–89.

31 Warren RP (1946) *All the King's Men*. Modern Library, New York, 1953, pp. 269–75.

32 Ibid., p. 343.

33 Ibid., p. 420.

34 Molière JBP (1666) The Physician in Spite of Himself. In: *The Plays of Molière*, vol. 5. Translated by Waller AR. John Grant, Edinburgh, 1926, pp. 154–5.

35 Fielding H (1749) The History of Tom Jones – a Foundling. In: Stephen S (ed.) (1882) *The Works of Henry Fielding*. Smith Elder, London, vol. 1, Book 7, Chapter 13, pp. 359–61.

36 Ibid., Book 8, Chapter 3, pp. 390–3.

37 Bashford HH (1911) *The Corner of Harley Street: being some familiar correspondence of Peter Harding MD*. Constable, London, 1913, pp. 66–70.

38 Mitchell SW, op. cit., p. 207.

39 Ibid., p. 267.

40 Ibid., p. 364.

41 Hill J (1987) The doctor as hero in nineteenth century British fiction. *The Pharos of Alpha Omega Alpha*. 50: 31–3.

42 Piercy M (1982) *Braided Lives*. Summit Books, New York, p. 189.

43 Orwell G (1946) How the Poor Die. In: Orwell G (1968) *Collected Essays, Journalism and Letters*, vol. 4. Secker and Warburg, London, pp. 223–33.

44 French M (1977) *The Women's Room*. Andre Deutsch, London, 1978, pp. 51–3.

45 Mitchell SW (1885) *In War Time*. Century Company, New York, 1913, p. 60.

46 Hasek J (1921–3) *The Good Soldier Svejk*. Translated by Parrott C. Penguin, Harmondsworth, 1981, pp. 69–77.

47 Wharton W (1978) *Birdy*. Jonathan Cape, London, 1979, pp. 24–5.

48 Ibid., p. 131.

49 Glasser RJ (1971) *365 Days*. George Braziller, New York, pp. 10–11.

50 Schneiderman LJ (1976) *Sea Nymphs by the Hour*. Authors' Guild Back-inprint.Com, Lincoln, NE, 2000, pp. 16–18.

51 Ibid., p. 36.

52 Le Sage AR (1715) *The Adventures of Gil Blas de Santillana*, vol. 1. Translated by Smollett T. World's Classics, Oxford University Press, London, 1907, pp. 116–17.

53 Martineau H (1839) *Deerbrook*. Virago Press, London, 1983, p. 297.

54 Ibid., pp. 318–23.

55 Hellerstein D (1986) Children of the Valley. In: Hellerstein D. *Battles of Life and Death*. Houghton Mifflin, Boston, MA, pp. 49–66.

56 Macharia WM, Leon G, Rowe BH, Stephenson BJ and Haynes RB (1992) An overview of interventions to improve compliance with appointment keeping for medical services. *JAMA*. **267**: 1813–17.

57 Pesata V, Pallija G and Webb AA (1999) A descriptive study of missed appointments. Families' perceptions of barriers to care. *J Ped Health Care*. **13**: 178–82.

58 Brown KA, Shetty V, Delarahim S, Belin T and Leathers R (1999) Correlates of missed appointments in orofacial surgery patients. *Oral Surgery, Oral Medicine, Oral Pathology, Oral Radiology and Endodontics* **87**: 405–10.

59 Hellerstein D (1986) The Battle for the Dead. In: Hellerstein D. *Battles of Life and Death*. Houghton Mifflin, Boston, MA, pp. 121–38.

60 Sheldon S (1994) *Nothing Lasts Forever*. HarperCollins, London, pp. 50–1.

61 Shem S (1978) *The House of God*. Richard Marek, New York, pp. 218–19.

62 Alexander H (2000) *Solemn Oath*. Bethany House Publishers, Minneapolis, MN, p. 277.

63 Hailey A (1984) *Strong Medicine*. Dell, New York, 1986, pp. 51–2.

64 Fitzgerald FS (1925) The Great Gatsby. In: Mizener A (ed.) (1963) *The Fitzgerald Reader*. Charles Scribner's Sons, New York, p. 183.

65 Rosenbaum EE (1988) *The Doctor* (also titled *A Taste Of My Own Medicine*). Ivy Books, New York, 1991, p. 88.

66 Plutarch (2nd century AD) Pericles. In: *Plutarch's Lives*, vol. 1. Translated by Dryden J. Modern Library, New York, 2001, p. 230.

67 Céline LF (1932) *Journey to the End of the Night*. Translated by Manheim R. New Directions, New York, 1983, p. 359.

68 Hellerstein D (1986) Fire in the Hills. In: Hellerstein D. *Battles of Life and Death*, Houghton Mifflin, Boston, MA, pp. 35–45.

69 Shem S, op. cit., pp. 37–8.

70 Thompson M (1955) *Not as a Stranger*. Michael Joseph, London, pp. 353–5.

71 Williams WC (1938) The Use of Force. In: *The Farmers' Daughters*. New Directions, New York, 1961, pp. 131–5.

72 Céline LF, op. cit., pp. 234–5.

73 Delany SR (1967) Corona. In: *Distant Stars*. Bantam Books, New York, 1981, pp. 65–86.

74 Mitchell SW (1885) *In War Time*. The Century Company, New York, 1913, pp. 242–3.

75 Ibid., pp. 323–6.

76 Levenkron S (1978) *The Best Little Girl in the World*. Penguin, London, 1988, pp. 63–80.

77 Williams M (1974) *Florence Copley of Romney*. Collins, Sydney.

78 Ibid., p. 39.

79 Ibid., p. 170.

80 Remarque EM (1945) *Arch of Triumph*. Translated by Sorell W and Lindley D. Appleton Century, New York, pp. 110–14.

81 Deeping W (1925) *Sorrell and Son*. Cassell, London, 1927, pp. 299–307.

82 Moynihan BGA (Lord Moynihan) (1936) *The Story of Those Who Deserted Medicine, Yet Triumphed.* University Press, Cambridge, p. 108.

83 Young FB (1928) *My Brother Jonathan.* Heinemann, London, p. 221.

84 Cronin AJ (1937) *The Citadel.* Gollancz, London, p. 136.

85 Simenon G (1941) The Country Doctor. In: Simenon G (1980) *The White Horse Inn and Other Novels.* Translated by Ellenbogen E. Hamish Hamilton, London, pp. 229–30.

86 Reade C (1877) *A Woman Hater.* Chatto and Windus, London, 1894, p. 226.

87 Glasser RJ (1973) *Ward 402.* Garnstone Press, London, 1974, pp. 192–7.

CHAPTER 11

The physician in court

Physicians appear in court, as physicians, for two major reasons: they act as expert witnesses, providing evidence on behalf of one of the parties in civil or criminal cases. More dramatically, they stand accused of malpractice, facing heavy fines, loss of reputation and deregistration. Doctors confronted by criminal charges relating to euthanasia and abortion will be discussed in Volume 3.

The doctor as expert witness

True leaders of the profession, who dislike vulgar publicity, keep away from the law as far as possible, so that lawyers casting around for 'medical experts' frequently finish up with third and fourth raters. They may even be forced to choose alcoholic physicians, who are no longer able to work in a regular medical occupation, and who become habitual witnesses, presumably because the required bouts of sobriety are relatively brief. Grisham's attorney Jake Brigance[1] spends many anxious hours agonizing over whether Dr Bass, a drunkard with psychiatric training, and a caricature of a key expert, will be fit to testify on the appropriate day.[1] At the trial, opposing council wastes no time before emphasizing the lowly professional status of this 'authority'.[2]

> 'Dr Bass, in your opinion, are you an expert in the field of psychiatry?' . . .
> 'Yes.' 'Have you ever taught psychiatry?' 'No.' 'Have you ever published
> any articles in psychiatry?' 'No.' 'Have you ever published any books
> on psychiatry?' 'No.' . . . 'What hospital positions do you . . . hold, as of
> today? 'None.'[2]

The witness is also asked whether he has ever been an office holder in a professional or scientific association, a question which he answers in the negative.[2] Grisham is not particularly sympathetic towards Dr Bass. Apart from the redundant and rhetorical question whether a person who has never published a journal article might have written an entire book, the doctor deserves his rough treatment.

Another type of expert, more difficult to denigrate and intimidate in the witness box, is the university professor who, instead of leading and guiding his colleagues, becomes a political opportunist and a negative role model. His professional status among his peers is minimal, while his academic achievements (such as they are) stem largely from the efforts of his assistants.[3] Whether from pecuniary motives or from a desire to revenge himself on his colleagues who refuse to recognize the importance of his work, this type now spends a good deal of time as an expert witness in medico-legal cases. McGee's Professor Christopher Jones,[3,4] who still occupies his chair, but supplements his income by giving evidence against his colleagues, is portrayed as an irritating pest. Jones' credibility suffers substantial damage when evidence is presented that in a recent grant application he resorted to a considerable degree of exaggeration. To the reader's great satisfaction, the opposing lawyer asks rhetorically: 'You embellished the truth for the sake of money?'

Three medical 'experts' give evidence in *Anatomy of a Murder*.[5] One is totally discredited, one is considered reliable by both sides while the third, despite his strongly held and controversial views, speaks with sufficient assurance to sway the jury. Dr Adelord Dompierre, a semi-retired practitioner and part-time physician to the county jail, has a most uncomfortable time on the stand.[6] The doctor, whose main occupation consists of treating the jail inmates for symptoms of acute drug and alcohol withdrawal, has been called upon to perform a vaginal examination to determine whether or not the victim has been raped. While giving evidence, Dompierre reveals that he has obtained some four or five vaginal swabs in ten years and that his knowledge of gynecology is rudimentary.[6]

Dr Homer Raschid, a pathologist, presents the autopsy findings and apart from a lapse into technical jargon, his presentation is straightforward and he emerges relatively unscathed.[7]

Dr Matthew Smith, on the other hand, the psychiatrist who testifies that the defendant is insane,[8] functions brilliantly during an intense and hostile cross-examination. He is asked why he has not performed certain personality tests.

> 'Because I felt they were not indicated . . . I may add, sir that I belong to the school of psychiatry that tends to stress individual study and appraisal rather than to that group that has sometimes lightly been referred to as the slot machine . . . school of psychiatry.'[8]

When the doctor is asked what particular part of his personality assessment is the most important, he does not fall into the trap of dissecting various factors from one another and then having to face a challenge on each character trait. He very cleverly declares that he cannot divide his opinion into discrete components. 'Separating . . . part from part would destroy the significance of individual parts like adding dimples or removing the smile from the Mona Lisa.'[8]

Litigation against doctors

Unlike medical expert witnesses who are interesting rather than exciting figures, the doctor as the defendant becomes a culprit or a victim, and the reader, especially the medical reader, becomes emotionally involved in the court drama.

Remarkably, malpractice suits, which have become a major industry in the real world,[9–11] are relatively rare in fictional literature. When litigation is mentioned, it features as a threat rather than an actual event. In one of the earliest hospital novels,[12] Freya Sullivan, who has been admitted for a breast biopsy, contemplates litigation within hours of climbing into her bed. 'They probably think that when it comes to ward patients they can get away with murder . . . If there's any scar . . . I'll sue the hospital or the doctor or both.'[13] (The biopsy proves malignant, Freya goes on to a radical mastectomy with its disfiguring results, but there is no further talk of litigation.)

Members of the Tabbernoy family in Green's *The Last Angry Man*[14] at least have some cause for threatening litigation. Dr Harry Hemitz, their ruthless and aggressive surgeon, breaks a needle while giving old Mrs Tabbernoy a postoperative injection and a further surgical operation is required to extract the pointed end from the old lady's posterior. Hemitz, who does not argue with his patients, is quite dismissive about the possibility of any legal action. His lawyer contacts the manufacturers, who freely admit that a small number of their needles are defective, and claim there is no way of testing them before they are used on a patient. The manufacturers and Dr Hemitz are insured but no malpractice suit eventuates.[14]

In Paretsky's *Toxic Shock*[15] the threat of a malpractice suit against a doctor is used as straightforward blackmail. Mrs Portis, a disgruntled patient and the mother of Amanda Portis, has clearly dreamt up her baseless accusation of sexual assault against Dr Lotty Herschel. The matter would normally not go any further but Gustav Humbolt, a scheming industrial tycoon,[15] has somehow 'discovered' this patient and uses her to threaten the doctor and her friend, Detective Victoria Warshawski.

> 'This is Mrs Portis, Ms Warshawski. Her daughter was a patient of Dr Herschel. Isn't that right Mrs Portis?' She nodded vigorously. 'My Mandy. And Dr Herschel did what she should have known better than to do, a grown woman with a little girl. Mandy was crying and screaming when she came out of the examining room, it took me days to get her settled down and find out what went on. But when I found out.' . . .[15]

Humbolt threatens to find other worried mothers whose daughters Dr Herschel has treated. He predicts that a jury in an indecent assault case would consider Dr Herschel, who is almost sixty and has never married, with suspicion. 'A jury would be bound to suspect her sexual preferences.'[15] Dr Herschel's version is that Amanda Portis, who was eight at the time, was vomiting a lot and that the child's mother walked out in a huff because she did not like the suggestion that the symptoms might be psychological in origin. In the end, the matter dies a natural death when Mrs Portis loses interest in bringing charges against Dr Herschel.[15]

Legal actions against physicians, some quite unjustified, may originate as the result of a casual remark by a colleague. Susan Cheever[16] illustrates this scenario with the case of Mrs Matilda Loomis, who has been subjected to a vaginal hysterectomy in a suburban hospital. When the uterus is found to contain an endometrial carcinoma, she is referred to Dr Macklin Riley, an oncologist at the 'Parkinson Hospital and Cancer Center' (*see also* pp 66 and 183). Mrs Loomis' daughter Kate personally delivers the pathology slides to Dr Riley who asks for some clinical details.[16]

> 'Was your mother taking any estrogens? Any pills to help with postmenopausal symptoms?' 'Yes, one called Premarin, I think . . . Why?' 'Estrogens are associated with this disease in postmenopausal women but this particular kind of tumor responds very well to treatment.'

Kate loses no time in picking up the clue and assigning blame. Her mother's cancer was obviously due to the pills prescribed by the family doctor.

'Are you saying those pills may have caused the cancer? Dr Gross prescribed pills which may have made this happen?'

Dr Riley, whose terminology 'Estrogens are associated with this disease' is almost mischievous, defends his colleague in an inept and half-hearted way.

'It's a very routine prescription and we can't really tell. We didn't know about the connection between estrogen and endometrial cancer until recently – and of course it might have happened anyway.' 'Still.' 'Yes it may have been a mistake.'[16]

Kate and her mother are not particularly litigious. The word 'malpractice' is not mentioned and the reader is left with the impression that there would have been no legal action even if the outcome had been unfavorable. In the event, Mrs Loomis is given a course of radiotherapy and survives.[17]

Victims of a hostile system

When a malpractice suit goes to court, the doctors are generally innocent of any wrongdoing, but the scales are weighted against them and they tend to lose. Many authors, including Plato,[18] express their disapproval of a legal system, which is inappropriate for this kind of case. Plato ridicules the entire concept of litigation against physicians in a lay court, where the non-medical participants can have no understanding of the subtleties involved in clinical practice. In such a court, Plato remarks sarcastically, the counsel for the plaintiff is likely to have the expertise and the prejudices of a cook while members of the bench have the mentality of little boys deprived of their dessert. The doctor who has recommended painful and unpleasant measures, and now stands accused of unnecessary cruelty, is of course found guilty in such an atmosphere, but the process is a farce from beginning to end.[18]

Rider Haggard's Doctor Therne,[19] who is dragged into court on a criminal charge and then threatened with a civil action after a fatal case of 'puerperal sepsis', is obviously innocent. The court actions are entirely inappropriate and based on false and malicious evidence supplied by a jealous senior colleague.[19]

The dynamics of medical litigation are particularly well described by Ravin whose novels constitute some of the most true to life accounts of contemporary teaching hospitals. In Ravin's works[20,21] the motivation for malpractice suits consists largely of greed and anger while the court proceedings are meaningless charades conducted precisely along 'Platonic'[18] principles. One of Ravin's cases concerns the late Mr Sloan, who had died in 'Manhattan Hospital' of ischemic heart disease.[20]

Mr Sloan did not have much heart left. At forty-three he had already wiped out most of its underside, part of the anterior wall and some of the back part . . . Every walk to the bathroom left him drained and breathless. He did not have to be told how close death was. . . . His wife, however, could not believe what she could not accept. He looked a little tired to her but he could not be dying. If he was dying, it was Dr Cohen's fault. She was possessed by a desperate fury. Bad things meant someone was to blame. She had taken her husband to Dr Cohen, paid his prices because he was supposed to be the best heart man in New York. But he was failing as wretchedly as her husband's heart . . . Mrs Sloan was overtly hostile to anything in white. Ryan noticed her sitting alone in the cafeteria staring at the interns and residents from her husband's floor as they relaxed at dinner. They were laughing and not acting at all gloomy about her husband who was lying upstairs . . . When her husband infarcted what remained of his heart . . . Mrs Sloan refused an autopsy but she did subpoena his chart. Then she sued Cohen for killing her husband . . . 'Some people just can't accept random misfortune.' Cohen told Ryan. 'They've got to blame someone.'[20]

Two other malpractice suits described by Ravin[21] are farcical and bear no relation whatever to the quality of medical care. In one of them, the father of a child that had been run over by a drunken driver is suing Dr Brendan O'Brien. The driver, John Lockhart, is an insulin-dependent diabetic, whose application for a driver's license has been signed by Dr O'Brien. The parents of the dead child are now claiming damages from the doctor, who is here explaining the concepts of 'deep pockets' to his secretary:

'John Lockhart pumps gas for a living. He's got, maybe ten dollars to his name, less after payday when he hits the bars. He goes out and gets loaded and runs over some poor kid . . . The family goes to sue Lockhart and discovers he's uninsured and there is nothing to go after in his bank account. So they get a lawyer who says to John, "Look, this isn't your fault. You weren't drunk. You were in insulin coma. This is all your doctor's fault." Now John is most happy to learn this. And the family is most happy and, most of all, the lawyer is happy because they can all sue me. And I've got deep pockets. I've got malpractice insurance' . . . 'I cannot believe you're being sued because your alcoholic patient ran down some child. Surely they cannot hope to win?' 'They cannot lose. Try this before a jury of twelve retired postal workers . . . They sit there looking at the bereaved father and they look at me, a doctor with deep pockets.'[21]

Another equally senseless case concerns a Mrs Barbara Roundtree, who has a malignant pleural effusion and subsequently dies. The widower sues the hospital and Dr Freudenberg, the attending physician, implying that Freudenberg

just dumped Mrs Roundtree in the hospital and he flew in and out of her room every day and charged her a bundle for the hospital visits, but abandoned her to the care of . . . young interns, fresh out of medical school.[21]

Dr Freudenberg is dead but 'due process' continues with Brendan O'Brien being cross-examined in court about a thoracentesis he had performed during his residency days.

'Now Dr O'Brien, what exactly is a thoracentesis?' 'A needle is passed between the ribs to drain fluid from between the lungs and the covering of the lungs called pleura.' 'And what are the potential complications of this procedure?' 'Pneumothorax and laceration of the lung are the major risks.' 'And pneumothorax is what in English?' 'Pneumothorax is English.' 'Well what does it mean?' 'It refers to air collecting between the lungs and the chest wall.' 'Pneumothorax can be fatal can it not?'[21]

The charade goes on. The lawyer wants to know why a thoracentesis had been performed.

'Her medical condition required it.' 'How did you know that?' 'I examined her.' 'Did Dr Freudenberg examine her with you?' 'No.' 'Why not?' 'He was in his office and there was no time to waste.'

The interrogation continues along these lines. In the end the hospital (Dr O'Brien's employer at the time of the event) settles for half a million dollars.[21]

Much of McGee's *Misconceptions*[3] is devoted to the lengthy and medically irrelevant malpractice trial of Dr Julia Kent, who stands accused of mishandling the delivery of a severely retarded child (Brendan Edwards, son of Tracey Edwards). The facts, which are not in dispute, are summarized in one page.[22] Towards the end of Tracey's pregnancy, Julia is aware of the child's small size, but there are no other worrying features. Tracey is admitted to hospital when contractions begin 'a day before term', and, as a believer in 'natural' childbirth, she spends most of the labor period under the shower. The nurses monitor fetal heart rates through two contractions every half-hour, and find no abnormality. When the membranes rupture and meconium-stained liquor and bradycardia are noted, Tracey is brought out from the shower recess, she is placed on a bed and the fetal heart rate is now monitored electronically and continuously. Episodes of cardiac deceleration are confirmed and Dr Kent is notified. She arrives at the hospital within fifteen minutes and forthwith proceeds to perform an easy forceps delivery. When little Brendan makes his appearance, he obviously suffers from severe neurological problems. Now, at the age of five, he has the mental age of a one-year-old, he is spastic and has daily epileptic seizures.[22]

Throughout the four-week trial, each individual step in Tracey's labor is minutely and repeatedly examined for evidence of 'negligence', even though it is quite clear to all concerned that Julia is a conscientious and knowledgeable obstetrician and that every one of her decisions is 'correct'. The witnesses are asked the same questions, and, predictably, answer them in accordance with declared 'party lines'. Both the plaintiff's expert witnesses express the view that labor should have been induced at thirty-eight weeks and that the fetal heart rate should have been monitored continuously.[23,24] Not so, says one of the defense witnesses. Induction was not indicated and continuous monitoring unnecessary.[25] Are the child's neurological problems due to birth-associated asphyxia? Two of the plaintiff's witnesses have no doubt they are.[24,26] Three defense witnesses are equally certain that they are not.[25,27,28]

One almost finds oneself in sympathy with Julia's lazy and pompous trial lawyer, appropriately named 'St Jude',* who displays a distinct lack of interest in the clinical details.[29] During his first meeting with Julia

---

* St Jude is the patron saint of hopeless causes.

St Jude had taken three prolonged phone calls on unrelated matters, buzzed his secretary for a cappuccino . . . and read the form guide for the mid-week horse races, while pretending to look in a drawer for a file. He had yawned when she had tried to explain the tests available in late pregnancy to assess fetal well-being and scratched his crotch when she described the difference between a healthy small baby and an unhealthy one. But worst of all, he had still not read the painstaking and detailed report she'd written about the events surrounding Tracey Edwards' pregnancy and delivery. His questions made it obvious he knew nothing of what had gone on. When she hesitantly challenged him . . . he had simply waved his hands dismissively. He'd seen it all before, he said, and could run these cases with his eyes closed.[29]

St Jude's slovenliness and laziness are inexcusable, but he is right on one point. This type of case is not won or lost according to clinical minutiae such as doctors are likely to prepare for lawyers. The game is played according to the law of charades with a predictable win for the side that raises the biggest laugh or (as in this case) springs the biggest surprise on its opponents.

Another baseless malpractice case forms the theme of Denker's *The Physicians*.[30] The story is that of an immensely wealthy and powerful business tycoon (John Stewart Reynolds) who pursues a fellow in neonatology (Christopher Grant) with relentless hatred, because the young doctor is perceived to have made an incorrect clinical decision. The patient, Reynolds' infant grandson and 'the only male heir in the Reynolds family', has neonatal jaundice because his Rh-negative mother (Reynolds' daughter) had become sensitized during a previous pregnancy to a black man. That pregnancy was terminated, but Reynolds' daughter, on the instructions of her father, says nothing about the matter to any of her current doctors.[31] Dr Grant, who has to decide whether or not to perform an exchange transfusion on the little boy, whose serum bilirubin is not spectacularly elevated,[30] decides to use phototherapy instead, and the child's jaundice promptly subsides. Unfortunately at the age of four months the 'future President of the United States'[30] is found to be mentally and physically handicapped.[32] John Reynolds has to blame someone for this disaster and decides it is all Dr Grant's fault. He declares vindictively:

> 'Before I'm through with you, you'll regret the day you decided to go into medicine. . . . I'm going to sue you for malpractice. Five million dollars. I don't give a damn if I don't collect a dime as long as I destroy you. Then try to get an appointment at any other hospital . . . You are finished as far as medicine is concerned in this country.'[32]

The case drags on for weeks with the presentation of much irrelevant material concerning animal data,[33] Dr Grant's political activities and sympathies[34] and his alleged inexperience.[35] The real question is barely touched upon during the trial. The doctor has, in good faith, chosen one of two clinical options (*see* pp 157–8). Both constitute recognized forms of treatment and both may have ended in a catastrophe. Does the poor outcome make Dr Grant guilty of malpractice?[10] Throughout the story, the author and the readers are on the side of the impetuous and idealistic young doctor whose career is permanently impaired by the court case[32] even though Reynolds terminates the action and offers to make a public apology.[31] The message of the entire book is that medical litigation, especially when the motive is revenge, is a useless and potentially harmful charade, from which no one profits except slick lawyers.

In *Doctor on Trial*,[36] which has a very similar plot (powerful father, drug-addicted daughter, fatal ectopic pregnancy, revengeful proceedings against a competent resident, ultimate exoneration), Denker makes the same point: legal arguments in courtrooms and at disciplinary hearings bear little relation to medical problems faced by physicians in their offices or in hospitals. At the final hearing of the State Board of Professional Conduct one of the medical members remarks: 'We've had too damned much legal maneuvering and too little medicine . . . I . . . vote to dismiss all charges'.[37]

Doctors who deserve to be sued

All this does not imply that there are no instances of incompetent or negligent behavior, which in real life should and would attract the prompt attention of the legal profession. Aesop's dishonest ophthalmologist,[38] who is involved in a court action as a plaintiff, behaves criminally rather than non-professionally. He steals his patient's valuables while her eyes are bandaged and she now refuses to pay his fee.[38] He obviously does not deserve to win.

In *The Verdict*[39] Barry Reed takes the side of the patient (Deborah Ruth Rosen), who is successful in her medical malpractice suit. Deborah, who had eaten a large meal one hour before admission, is given a general rather than a spinal anesthetic for her caesarean section, she becomes anoxic due to inhalation of vomitus, and she sustains severe brain damage. The defendants are Dr Towler, a prominent gynecologist, a chief of anesthesiology and a prestigious Boston teaching hospital. Towler, despite his 'striking silver hair' and his demeanor, which suggests that he has 'other, more important appointments', is not impressive when giving evidence. He quibbles even in response to straightforward questions. When asked whether he was Deborah Ruth's doctor, Towler replies:

> 'She was referred to me. Her regular physician was Dr Sheldon Rabb.' . . .
> 'But when she was referred to you, she became your patient, did she not? You were her physician, were you not?' 'She was sent to me primarily on a consult.'[40]

This sort of nit-picking does not make a good impression. When Towler is asked at what time he was notified that Deborah Ruth was coming in, he becomes garrulous and is politely but firmly put in his place:

> 'As I recall, it was about four, four fifteen in the morning. I'd just finished a difficult caesarean and fortunately, I was in the hospital when my service –' 'Thank you, Doctor, but just the time.'[41]

The anesthetist's original error of judgement is compounded by criminal behavior on the part of one of his colleagues who alters the hospital records to make 'one hour' look like 'nine hours'. Largely on the basis of this attempted fraud, the jury finds in favor of the plaintiff, who is awarded a large sum of money.[39]

Multiple instances of medical malpractice apparently go unpunished even though some would have been actionable even in the nineteenth century. When Dr Charles Bovary operates on 'Hippolyte's' clubfoot[42] he certainly does not have the patient's 'informed consent' to the procedure, which is bungled so badly that it ends in a mid-thigh amputation. The thought does indeed occur to Bovary that the patient might sue, and he presents Hippolyte with two artificial legs (one for work, one for special occasions). If Hippolyte entertains any notions of litigation, this act of 'generosity' evidently dispels them.[42]

Dr Richard Mahony, who has mishandled a teenager's fractured femur, is now threatened with legal action by the outraged father.[43]

> 'You've got a boy of your own haven't you? What would you say, I'd like to know, if a bloody fraud calling himself a doctor had been and made him a cripple for life? . . . As fine a young chap as ever you see, tall and upstanding. And now . . . he'll never walk straight again but'll have to hobble on crutches with one leg four inches shorter than the other . . . But I'll settle you! . . . I'll put a stop to your going round maiming other people's children . . . I'll take it into court, by Jesus I will!'[43]

In the end there is no court case (except in Richard's wild nightmares). A more competent surgeon takes over the boy's management and he is able to 're-break and reset the limb'. Richard makes a suicide gesture and soon afterwards leaves 'Barambogie', where he is regarded as an eccentric and incompetent fool.[43]

Dr Feuermann in Schnitzler's *Professor Bernhardi*,[44] who dabbles in gynecology, faces a charge of culpable negligence because one of his patients has died under his care through 'a series of unfortunate accidents'. Feuermann, who lacks adequate training, is shown as a histrionic poltroon,[44] but his former chief, the Professor of Gynecology, assures Feuermann's colleagues that he will do everything in his power to have him exonerated.

Dr Bergelon, Simenon's *Country Doctor*,[45] and his consultant handle a confinement with extraordinary negligence. The mother and the infant both die (*see* pp 80 and 232) and the widower reacts by lodging an official complaint at the Public Prosecutor's Office and threatening Bergelon with violence. There is no prosecution and no violence. The widower and the doctor get drunk together[45] and in the end it is the widower who leaves town while the doctor takes over the abandoned mistress.[46]

Taggert Hodge in John Gardner's *The Sunlight Dialogues*[47] watches helplessly as two psychiatric attendants seize his schizophrenic wife 'roughly as if she were a criminal and forced her to her knees' (twice) in front of the doctor who wants to demonstrate that she has to obey him implicitly. The 'crazy' woman has enough sense to say 'You're not supposed to use force against me', but all Hodge can think of is whether or not to take her out of that particular institution. The thought of litigation against this outrageous behavior does not even occur to him.[47]

These incompetent malefactors are all punished, reprimanded or ridiculed but not taken to court. Bovary's wife comes to despise her husband,[42] she goes on to betray him and ultimately to destroy him.[48] Richard Mahony disintegrates physically and mentally.[43] Feuermann is acquitted but no patient comes near him.[49] Dr Bergelon's punishment consists of imprisonment in a stale marriage and in having to practice, for the rest of his life, the type of medicine he detests.[45,46] Gardner's brutal psychiatrist is ridiculed. A colleague asks him: 'Do you really believe you're God?'[47]

Presumably, legal action against a priestly figure[50] is considered incongruous. The fictional medical practitioner who offends against accepted codes of behavior receives poetic justice, but he is not punished in an ordinary court of law.

William Carlos Williams' Dr James Rivers,[51] who engages in medical malpractice on a heroic scale, is something of an exception; he seems to escape any form of retribution. *Old Doc Rivers* is a drug addict who disappears at crucial times, and whose surgical adventures sound reckless even by the standards applicable in a small New Jersey town during the first two decades of the twentieth century. He should have had his license revoked long before his eventual retirement,[51] but neither his outraged colleagues nor the families of his dead patients ever initiate any moves in that direction. Somehow, this colorful Falstaff-like figure in colorless surroundings is beyond correctional measures and mere litigation[51] (*see* also Book II, Chapter 7).

Summary

The testimony of doctors appearing as expert witnesses tends to be unimpressive in form and content, possibly because the leaders of the medical profession avoid legal proceedings as long as they can. The doctor as the defendant in a malpractice suit is the victim of a hostile system with the cards stacked heavily against him regardless of the quality of his medical practice. Many medical miscreants are punished by extrajudicial measures rather than in a court of law.

References

1 Grisham J (1989) *A Time to Kill*. Island Books (Dell Publishing), New York, 1992, p. 228.

2 Ibid., p. 439.

3 McGee T (2003) *Misconceptions*. Pan Macmillan, Sydney, p. 138.

4 Ibid., p. 382.

5 Traver R (1958) *Anatomy of a Murder*. Dell, New York, 1959.

6 Ibid., pp. 352–7.

7 Ibid., pp. 263–71.

8 Ibid., pp. 432–8.

9 Brennan TA, Sox CM and Burstin HR (1996) Relation between negligent adverse events and the outcomes of medical malpractice litigation. *N Engl J Med*. **335**: 1963–7.

10 Mohr JC (2000) American medical malpractice: litigation in historical perspective. *JAMA*. **283**: 1731–7.

11 Studdert DM and Brennan TA (2001) No-fault compensation for medical injuries: the prospect for error prevention. *JAMA*. **286**: 217–23.

12 Fearing K (1939) *The Hospital*. Ballantine Books, New York.

13 Ibid., pp. 22–3.

14 Green G (1956) *The Last Angry Man*. Charles Scribner's Sons, New York, pp. 324–9.

15 Paretsky S (1988) *Toxic Shock* (also titled *Blood Shot*). Penguin, London, 1990, pp. 313–16.

16 Cheever S (1987) *Doctors and Women*. Methuen, London, 1988, pp. 13–14.

17 Ibid., p. 239.

18 Plato (4th century BC) *Gorgias*. Translated by Lamb WRM. Loeb's Classical Library, Heinemann, London, 1967, p. 515.

19 Haggard HR (1898) *Doctor Therne*. Hodder and Stoughton, London, 1923, pp. 81–117.

20 Ravin N (1981) *MD*. Delacorte Press, Seymour Lawrence, New York, pp. 346–7.

21 Ravin N (1989) *Mere Mortals*. MacDonald, London, 1990, pp. 290–305.

22 McGee T, op. cit., p. 57.

23 Ibid., p. 383.

24 Ibid., pp. 405–7.

25 Ibid., p. 436.

26 Ibid., p. 360.

27 Ibid., p. 427.

28 Ibid., p. 431.

29 Ibid., p. 244.

30 Denker H (1975) *The Physicians: a novel of malpractice*. WH Allen, London, pp. 23–33.

31 Ibid., pp. 378–81.

32 Ibid., pp. 58–63.

33 Ibid., p. 291.

34 Ibid., p. 250.

35 Ibid., p. 225.

36 Denker H (1992) *Doctor on Trial*. William Morrow, New York.

37 Ibid., p. 348.

38 Aesop (approx. 570 BC) *The Complete Fables*. Translated by Temple O and Temple R. Penguin, London, 1998, p. 69.

39 Reed B (1980) *The Verdict*. Simon and Schuster, New York.

40 Ibid., pp. 157–8.

41 Ibid., p. 161.

42 Flaubert G (1857) *Madame Bovary*. Translated by Steegmuller F. Modern Library, New York, 1982, pp. 196–210.

43 Richardson HH (1917–29) *The Fortunes of Richard Mahony*. Penguin, London, 1990, pp. 716–37.

44 Schnitzler A (1912) *Professor Bernhardi*. Translated by Landstone H. Faber and Gwyer, London, 1927, pp. 36–45.

45 Simenon G (1941) The Country Doctor. In: Simenon G. *The White Horse Inn and Other Novels*. Translated by Ellenbogen E. Hamish Hamilton, London, 1980, pp. 227–36.

46 Ibid., pp. 323–5.

47 Gardner J (1972) *The Sunlight Dialogues*. Ballantine Books, New York, 1973, pp. 254–7.

48 Flaubert G, op. cit., pp. 386–8.

49 Schnitzler A, op. cit., p. 136.

50 Norris CB (1969) The Image of the Physician in Modern American Literature. PhD dissertation, University of Maryland.

51 Williams WC (1932) Old Doc Rivers. In: *The Doctor Stories*. New Directions, New York, 1984, pp. 13–41.

Conclusions

The principal message emerging from this study is the astonishing continuity of the doctor–patient relationship, as described in fictional literature, across geographic and historical boundaries. When this relationship is suboptimal, the patients' complaints of two thousand years ago seem almost identical with those heard in the twenty-first century.

The incongruity of medical fees and the patients' resentment against them are mentioned in classical and biblical literature. The constant and conflicting demands for the doctor's time were evidently a problem in the seventeenth and eighteenth centuries and continue to plague the resident staff in contemporary hospital novels. Some of Plato's doctors, like their modern successors, lacked communication skills. While the white coat is a relatively modern invention, the doctor's mode of dress has been a subject for discussion since the time of Hippocrates. Doctors used medical jargon, particularly exotic and foreign terms, in Roman times, irritating some of their patients while impressing others.

Despite the massive changes in the perception of the etiology of diseases, and the profound improvement in treatment, the basic relationship between the patient, who wants help, and the doctor, who is willing and able to provide such help, remains unchanged. Questions concerning the degree of the doctor's emotional involvement, and whether or not the patients should be provided with 'the truth', are likely to remain unanswerable.

The idealistic notion that all patients, regardless of their social status, should be treated equally is manifestly impractical and is treated as such over the centuries.

The resentment against the doctor's perceived greed, his arrogance and his failure to deliver, rarely turns into open confrontation except in the case of patients with restricted responsibilities, such as children, psychotics and inebriates. Litigation is perceived as a threat rather than an actual event. When a case actually goes to court, the doctor is portrayed as a victim of a hostile system.

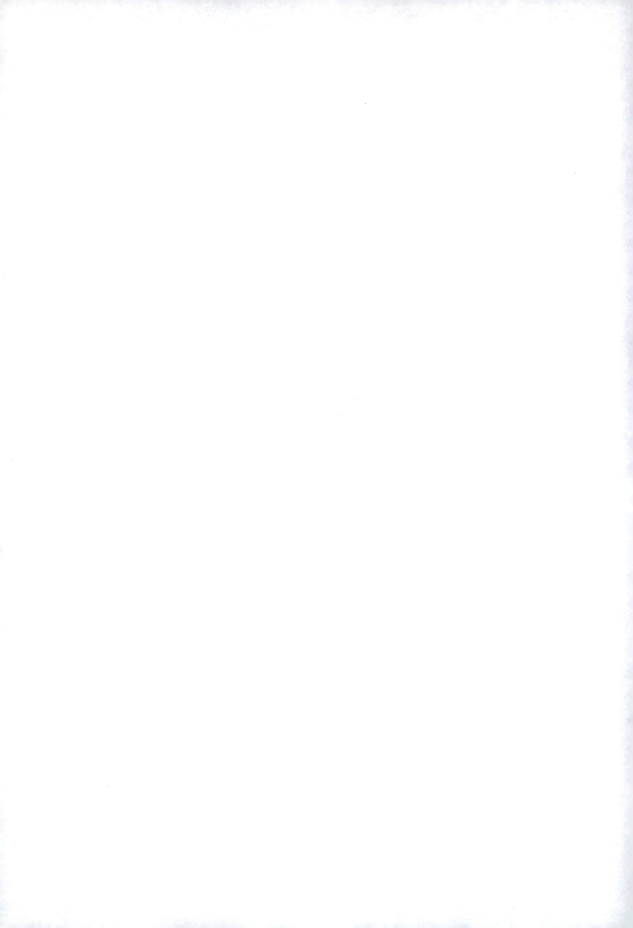

Bibliography

Primary sources

The dates in round brackets refer to the original publication of the work being quoted. An additional unbracketed date refers to the date of publication of the edition being used. The volume and page numbers refer to the publication being cited. The numbers in square brackets refer to the pages where the relevant citations appear in this book. For instance, Alcott's *Hospital Sketches* was first published in 1863, the edition being used for citation appeared in 1988, where the relevant extracts are found on pages 26–39. They are cited on pages 81 and 91 in this book.

Aesop (approx. 570 BC) *The Complete Fables*. Translated by Temple O and Temple R. Penguin, London, 1998, 262 pp.; p. 69 [p. 6, p. 246], p. 184 [p. 89, pp. 129–30].

Aiken, Conrad (1932) Silent Snow, Secret Snow. In: *Conrad Aiken, Collected Short Stories*. Schocken Books, New York, 1982, 566 pp.; pp. 216–35 [pp. 105–6].

Alcott, Louisa May (1863) Hospital Sketches. In: *Alternative Alcott*. Showalter, Elaine (ed.). Rutgers University Press, New Brunswick, 1988, 462 pp.; pp. 26–39 [p. 81, p. 91].

Alexander, Hannah (2000) *Solemn Oath*. Bethany House, Minneapolis, MN, 351 pp.; pp. 149–157, pp. 231–4, p. 277 [p. 158].

Ambler, Eric (1974) *Doctor Frigo*. Fontana Collins, Glasgow, 1976, 245 pp.; pp. 132–3, [p. 108], pp. 163–4 [pp. 137–8].

Amis, Kingsley (1974) *Ending Up*. Jonathan Cape, London, 176 pp.; pp. 8–10, pp. 76–80, pp. 84–5, pp. 161–3 [pp. 86–7].

Anonymous (1978) Doctor, Doctor, Come Here Quick. In: Turner, Ian, Factor, June and Lowenstein, Wendy. *Cinderella Dressed in Yella*. Heinemann Educational, Richmond, Victoria, Australia, 73 pp.; p. 15 [p. 121].

Anonymous (1987) Miss Polly had a Dolly. In: Pooley, Sarah. *A Day of Rhymes*. Knopf, New York, 75 pp.; p. 65 [p. 25].

Anonymous (1978) Miss Polly had a Dolly. In: Turner, Ian, Factor, June and Lowenstein, Wendy. *Cinderella Dressed in Yella*. Heinemann Educational, Richmond, Victoria, Australia, 173 pp.; p. 32 [p. 25].

Anonymous (15th century) *The Dance of Death*. Warren, Florence (ed.) Early English Text Society, Kraus Reprint Co., New York, 1971, vol. 181, 118 pp.; pp. 53–5 [p. 23].

Apuleius, Lucius (2nd century AD) *The Transformations of Lucius* (also titled *The Golden Ass*). Translated by Graves, Robert. Penguin, Harmondsworth, 1950, 298 pp.; pp. 246–7 [p. 6].

Aristophanes (388 BC) *The Plutus*. Translated by Rogers, Benjamin Buckley. Loeb's Classical Library, Heinemann, London, 1963, vol. III, 471 pp.; p. 399 [p. 23].

Ariyoshi, Sawako (1967) *The Doctor's Wife*. Translated by Hironaka, Wakako and Kostant, Ann Siller. Kodansha, Tokyo, 1989, 174 pp.; p. 76 [p. 7, p. 42].

Arlen, Michael (1924) *The Green Hat*. George H Doran, New York, 350 pp.; p. 221 [p. 105, p. 195].

Arnold, Matthew (1867) A Wish. In: Tinker, Chauncey Brewster and Lowry, Howard Foster (eds). Arnold Poetical Works, Oxford University Press, London, 1966, 509 pp.; pp. 249–51 [p. 111, p. 123].

Ashton, Helen (1930) *Doctor Serocold*. Penguin, London, 1936, 256 pp.; p. 10 [pp. 112–13, p. 145, p. 162].

Auden, Wystan Hugh (1972) The Art of Healing, In Memoriam David Protetch MD. In: Auden, Wystan Hugh. *Epistle to a Godson and Other Poems*. Faber and Faber, London, 72 pp.; pp. 13–15 [p. 10, p. 113, p. 128].

Auden, Wystan Hugh (1936) Miss Gee. In: Auden, Wystan Hugh. *Selections by the Author*. Penguin, Harmondsworth, 1970, 70 pp.; pp. 43–5 [p. 82, p. 110].

Babylonian Talmud (approx. 450 AD) Baba Kamma. Translated by Kirzner EW. Epstein I (ed.). Soncino Press, London, 1964, p. 85a [p. 33].

Balzac, Honoré de (1833) *The Country Doctor*. Translated by Marriage, Ellen. Dent, London, 1923, 287 pp.; p. 32 [p. 40, p. 92].

Balzac, Honoré de (1847) *Cousin Pons*. Translated by Hunt, Herbert J. Penguin, Harmondsworth, 1968, 354 pp.; p. 117 [p. 173, p. 190], pp. 172–3 [p. 43].

Balzac, Honoré de (1840) *Pierrette*. Translated by Ives, George B. George Barrie and Sons, Philadelphia, PA, 1897, 338 pp.; pp. 215–16 [p. 115, p. 175].

Balzac, Honoré de (1831) *The Wild Ass's Skin*. Translated by Marriage, Ellen. Dent, London, 1960, 239 pp.; pp. 199–201 [pp. 73–4].

Barnes, Djuna (1936) *Nightwood*. Faber and Faber, London, 1985, 239 pp.; p. 13, p. 29, pp. 54–8, p. 117–21, p. 164, p. 232 [p. 6].

Bashford, Henry Howarth (1911) *The Corner of Harley Street: being some familiar correspondence of Peter Harding MD*. Constable, London, 1913, 271 pp.; p. 13, p. 14, pp. 66–70, p. 74, pp. 76–7, p. 78, p. 201, p. 260 [p. 8, p. 35, p. 61, p. 112, pp. 131–2, p. 207, p. 221].

Baum, Vicki (1929) *Grand Hotel*. Translated by Creighton, Basil. Geoffrey Bles, London, 1930, 315 pp. [p. 8].

Baum, Vicki (1939) *Nanking Road* (also titled *Shanghai '37*). Translated by Creighton, Basil. Geoffrey Bles, London, 807 pp. [p. 4].

Beaumont, Francis and Fletcher, John (1621) The Tragedy of Thierry and Theodoret. In: *The Dramatic Works in the Beaumont and Fletcher Canon*. Cambridge University Press, Cambridge, 1976, vol. III, 612 pp.; Act II, Scene I, p. 397 [p. 8].

Beauvoir, Simone de (1964) *A Very Easy Death*. Translated by O'Brian, Patrick. Andre Deutsch and Weidenfeld and Nicolson, London, 1966, 106 pp.; pp. 21–2 [p. 72, p. 194].

Beckett, Samuel (1934) A Case in a Thousand. In: Gontarski SE (ed.) *Samuel Beckett: The Complete Short Prose 1929–1989*. Grove Press, New York, 1995, 294 pp.; pp. 18–24 [p. 7, pp. 157–8].

Bellaman, Henry (1940) *Kings Row*. Dymocks, Sydney, 1945, 504 pp.; pp. 254–5, pp. 395–415 [p. 6, p. 145].

Bellaman, Henry and Bellaman, Katherine (1948) *Parris Mitchell of Kings Row*. Simon and Schuster, New York, 333 pp.; p. 60 [p. 146].

Belloc, Hilaire (1940) *Selected Cautionary Verses*. Penguin, Harmondsworth, 1973, 185 pp.; pp. 23–4 [p. 24].

Bellow, Saul (1956) *Seize the Day*. Penguin, New York, 1996, 118 pp.; pp. 66–9 [p. 6].

Bennett, Arnold (1926) Lord Raingo. In: *The Arnold Bennett Omnibus Book*. Books for Libraries Press, Plainview, NY, 1975, 409 pp.; pp. 372–410 [pp. 134–5].

Bennett, Arnold (1908) *The Old Wives' Tale*. Hodder and Stoughton, London, 1964, 544 pp.; p. 453, pp. 461–3, pp. 465–6, p. 489 [p. 85, p. 149].

Bennett, Arnold (1923) *Riceyman Steps*. Cassell, London, 1947, 319 pp.; pp. 213–20, p. 230, pp. 245–64, pp. 265–70, pp. 271–81, p. 308 [p. 39, p. 73, pp. 153–4, p. 213].

Bernhard, Thomas (1978) Breath – A Decision. In: Bernhard T. *Gathering Evidence*. Translated by McLintock, David. Alfred A Knopf, New York, 1985, 340 pp.; pp. 240–1 [p. 73, p. 196, p. 209].

Bernhard, Thomas (1981) In the Cold. In: Bernhard T. *Gathering Evidence*. Translated by McLintock, David. Alfred A Knopf, New York, 1985, 340 pp.; p. 301 [p. 196].

Bernières, Louis de (1994) *Captain Corelli's Mandolin*. Vintage, London, 1998, 434 pp.; p. 119 [p. 4, p. 145].

The Bible, Revised Standard Version, Oxford University Press, New York, 1977.

   II Chronicles (approx. 4th century BC), 21: 18–19 [p. 111].

   Deuteronomy (approx. 7th century BC), 23: 18 [p. 32].

   Job (7th–4th century BC), 13: 4 [p. 201].

   II Kings (6th century BC), 5: 11 [p. 61].

   Luke (1st century AD), 8: 43 [p. 44].

   Mark (1st century AD), 5: 25–6 [p. 44].

   Matthew (1st century AD), 27: 24 [p. 110].

Blodgett, Ruth (1932) *Home is the Sailor*. Harcourt Brace, New York, 349 pp.; p. 289 [pp. 58–9].

Brand, Max (Frederick Faust) (1941) *Young Dr Kildare*. Ian Henry, Hornchurch, UK, 1977, 158 pp. [p. 149].

Brieux, Eugene (1902) Damaged Goods. In: *Three Plays by Brieux*. Translated by Pollock, John. Brentanos, New York, 1911, 333 pp.; pp. 185–254 [p. 153, p. 213].

Bronte, Charlotte (1853) *Villette*. Penguin, Harmondsworth, 1983, 622 pp.; pp. 161–5 [p. 184].

Bulwer-Lytton, Edward George Earle (Pisistratus Caxton, pseudonym) (1859) *What Will He Do With It?* Routledge and Sons, London, undated, vol. 1, 415 pp.; p. 211 [p. 129].

Burgess, Anthony (1960) *The Doctor is Sick*. Heinemann, London, 1968, 260 pp.; pp. 1–3 [p. 107].

Busch, Frederick (1984) A History of Small Ideas. In: Busch, Frederick. *Too Late American Boyhood Blues*. David R Godine, Boston, MA, 275 pp.; pp. 150–70 [pp. 37–8].

Busch, Frederick (1984) Rise and Fall. In: Busch, Frederick. *Too Late American Boyhood Blues*. David R Godine, Boston, MA, 275 pp.; p. 26, p. 41 [p. 114, p. 146].

Busch, Frederick (1979) *Rounds*. Farrar, Straus and Giroux, New York, 243 pp.; p. 38, pp. 80–81 [p. 67, p. 147].

Buzacott, Martin (1987) *Charivari*. Picador, Sydney, 251 pp.; pp. 200–6 [p. 156, p. 190].

Cable, George Washington (1885) *Dr Sevier*. James R Osgood and Company, Boston, MA, 473 pp., pp. 6–19, p. 102 [p. 41, p. 99, pp. 205–6].

Caldwell, Taylor (1968) *Testimony of Two Men*. Collins, London, 1990, 476 pp.; p. 348 [p. 34].

Camus, Albert (1947) *The Plague*. Translated by Gilbert, Stuart. Penguin, Harmondsworth, 1960, 252 pp.; pp. 75–6 [p. 64].

Cao Xue Qin (also spelt Tsao Hsueh Chin) (1791) *The Story of the Stone* (also titled *The Dream of the Red Chamber*). Translated by Hawkes, David. Penguin, Harmondsworth, 1973, 540 pp.; pp. 217–28 [p. 88].

Capek, Karel (1929) Giddiness. Translated by Selver, Paul. In: Capek, Karel. *Tales From Two Pockets*. Allen and Unwin, London, 1967, 215 pp. 177–83 [p. 163].

Capote, Truman (1966) In *Cold Blood, A True Account of a Multiple Murder and its Consequences*. Random House, New York, 343 pp.; p. 7, p. 29 [pp. 162–3].

Carossa, Hans (1931) *Doctor Gion*. Translated by Scott, Agnes Neill. Robert O Ballou, New York, 1933, 319 pp.; p. 16 [p. 122].

Céline, Louis Ferdinand (Louis-Ferdinand Destouches) (1932) *Journey to the End of the Night*. Translated by Manheim, Ralph. New Directions, New York, 1983, 446 pp.; pp. 209–11, pp. 227–8, pp. 234–5, p. 322, p. 353, p. 359 [p. 25, p. 31, pp. 42–3, p. 189, p. 227, p. 228].

Chandler, Raymond (1949) *The Little Sister*. Houghton Mifflin, Boston, MA, 249 pp.; p. 31, p. 53, pp. 134–5, pp. 235–6 [p. 4, p. 53, p. 195].

Chandler, Raymond (1953) *The Long Good-Bye*. Pan, London, 1979, 285 pp.; pp. 102–3 [p. 73, p. 195–6].

Chaucer, Geoffrey (approx. 1390) The Canterbury Tales. In: Fisher, John H (ed.) *The Complete Poetry and Prose of Geoffrey Chaucer*. Holt, Rinehart and Winston, New York, 1977, 1032 pp.; pp. 17–18 [p. 23, p. 24, p. 160].

Cheever, Susan (1987) *Doctors and Women*. Methuen, London, 1988, 240 pp.; pp. 13–14, p. 18, p. 21, pp. 43–5, pp. 182–7, p. 190, p. 197, pp. 210–13, p. 219, p. 229, pp. 236–8, p. 239 [p. 11, pp. 66–7, p. 76, pp. 182–3, pp. 241–2].

Chekhov, Anton Pavlovich (1888) An Awkward Business. In: *The Oxford Chekhov*. Translated by Hingley, Ronald. Oxford University Press, London, 1980, vol. 4, 287 pp.; pp. 99–115 [p. 100].

Chekhov, Anton Pavlovich (1898) A Case History. In: *The Oxford Chekhov*. Translated by Hingley, Ronald. Oxford University Press, London, 1975, vol. 9, 328 pp.; pp. 69–78 [p. 104].

Chekhov, Anton Pavlovich (1887) The Enemies (also titled Two Tragedies; also titled Antagonists). In: Chekhov, Anton Pavlovich. *Short Stories*. Translated by Fen, Elisaveta. Folio Society, London, 1974, 259 pp.; pp. 58–72 [p. 42].

Chekhov, Anton Pavlovich (1887–9) Ivanov. In: *The Oxford Chekhov*. Translated by Hingley, Ronald. Oxford University Press, London, 1967, vol. 2, 362 pp.; p. 170, p. 174, p. 191, p. 200, pp. 207–8, pp. 226–7 [pp. 177–8, p. 190].

Chekhov, Anton Pavlovich (1896) The Seagull. In: *The Oxford Chekhov*. Translated by Hingley, Ronald. Oxford University Press, London, 1967, vol. 2, 362 pp.; p. 250, pp. 270–1 [p. 178].

Chekhov, Anton Pavlovich (1900–1) Three Sisters. In: *The Oxford Chekhov*. Translated by Hingley, Ronald. Oxford University Press, London, 1964, vol. 3, 343 pp.; pp. 71–139, pp. 74–7, p. 113, p. 130 [p. 6, p. 194].

Chekhov, Anton Pavlovich (1892) Ward Number Six. In: *The Oxford Chekhov*. Translated by Hingley, Ronald. Oxford University Press, London, 1971, vol. 6, 316 pp.; p. 134 [p. 2].

Choromanski, Michael (1932) *Jealousy and Medicine*. Translated by Arthurton-Barker E. New Directions, Norfolk, CT, 1964, 216 pp.; p. 20, p. 38 [p. 129].

Clark, Brian (1972) *Whose Life Is It Anyway*. Amber Lane Press, Ashover, UK, 1978, 80 pp.; p. 11, p. 34, p. 52 [pp. 109–10, p. 137, p. 207].

Cobb, Irvin S (1915) Speaking of Operations. In: Zevin, Benjamin David (ed.) *Cobb's Cavalcade*. World Publishing Company, Cleveland, OH, 1945, 466 pp.; pp. 17–37 [p. 46, p. 55, p. 109].

Cohen, Anthea (1982) *Angel of Vengeance*. Quartet Crime, London, 160 pp.; pp. 85–9 [pp. 218–19].

Collins, Wilkie (1868) *The Moonstone*. Perennial Classics, Harper and Row, New York, 1965, 462 pp.; pp. 211–12 [p. 103, p. 126].

Conrad, Joseph (1902) *Heart of Darkness*. Penguin, London, 1988, 120 pp.; pp. 37–8 [p. 160].

Corris, Peter (1999) *The Other Side of Sorrow*. Bantam Books, Sydney, 216 pp.; pp. 105–11 [p. 8].

Cozzens, James Gould (1933) *The Last Adam*. Harcourt Brace and Company, New York, 301 pp.; p. 23, p. 35, pp. 36–40, p. 42, p. 66, p. 106, pp. 150–2, pp. 164–6, p. 215, p. 232, p. 249, pp. 251–5, pp. 284–9, p. 298 [p. 1, p. 11, p. 41, pp. 80–1, p. 101, p. 163].

Crichton, Michael (Jeffery Hudson, pseudonym) (1968) *A Case of Need*. Signet, New York, 1969, 416 pp.; p. 51, p. 90 [p. 73, p. 144].

Cronin, Archibald Joseph (1937) *The Citadel*. Gollancz, London, 446 pp.; p. 56, p. 68, p. 95, p. 136, pp. 140–9, pp. 376–80 [p. 76, pp. 113–14, p. 150, p. 154, p. 157, p. 233].

Cuthbert, M (1998) *The Silent Cradle*. Simon and Schuster, London, 353 pp.; pp. 78–9 [p. 99].

Danby, Frank (Julia Frankau) (1887) *Dr Phillips: a Maida Vale idyll*. Garland Publishing, New York, 1984, 342 pp; pp. 27–30, pp. 32–4, p. 71, pp. 95–7, pp. 186–7, pp. 276–86 [p. 7, p. 41, p. 103, p. 112].

Daudet, Léon (1894) *Les Morticoles*. Fasquelle, Paris, 1956, 360 pp.; pp. 94–7, p. 115, pp. 142–6, p. 153, pp. 258–9 (French) [p. 3, pp. 79–80, pp. 123–4, p. 150, p. 192, p. 196].

Davies, Robertson (1951) A Mixture of Frailties. In: Davies, Robertson. *The Salterton Trilogy*. Penguin, London, 1986, 775 pp.; pp. 717–25 [p. 82].

Davies, Robertson (1951) Tempest-Tost. In: Davies, Robertson. *The Salterton Trilogy*. Penguin, London, 1986, 775 pp.; p. 240 [p. 60].

Davies, Robertson (1994) *The Cunning Man*. Viking, London, 1994, 469 pp.; pp. 26–7 [p. 11].

Dawson, William James (1900) John Carson's Wife. In: *The Doctor Speaks*. Grant Richards, London, 334 pp.; pp. 133–47 [p. 148].

Deeping, Warwick (1925) *Sorrell and Son*. Cassell, London, 1927, 394 pp.; pp. 299–307 [pp. 231–2].

Delany, Samuel R (1967) Corona. In: *Distant Stars*. Bantam Books, New York, 1981, 352 pp.; pp. 65–86 [p. 228].

Denker, Henry (1992) *Doctor on Trial*. William Morrow, New York, 352 pp.; p. 38, p. 348 [p. 2, p. 246].

Denker, Henry (1975) *The Physicians: a novel of malpractice*. WH Allen, London, 384 pp.; 23–33, pp. 58–63, p. 225, p. 291, pp. 378–81 [pp. 245–6].

Dickens, Charles (1852–3) *Bleak House*. Collins, London, 1953, 799 pp.; p. 796 [p. 38].

Dickens, Charles (1849–50) *David Copperfield*. Signet Books, New York, 1962, 879 pp.; pp. 21–4 [p. 216].

Dickens, Charles (1837) *Pickwick Papers*. Signet Classics, New American Library, New York, 1964, 888 pp.; p. 726 [p. 5, p. 216].

Dickens, Charles (1859) *A Tale of Two Cities*. Oxford University Press, London, 1988, 524 pp.; pp. 394–406 [p. 216].

Dillon, Thomas Patrick and Leary, Nolan (1940) The Doctor from Dunmore. In: Fowler, Henry George. *Curtain Up: ten short modern plays*. Melbourne University Press, Carlton, Victoria, 1957, 242 pp.; pp. 117–43 [p. 28, p. 110].

Dix, John (1846) *Pen and Ink Sketches of Poets, Preachers and Politicians*. David Bogue, London, 275 pp.; pp. 174–81 [p. 78].

Doctor X (Alan Edward Nourse) (1965) *Intern*. Harper and Row, New York, 404 pp.; p. 87 [p. 64].

Dooling, Richard (1991) *Critical Care*. William Morrow, New York, 248 pp.; pp. 93–104 [p. 150, pp. 209–10].

Dostoyevsky, Fyodor (1880) *The Brothers Karamazov*. Translated by Magarshak, David. Penguin, Harmondsworth, 1978, 2 vols, 913 pp., vol. 1, pp. 211–12, vol. 2, pp. 603–16, p. 633, pp. 655–9, pp. 789–95 [p. 25, p. 58, p. 193].

Douglas, Lloyd C (1929) *Magnificent Obsession*. George Allen and Unwin, London, 1944, 314 pp.; pp. 38–47, pp. 187–221, pp. 296–304 [p. 149[.

Doyle, Arthur Conan (1894) Behind the Times. In: Doyle, Arthur Conan. *Round the Red Lamp*. John Murray, London, 1934, 328 pp.; pp 1–8 [p. 90, p. 161].

Doyle, Arthur Conan (1894) The Curse of Eve. In: Doyle, Arthur Conan. *Round the Red Lamp*. John Murray, London, 1934, 328 pp.; pp. 89–108 [p. 35, p. 58].

Doyle, Arthur Conan (1894) A False Start. In: Doyle, Arthur Conan. *Round The Red Lamp*. John Murray, London, 1934, 328 pp.; pp. 65–88 [p. 31, p. 36].

Drabble, Margaret (1965) *The Millstone*. Weidenfeld and Nicolson, London, 199 pp.; p. 127, pp. 138–43 [p. 77, p. 161].

Drabble, Margaret (1987) *The Radiant Way*. Weidenfeld and Nicolson, London, 396 pp.; pp. 132–3 [100].

Dreiser, Theodore (1919) The Country Doctor. In: Dreiser, Theodore. *Twelve Men.* Constable, London, 1930, 320 pp.; pp. 102–22 [p. 39, p. 92].

Dryden, John (1699) To My Honour'd Kinsman, John Driden, of Chesterton in the County of Huntingdon, Esquire. In: Dearing VA. *The Works of John Dryden.* University of California Press, Berkeley, 2000, vol. 7, 991 pp., p. 199 [p. 190].

Duhamel, Georges (1928) *Les Sept Dernières Plaies.* Mercure de France, Paris, 295 pp.; pp. 25–31 [p. 3, pp. 219–20].

Dumas, Alexandre (1848) *The Lady of the Camellias.* Translated by Gosse E. Alan Sutton, Gloucester, UK, 1986, 186 pp.; p. 178 [p. 147, p. 152].

Edson, Margaret (1993) *Wit.* Faber and Faber, New York, 1999, 85 pp.; p. 23, pp. 26–7, pp. 55–7 [pp. 73–4, p. 102].

Eliot, George (Mary Ann Evans) (1871–2) *Middlemarch.* Penguin, London, 1988, 908 pp.; pp. 118–20, p. 321, p. 327, pp. 459–61, pp. 484–5 [p. 3, p. 46, pp. 121–2, p. 126, p. 214].

Ellis AE (Derek Lindsay) (1958) *The Rack.* Penguin Books, London, 1988, 357 pp.; p. 30, p. 33, pp. 35–6, pp. 57–60, pp. 62–6, pp. 64–7, pp. 71–3, pp. 83–4, pp. 97–8, pp. 99–100, pp. 140–1, pp. 173–5, p. 230, pp. 242–3, p. 258, pp. 259–60, pp. 260–1, p. 264, pp. 342–3, pp. 349–51, pp. 352–7 [p. 12, p. 13, pp. 40–1, p. 56, p. 59, p. 72, p. 83, pp. 88–9, p. 106, p. 111, p. 144, pp. 160–1, pp. 197–9, pp. 208–9].

Ellison, Harlan (1957) Wanted in Surgery. In: Ellison, Harlan. *The Fantasies of Harlan Ellison.* Gregg Press, Boston, MA, 316 pp.; pp. 120–52 [p. 175].

Faulkner, William (1930) *As I Lay Dying.* Vintage Books, New York, 1985, 267 pp., p. 44, p. 204, p. 237, p. 260 [p. 41, p. 64].

Faulkner, William (1939) *The Wild Palms.* Random House, New York, 339 pp.; p. 4, pp. 12–14, pp. 40–4, pp. 84–5, p. 219, pp. 241–9, pp. 279–89, p. 293, p. 297, pp. 298–301, p. 321 [pp. 178–9].

Fearing, Kenneth (1939) *The Hospital.* Ballantine Books, New York, 1939, 144 pp.; p. 7, p. 16, pp. 22–3 [p. 9, pp. 192–3].

Fielding, Henry (1749) The History of Tom Jones – A Foundling. In: Stephen S (ed.) *The Works of Henry Fielding.* Smith Elder, London, 1882, vol. 1, 467 pp., Book 7, Chapter 13, pp. 359–61, Book 8, Chapter 3, pp. 390–3 [pp. 122–3, p. 221].

Fitzgerald, F Scott (1925) The Great Gatsby. In: Mizener, Arthur (ed.) *The Fitzgerald Reader.* Charles Scribner's Sons, New York, 1963. 509 pp.; p. 183 [p. 226].

Fitzgerald, F Scott (1935) One Interne. In: Fitzgerald, Scott. *Taps at Reveille.* Charles Scribner's Sons, New York, 407 pp.; pp. 294–313 [p. 5, pp. 108–9].

Fitzgerald, F Scott (1934) *Tender is the Night.* Penguin, Harmondsworth, 1998, 358 pp.; pp. 202–4, pp. 262–3 [p. 3, p. 176].

Flaubert, Gustave (1857) *Madame Bovary.* Translated by Steegmuller, Francis. Modern Library, New York, 1982, 396 pp.; pp. 68–9, pp. 196–210, pp. 291–305, pp. 386–8 [p. 2, p. 3, p. 157, p. 247].

Franzen, Jonathan (2001) *The Corrections.* Fourth Estate, London, 2002, 653 pp.; p. 364 [p. 76].

Frede, Richard (1960) *The Interns.* Corgi, London, 1965, 346 pp.; pp. 19–37, p. 59 [p. 64, p. 78, p. 208].

Frede, Richard (1985) *The Nurses*. WH Allen, London, 1986, 507 pp.; p. 86 [p. 109].

French, Marilyn (1977) *The Women's Room*. Andre Deutsch, London, 1978, 471 pp.; pp. 51–3 [p. 222].

Freud, Sigmund (1913) On Beginning the Treatment. Further Recommendations in the Technique of Psychoanalysis. In: Strachey, James (ed.) *The Standard Edition of the Complete Psychological Works of Sigmund Freud*. Hogarth Press, London, 1958, vol. 12, pp. 131–3 [p. 33, p. 41].

Galen (2nd century AD) The Affections and Errors of the Soul. In: *Galen, Selected Works*. Translated by Singer, Peter N. Oxford University Press, Oxford, 1997, 448 pp.; p. 108 [p. 143].

Galsworthy, John (1906) *The Man of Property*. Penguin, Harmondsworth, 1951, 317 pp.; p. 101 [p. 4].

Gardner, John (1972) *The Sunlight Dialogues*. Ballantine Books, New York, 1973, 746 pp.; pp. 254–7 [p. 247].

Gaskell, Elizabeth (1864–6) *Wives and Daughters*. Oxford University Press, Oxford, 1987, 740 pp.; p. 45, pp. 31–54 [p. 3, p. 8].

Gay, John (1727) The Sick Man and the Angel (Fable 27). In: Gay, John. *Fables*. Scolar Press, Menston, England, 1969, vol. 1, 173 pp.; p. 90 [p. 24].

Gibbons, Kaye (1993) *Charms For an Easy Life*. Abacus, London, 1994, 254 pp.; pp. 85–8 [p. 164].

Gide, André (1914) *The Vatican Caves* (also titled *The Vatican Cellars*). Translated by Bussy, Dorothy. Penguin, Harmondsworth (with *Strait is the Gate*), 1965, 360 pp.; p. 150 [p. 33].

Gilman, Charlotte Perkins (1892) *The Yellow Wallpaper*. Bauer, Dale M (ed.). Bedford Books, Boston, MA, 1998, 377 pp.; pp. 41–59 [p. 165].

Gilman, Charlotte Perkins (1935) *The Living of Charlotte Perkins Gilman: an autobiography*. University of Wisconsin Press, Madison, WI, 1991, 341 pp.; pp. 118–21 [p. 165].

Glasgow, Ellen (1925) *Barren Ground*. Virago, London, 1986, 409 pp.; p. 89, p. 262 [p. 33].

Glasser, Ronald J (1971) *365 Days*. George Braziller, New York, 242 pp.; pp. 10–11 [p. 223].

Glasser, Ronald J (1973) *Ward 402*. Garnstone Press, London, 1974, 240 pp.; pp. 135–45, pp. 192–7 [p. 62, pp. 166–7, p. 233].

Goldsworthy, Peter (1992) *Honk If You Are Jesus*. Angus and Robertson, Sydney, 290 pp.; pp. 48–9 [p. 146].

Goldsworthy, Peter (2003) *Three Dog Night*. Penguin, Melbourne, 342 pp.; pp. 82–4, p. 135 [pp. 183–4].

Gordon, Noah (1969) *The Death Committee*. The Book Society, London, undated, 361 pp.; p. 35, pp. 38–41, p. 332 [p. 46, p. 209].

Gordon, Noah (1986) *The Physician*. Simon and Schuster, New York, 604 pp.; p. 306 [p. 205].

Green, Gerald (1956) *The Last Angry Man*. Charles Scribner's Sons, New York, 494 pp.; pp. 2–9, p. 35, pp. 46–8, p. 152, p. 188, p. 308, p. 322, pp. 324–9, p. 344, p. 349, p. 368, p. 384, pp. 423–4 [pp. 36–7, pp. 72–3, p. 146, p. 147, p. 176, p. 241].

Greene, Graham (1961) *A Burnt-Out Case*. Heinemann and The Bodley Head, London, 1974, 236 pp.; p. 15 [p. 42].

Greene, Graham (1965) Doctor Crombie. In: Greene, Graham, *Collected Stories*. The Bodley Head and William Heinemann, London, 1972, 561 pp.; pp. 128–35 [p. 161].

Greene, Graham (1973) *The Honorary Consul*. Simon and Schuster, New York, 315 pp.; p. 83 [p. 106].

Grisham, John (1989) *A Time to Kill*. Island Books (Dell Publishing), New York, 1992, 515 pp.; p. 228, p. 439 [p. 239].

Guibert, Hervé (1990) *To the Friend who did not Save my Life*. Translated by Coverdale, Linda. Quartet Books, London, 1991, 246 pp.; pp. 23–5, pp. 38–9 [p. 128, p. 157].

Guterson, David (1999) *East of the Mountains*. Bloomsbury, London, 279 pp.; pp. 74–5 [p. 92].

Haggard, H Rider (1898) *Doctor Therne*. Hodder and Stoughton, London, 1923, 252 pp.; pp. 81–117 [p. 242].

Hailey, Arthur (1984) *Strong Medicine*. Dell, New York, 1986, 445 pp.; pp. 51–2 [p. 226].

Hammurabi (23rd century BC) Code of Laws. In: Johns, Claude Hermann Walter. *The Oldest Code of Laws in the World*. T and T Clark, Edinburgh, 1903, 88 pp. pp. 45–7 [p. 23].

Hardy, Thomas (1886–7) *The Woodlanders*. Oxford University Press, Oxford, 1988, 305 pp.; pp. 77–8 [pp. 174–5, pp. 194–5].

Hasek, Jaroslav (1921–3) *The Good Soldier Svejk*. Translated by Parrott, Cecil. Penguin, Harmondsworth, 1981, 752 pp.; pp. 69–77 [p. 222].

Hecht, Ben (1959) Miracle of the Fifteen Murderers. In: *A Treasury of Ben Hecht*. Crown Publishers, New York, 397 pp.; pp. 189–203 [p. 129, p. 207].

Heller, Joseph (1962) *Catch 22*. Dell Publishing Co., New York, 1974, 463 pp.; pp. 33–41 [pp. 24–5].

Heller, Joseph (1974) *Something Happened*. Jonathan Cape, London, 569 pp.; pp. 531–2 [p. 191].

Hellerstein, David (1986) The Battle for the Dead. In: Hellerstein, David. *Battles of Life and Death*. Houghton Mifflin, Boston, MA, 264 pp.; pp. 121–38 [pp. 224–5].

Hellerstein, David (1986) Children of the Valley. In: Hellerstein, David. *Battles of Life and Death*. Houghton Mifflin, Boston, MA, 264 pp.; pp. 49–66 [p. 224].

Hellerstein, David (1986) Fire in the Hills. In: Hellerstein, David. *Battles of Life and Death*. Houghton Mifflin, Boston, MA, 264 pp.; pp. 35–45 [p. 227].

Hellerstein, David (1986) Touching. In: Hellerstein, David. *Battles of Life and Death*. Houghton Mifflin, Boston, MA, 264 pp.; pp. 69–73 [p. 76].

Hemingway, Ernest (1924) The Doctor and the Doctor's Wife. In: *The Complete Short Stories of Ernest Hemingway*. Scribner Paperback Edition, Simon and Schuster, New York, 1998, 650 pp.; pp. 73–6 [p. 2].

Hemingway, Ernest (1929) *A Farewell to Arms*. Jonathan Cape, London, 349 pp.; p. 349 [p. 157].

Hemingway, Ernest (1933) God Rest You Merry, Gentlemen. In: *The Complete Short Stories of Ernest Hemingway*. Scribner Paperback Edition, Simon and Schuster, New York, 1998, 650 pp.; pp. 298–301 [pp. 155–6].

Hemingway, Ernest (1927) In Another Country. In: *The Complete Short Stories of Ernest Hemingway*. Scribner Paperback Edition, Simon and Schuster, New York, 1998, 650 pp.; pp. 206–10 [pp. 130–1].

Henry O (Porter, William Sidney) (1910) Let Me Feel Your Pulse. In: Henry O. *Roads of Destiny and Other Stories*. Hodder and Stoughton, London, 1974, 504 pp.; pp. 174–86 [p. 44].

Herrick, Robert (1900) *The Web of Life*. Macmillan, London, 356 pp.; p. 7, pp. 117–20 [p. 8, p. 27, p. 71].

Hierocles and Philagrius (3rd century AD) *The Philogelos*. Translated by Baldwin, Barry. Gieben, Amsterdam, 1983, 134 pp.; p. 34 [p. 83].

Hippocrates (5th century BC) *Epidemics III*. Translated by Jones WHS. Loeb's Classical Library, Heinemann, London, 1923, vol. 1, 361 pp., Case VIII, p. 233 [p. 4, pp. 10–11, p. 111].

Hoffman, Ernst Theodor Amadeus (1818) Rath Krespel. In: Bleiler, Everett Franklin (ed.) *The Best Tales of Hoffman*. Translated by Bealby, John Thomas. Dover Publications, New York, 1967, 419 pp.; p. 232 [p. 147, p. 152].

Holmes, Oliver Wendell (1871) The Young Practitioner. In: Holmes, Oliver Wendell. *Medical Essays 1842–1882, Holmes' Works*. Houghton Mifflin, Boston, MA, 1892, vol. 9, 445 pp.; pp. 370–95 [p. 128].

Howard, Sidney (1932) The Late Christopher Bean. In: Warnock, Robert. *Representative Modern Plays*. Scott Foresman and Company, Chicago, 1952, 758 pp.; pp. 118–24 [p. 37].

Howells, William Dean (1881) *Dr Breen's Practice*. James Osgood, Boston, MA, 272 pp.; p. 107 [pp. 184–5].

Huyler, Frank (1999) Sugar. In: Huyler, Frank. *The Blood of Strangers*. University of California Press, Berkeley, CA, 154 pp.; 127–31 [p. 115].

Ibsen, Henrik (1879) A Dolls House. In: Ibsen, Henrick. *A Dolls House and Other Plays*. Translated by Peter Watts. Penguin, London, 1965, pp. 191–2 [p. 5].

Ibsen, Henrik (1884) The Wild Duck. In: Ibsen, Henrik. *Three Plays*. Translated by Ellis-Fermor, Una. Penguin, Harmondsworth, 1957, 368 pp.; p. 207, pp. 243–58 [p. 5].

Irving, John (1985) *Cider House Rules*. Bantam Books, New York, 1986, 587 pp.; pp. 55–67 [p. 76].

Irving, John (2001) *The Fourth Hand*. Bloomsbury, London, 416 pp.; p. 31, p. 169 [p. 60].

James, Henry (1881) *Washington Square*. Bantam Books, New York, 1959, 162 pp.; pp. 1–5, p. 125 [p. 13, pp. 146–7, p. 213].

James, Henry (1902) *The Wings of the Dove*. Signet Classics, New York, 1964, 512 pp.; pp. 81–97, pp. 165–70, p. 304, pp. 400–37 [p. 34, pp. 92–3, p. 129].

James PD (1971) *Shroud for a Nightingale*. Sphere Books, London, 1988, 300 pp.; pp. 277–8 [p. 215].

Kafka, Franz (1919) A Country Doctor. In: Kafka, Franz. *Wedding Preparations (In the Country) and Other Stories*. Translated by Muir, Willa and Muir, Edwin. Penguin, Harmondsworth, 1978, 190 pp.; pp. 119–24 [p. 7, p. 121].

Kellogg, Marjorie (1968) *Tell Me That You Love Me, Junie Moon*. Popular Library, New York, 191 pp.; pp. 39–41 [p. 208].

Kingsley, Charles (1857) *Two Years Ago*. Macmillan and Co., London, 1884, 495 pp.; pp. 303–4 [p. 64, p. 154].

Kingsley, Sidney (1933) Men in White. In: Kingsley, Sidney. *Five Prizewinning Plays*. Ohio State University Press, Columbus, OH, 1995, 407 pp.; p. 37, p. 67 [p. 36].

Kipling, Rudyard (1910) A Doctor of Medicine. In: Kipling, Rudyard. *Rewards and Fairies*. Macmillan, London, 1960, 338 pp.; pp. 253–76 [p. 143, p. 144].

Kipling, Rudyard (1932) The Tender Achilles. In: Kipling, Rudyard. *Limits and Renewals*. Macmillan, London, 400 pp.; pp. 343–67 [p. 82, p. 84].

Kopit, Arthur L (1978) *Wings*. Hill and Wang, New York, 78 pp.; pp. 29–41 [p. 107].

Kornbluth CM (1950) The Little Black Bag. In: Conklin, Groff and Fabricant, Noah Daniel (eds) *Great Science Fiction About Doctors*. Collier Books, New York, 1963, 412 pp.; pp. 165–95 [p. 9].

Lacy, John (1672) *The Dumb Lady or The Farriar Made Physician*. Thomas Dring, London, 83 pp.; p. 13 [p. 72].

Lathen, Emma (Dominic RB, pseudonym) (1980) *The Attending Physician*. Macmillan, London, 220 pp.; p. 10, p. 34, p. 123 [p. 28].

Lapierre, Dominique (1985) *City of Joy*. Translated by Spink, Kathryn. Arrow Books, London, 1991, 518 pp., pp. 335–45 [p. 41].

Leavitt, David (1989) *Equal Affections*. Penguin, London, 268 pp.; p. 29, pp. 173–4 [p. 91].

Lee, Harper (1960) *To Kill a Mockingbird*. Popular Library, New York, 1962, 284 pp.; pp. 82–3 [p. 84].

Le Sage, Alain-René (1715) *The Adventures of Gil Blas de Santillana*. Translated by Smollett, Tobias. Oxford University Press, London, 1907, vol. 1, pp. 100–15, pp. 116–17 [p. 13, p. 160, p. 224].

Levenkron, Steven (1979) *The Best Little Girl in the World*. Penguin, London, 1988, 229 pp.; pp. 63–89 [p. 45, p. 55, pp. 228–9].

Levenkron, Steven (1997) *The Luckiest Girl in the World*. Scribner, New York, 188 pp.; p. 73 [p. 74].

Lewis, Sinclair (1924) *Arrowsmith*. Signet Books, New York, 1961, 438 pp., pp. 16–17, pp. 23–30, p. 42, pp. 82–5 [p. 1, p. 3, p. 42, pp. 158–9, pp. 164–5].

Lewis, Sinclair (1920) *Main Street*. Harcourt Brace and Company, New York, 1948, 486 pp.; pp. 176–9 [p. 39, p. 64].

Lewisohn, Ludwig (1928) *The Island Within*. Harper and Brothers, New York, 350 pp.; pp. 215–17 [p. 32].

Lightman, Alan (2000) *The Diagnosis*. Pantheon Books, New York, 369 pp.; pp. 107–14, pp. 116–17, pp. 119–20, pp. 180–2, pp. 200–1, p. 272, p. 324, p. 367, p. 368 [p. 54, pp. 102–3, p. 111, p. 113, p. 134, p. 152].

Lucian of Samosata (2nd century AD) *Disowned*. Translated by Harmon AM. In: *Lucian*. Loeb's Classical Library, Heinemann, London, 1972, vol. 5, 537 pp.; p. 487, pp. 477–525 [p. 189].

Lurie, Alison (1974) *The War Between the Tates*. Heinemann, London, 314 pp.; pp. 57–70, pp. 115–17 [p. 53, p. 76, p. 125].

Maartens, Maarten (1906) *The Healers*. Constable, London, 379 pp.; pp. 82–3 [p. 30, p. 160].

Malègue, Joseph (1932) *Augustin, ou, Le maître est là*. Spes, Paris, 1935, vol. 2,

510 pp.; p. 20, pp. 117–19, pp. 213–30, pp. 277–83, pp. 323–9, pp. 341–51, pp. 380–5, pp. 415–22, p. 489 (French) [p. 3, p13, p. 76, p. 105, pp. 199–201].

Malory, Thomas (1485) *Le Morte D'Arthur (1485)*. Dent, London, 1938, vol. 1, 401 pp.; pp. 40–2 [p. 4].

Mann, Thomas (1901) *Buddenbrooks*. Translated by Lowe-Porter HT. Penguin, Harmondsworth, 1957, 587 pp.; pp. 28–9, p. 54, pp. 429–39 [pp. 89–90, p. 162, pp. 216–17].

Mann, Thomas (1947) *Doctor Faustus*. Translated by Lowe-Porter HT. Secker and Warburg, London, 1949, 510 pp.; pp. 475–6 [p. 27, p. 44].

Mann, Thomas (1924) *The Magic Mountain*. Translated by Lowe-Porter HT. Penguin, Harmondsworth, 1960, 716 pp.; pp. 174–81, p. 203, pp. 203–19 [p. 3, p. 55, p. 56, p. 105, p. 124].

Manzoni, Alessandro (1827) *The Betrothed*. Translated by Penman, Bruce. Penguin, Harmondsworth, 1983, 719 pp.; p. 609 [pp. 26–7].

Marlowe, Christopher (1590) Tamburlaine Part II. In: Marlowe, Christopher. *Plays*. Dent, London, 1947, 488 pp.; Act V, Scene III, p. 115 [p. 167].

Marquis, Don (Donald Robert Perry) (1939) Country Doctor. In: Marquis, Don. *The Best of Don Marquis*. Garden City Books, Garden City, NY, 670 pp.; pp. 444–63 [p. 150].

Martin du Gard, Roger (1940) *Summer 1914*. Translated by Gilbert, Stuart. John Lane, The Bodley Head, London, 1078 pp. [p. 192].

Martin du Gard, Roger (1922–9) *The Thibaults*. Translated by Gilbert, Stuart. John Lane, The Bodley Head, London, 1939, 889 pp.; pp. 323–37, p. 529, p. 576 [p. 8, p. 130, p. 151, p. 192].

Martineau, Harriet (1839) *Deerbrook*. Virago Press, London, 1983, 523 pp., p. 44, pp. 173–8, p. 297, pp. 318–23, p. 426 [p. 2, p. 36, p. 63, p. 90, p. 126, p. 224].

Maugham, W Somerset (1940) Lord Mountdrago. In: Maugham, W Somerset. *Collected Short Stories, vol. II*. Pan Books, London, 1975, 478 pp.; pp. 268–89 [p. 220].

Maugham, W Somerset (1919) *The Moon and Sixpence*. Penguin, Harmondsworth, 1953, 217 pp.; pp. 198–212 [pp. 39–40, pp. 127–8, p. 190].

Maugham, W Somerset (1915) *Of Human Bondage*. Signet Classics, New York, 1991, 680 pp.; pp. 438–42, p. 521, pp. 595–6 [p. 3, p. 9, p. 114, p. 128, p. 131].

Maugham, W Somerset (1909) Penelope. In: Maugham, W Somerset. *The Collected Plays*. Heinemann, London, 1960, vol. 1, 110 pp.; Act II, p. 40 [p. 30].

Maugham, W Somerset (1947) Sanatorium. In: Maugham, W Somerset. *Sixty-Five Short Stories*. Heinemann/Octopus, London, 1976, 937 pp.; pp. 541–56 [p. 56].

Maugham, W Somerset (1933) The Vessel of Wrath. In: Maugham, W Somerset. *Collected Short Stories, vol. II*, Pan Books, London, 1975, 478 pp.; pp. 9–46 [p. 42].

Mauriac, Francois (1925) *The Desert of Love*. Translated by Hopkins, Gerard. Eyre and Spottiswoode, London, 1949, 279 pp.; p. 11, p. 31, p. 50, p. 51, p. 58, p. 60, p. 63 [p. 2, p. 8, p. 9, p. 11, p. 74, p. 144].

Mauriac, Francois (1927–35) *Thérèse*. Translated by Hopkins, Gerard. Penguin, Harmondsworth, 1959, 318 pp.; p. 312 [pp. 64–5].

Maurois, André (Émile Herzog) (1921) *Colonel Bramble*. Translated by Wake, Thurfrida. Jonathan Cape, London, 1937, 256 pp.; p. 222 [p. 251].

McCarthy, Mary (1954) *The Group*. Signet, New York, 1964, 397 pp.; p. 139, 240–1, 286, 358 [p. 111, p. 158, p. 166].

McCarthy, Mary (1942) *The Company She Keeps*. Penguin, Harmondsworth, 1975, 224 pp.; pp. 185–6 [p. 60].

McCullers, Carson (1953) *Clock Without Hands*. Houghton Mifflin, Boston, MA, 1963, 241 pp.; p. 5, pp. 61–3 [p. 13, p. 74, pp. 101–2, p. 110, pp. 132–3].

McCullers, Carson (1943) *The Heart is a Lonely Hunter*. Cresset Press, London, 1953, 350 pp.; p. 138 [p. 65].

McGee, Tess (2003) *Misconceptions*. Pan Macmillan, Sydney, 462 pp.; p. 57, p. 138, p. 244, p. 360, pp. 382–3, pp. 405–7, p. 427, p. 431, p. 436 [pp. 239–40, pp. 244–5].

Melville, Herman (1850) *White Jacket*. LC Page, Boston, MA, 1892, 374 pp.; pp. 232–49 [p. 5].

Middleton, Thomas (1662) Anything for a Quiet Life. In: Bullen AH (ed.) *The Works of Thomas Middleton*. JC Nimmo, London, 1885, 453 pp., vol. V, Act II, Scene 4, pp. 281–2 [p. 122].

Miller, Arthur (1968) *The Price*. Secker & Warburg, London, 116 pp.; p. 17, p. 72, pp. 81–2 [p. 29].

Milne AA (Alan Alexander) (1924) The Dormouse and the Doctor. In: Milne AA. *When We Were Very Young*. Methuen, London, 1977, 100 pp.; pp. 66–7 [p. 164].

Mitchell, S Weir (1901) *Circumstance*. Century Company, New York, 1902, 495 pp.; p. 42, p. 48, pp 126–31, p. 207, p. 267, p. 364 [p. 113, p. 216, p. 221].

Mitchell, S Weir (1885) *In War Time*. Century Company, New York, 1913, 423 pp.; p. 14, p. 57, pp. 60–1, p. 81, pp. 98–103, p. 163, pp. 242–3, pp. 323–6, p. 371 [p. 53, p. 55, pp. 126–7, p. 155, p. 174, p. 222, p. 228].

Molière, Jean-Baptiste (1673) The Hypochondriack. In: *Molière's Comedies*. Translated by Baker, Henry and Miller, James. Dent, London, 1961, vol. 2, 472 pp.; pp. 469–71 [p. 5, p. 159].

Molière, Jean-Baptiste (1665) Love's The Best Doctor. In: *The Plays of Molière*. Translated by Waller, Alfred Rayney. John Grant, Edinburgh, 1907, vol. 4, 336 pp.; pp. 291–7 [p. 5, p. 6].

Molière, Jean-Baptiste (1666) The Physician in Spite of Himself. In: *The Plays of Molière*. Translated by Waller, Alfred Rayney. John Grant, Edinburgh, 1907, vol. 5, 435 pp.; pp. 154–5 [p. 72, p. 221].

Montaigne, Michel de (1580–1588) *Essays*. Translated by Trechmann EJ. Oxford University Press, London, 1927, vol. 2, 614 pp.; pp. 564–6 [p. 189].

Mortimer, John (1985) *Paradise Postponed*. Penguin, Harmondsworth, 1986, 447 pp.; p. 47, p. 113, p. 140 [p. 138].

Munthe, Axel (1929) *The Story of San Michele*. John Murray, London, 1950, 431 pp.; p. 176, pp. 188–9 [p. 29, pp. 131–2].

Nourse, Alan Edward (1978) *The Practice*. Futura Publications, London, 1979, 574 pp.; pp. 219–20, pp. 378–80 [p. 34, pp. 61–2].

Oates, Joyce Carol (1971) The Metamorphosis. In: Oates, Joyce Carol. *Marriages and Infidelities*. Vanguard Press, New York, 1972, 497 pp.; p. 372 [p. 109].

O'Brian, Patrick (1992) *The Truelove*. WW Norton, New York, 256 pp.; pp. 15–35 [p. 101, p. 185, p. 217].

O'Brien, Edna (1965) *August Is A Wicked Month*. Jonathan Cape, London, 221 pp.; pp. 219–20 [p. 106].

O'Connor, Flannery (1964) Revelation. In: O'Connor, Flannery. *Collected Works*. Library of America, New York, 1988, 1281 pp.; p. 634 [p. 45, p. 62].

O'Hara, John (1935) The Doctor's Son. In: O'Hara, John. *Collected Stories*. MacShane, Frank (ed.). Random House, New York, 1984, 414 pp.; pp. 8–9 [p. 64].

Olsen, Tillie (1962) *Tell Me a Riddle*. Virago, London, 1990, 335 pp.; pp. 84–5 [p. 196].

O'Neill, Eugene (1928) Strange Interlude. In: O'Neill, Eugene. *Complete Plays*. Library of America, New York, 1988, vol. 2, 1092 pp., p. 642, p. 660, p. 724 [p. 44, p. 104, p. 191].

Orwell, George (Blair, Eric Arthur) (1946) How the Poor Die. In: Orwell, George. *Collected Essays, Journalism and Letters*. Secker and Warburg, London, 1968, vol. 4, 555 pp.; pp. 223–33 [p. 222].

Osler, William (1889) *Aequanimitas*. HK Lewis, London, 1920, 474 pp.; p. 5 [p. 73, p. 173].

Osler, William (1906) Unity Peace and Concord. In: Osler, William. *Aequanimitas*. HK Lewis, London, 1920, 474 pp.; pp. 447–465 [p. 81].

Ozick, Cynthia (1971) The Doctor's Wife. In: Ozick, Cynthia. *The Pagan Rabbi and Other Stories*. Penguin, New York, 1991, 270 pp.; p. 181 [p. 37].

Palmer, Michael (1982) *The Sisterhood*. Bantam Books, New York, 1995, 343 pp.; p. 14 [p. 36].

Paretsky, Sara (1988) *Toxic Shock* (also titled *Blood Shot*). Penguin, London, 1990, 320 pp.; pp. 313–16 [p. 241].

Pasternak, Boris (1957) *Doctor Zhivago*. Translated by Hayward, Max and Harari, Manya. Pantheon, New York, 1958, 558 pp.; pp. 67–9, pp. 102–5 [p. 74, p. 114, pp. 136–7].

Percy, Walker (1961) *The Moviegoer*. Noonday Press, New York, 1977, 241 pp.; pp. 152–4 [p. 124, p. 164].

Percy, Walker (1987) *The Thanatos Syndrome*. Farrar Straus Giroux, New York, 372 pp.; p. 13, p. 363 [p. 91, p. 124].

Petrarch, Francesco (1355) Invective Contra Medicum. In: *Petrarch, Works*. Gregg Press, Ridgewood, NJ, 1965, vol. 2, 1200–33 (Latin) [p. 129, p. 134].

Phelps, Elizabeth Stuart (1882) *Doctor Zay*. Feminist Press, New York, 1987, 321 pp.; pp. 51–2 [p. 99, p. 100].

Piercy, Marge (1982) *Braided Lives*. Summit Books, New York, 443 pp.; p. 189 [p. 222, p. 226].

Pindar (approx. 474 BC) Pythian Odes. In: *The Odes of Pindar*. Translated by Sandys, John. Loeb's Classical Library, Heinemann, London, 1946, 635 pp.; pp. 189–91 [p. 23].

Plath, Sylvia (1963) *The Bell Jar*. Bantam Books, New York, 1972, 216 pp.; pp. 189–90 [p. 59].

Plath, Sylvia (1965) Lady Lazarus. In: Plath, Sylvia. *Ariel*. Faber and Faber, London, 1976, p. 18 [p. 45, p. 193, p. 194].

Plato (4th century BC) *Gorgias*. Translated by Lamb (Walter Rangeley Maitland). Loeb's Classical Library, Heinemann, London, 1967, vol. III, 536 pp.; p. 291, p. 515 [p. 71, p. 242].

Plato (4th century BC) Protagoras. Translated by Jowett, Benjamin. In: Buchanan,

Scott (ed.) *The Portable Plato*. Penguin, Harmondsworth, 1979, 696 pp.; p. 103 [p. 8, p. 9, p. 104].

Plato (4th century BC) The Republic. Translated by Jowett, Benjamin. In: Buchanan, Scott (ed.) *The Portable Plato*. Penguin, Harmondsworth, 1979, 696 pp.; pp. 396–7 [p. 22, p. 145].

Pliny the Elder (Gaius Plinius Secundus) (1st century AD) *Natural History*. Translated by Holland, Philemon. Southern Illinois University Press, 1962, Book 29, 496 pp.; pp. 294–7 [p. 23, p. 122, p. 123, p. 134, pp. 159–60, p. 189, p. 192].

Plutarch (2nd century AD) Pericles. In: *Plutarch's Lives*. Translated by Dryden, John. Modern Library, New York, 2001, p. 230 [p. 227].

Proust, Marcel (1913–22) *Remembrance of Things Past*. Translated by Moncrieff, CK Scott and Kilmartin, Terence. Penguin, Harmondsworth, 1985, vol. 1, 1197 pp.; p. 467, p. 536–7 [p. 112, p. 152].

Proust, Marcel (1913–22) *Remembrance of Things Past*. Translated by Moncrieff, CK Scott and Kilmartin, Terence. Penguin, Harmondsworth, 1987, vol. 2, 1040 pp.; p. 308, p. 316, pp. 323–8, p. 333, p. 335, pp. 354–5 [p. 1, p. 3, p. 8, p. 30, pp. 164–5, p. 166, p. 168].

Pushkin, Alexander S (1830) The Postmaster. Translated by Keane T. In: Yarmolinsky, Avraham (ed.) *The Poems, Prose and Plays of Alexander Pushkin*. Modern Library, New York, 1936, 896 pp.; p. 523 [p. 218].

Puzo, Mario (1968) *The Godfather*. Fawcett, Greenwich, CT, 446 pp.; pp. 45–6 [p. 82–3].

Pym, Barbara (1980) *A Few Green Leaves*. EP Dutton, New York, 250 pp.; pp. 2–17 [p. 109, p. 147].

Ravin, Neil (1987) *Evidence*. Charles Scribner's Sons, New York, 292 pp.; pp. 151–8 [p. 26].

Ravin, Neil (1983) *Informed Consent*. GP Putnam's Sons, New York, 303 pp.; pp. 79–84 [p. 3, pp. 56–7].

Ravin, Neil (1981) *MD*. Delacorte Press/Seymour Lawrence, New York, 404 pp.; pp. 28–31, pp. 66–7, pp. 155–7, p. 333, pp. 346–7 [p. 3, p. 64, pp. 114–15, p. 137, pp. 242–3].

Ravin, Neil (1989) *Mere Mortals*. MacDonald, London, 1990, 420 pp.; p. 27. p. 48, pp. 290–305 [p. 29, pp. 243–4].

Ravin, Neil (1985) *Seven North*. EP Dutton/Seymour Lawrence, New York, 371 pp.; pp. 110–16 [p. 3, p. 115].

Reade, Charles (1863) *Hard Cash*. Chatto and Windus, London, 1894, 625 pp.; pp. 31–3, p. 180, pp. 210–11 [p. 13, pp. 29–30, p. 54, p. 123].

Reade, Charles (1877) A Woman Hater. In: *Reade's Novels*. Chatto and Windus, London, 1894, 398 pp.; p. 226 [p. 233].

Reed, Barry (1980) *The Verdict*. Simon and Schuster, New York, 282 pp.; pp. 157–8, p. 161 [pp. 246–7].

Remarque, Erich Maria (1945) *Arch of Triumph*. Translated by Sorell, Walter and Lindley, Denver. Appleton Century, New York, 455 pp.; p. 48, pp. 110–14 [p. 4, p. 60, pp. 230–1].

Rhinehart, Luke (1971) *The Dice Man*. Panther Books, London, 1975, 431 pp.; pp. 37–42 [pp. 83–4].

Richardson, Henry Handel (Ethel Florence Lindesay Robertson) (1917–29) *The*

Fortunes of Richard Mahony. Penguin, London, 1990, 841 pp.; p. 138, pp. 165–7, pp. 188–9, p. 205, pp. 273–4, pp. 304–10, p. 680, pp. 716–37 [p. 30, p. 36, p. 44, p. 79, p. 132, p. 166, p. 185, p. 247].

Richardson, Samuel (1747–8) The History of Clarissa Harlowe. In: Stephen, Leslie (ed.) *The Works of Samuel Richardson*. Henry Sotheran, London, 1883, vol. 7, 520 pp.; pp. 377–8, p. 397, p. 398; vol. 8, 540 pp.; pp. 111–14 [p. 33, p. 38, pp. 44–5, p. 76, p. 190].

Rinehart, Mary R (1935) *The Doctor*. Farrar and Rinehart, New York, 506 pp.; pp. 12–14, pp. 19–21, p. 41, pp. 99–100, p. 408 [p. 36, pp. 84–5, p. 147, pp. 213–14].

Roe, Francis (1989) *Doctors and Doctors' Wives*. Constable, London, 336 pp.; pp. 35–8 [p. 207].

Rosenbaum, Edward E (1988) *The Doctor* (also titled *A Taste Of My Own Medicine*). Ivy Books, New York, 1991, 182 pp.; p. 37, p. 88 [p. 109, p. 226].

Runyon, Damon (1946) Why Me? In: Runyon, Damon. *Short Takes*. Somerset Books, New York, 435 pp.; pp. 364–6 [p. 191].

Russell, Robert (1985) *While You're Here, Doctor*. Souvenir Press, London, 254 pp.; pp. 8–11, p. 66, pp. 109–15, pp. 202–5, p. 225 [p. 2, p. 57, p. 115, p. 145, p. 219].

Sanders, Lawrence (1973) *The First Deadly Sin*. Berkley Books, New York, 1974, 576 pp.; pp. 61–2, p. 83, p. 87, p. 102 [p. 12, p. 13, p. 43, pp. 57–8].

Sava, George (1979) *No Man is Perfect*. Robert Hale, London, 256 pp.; p. 39 [p. 82].

Sayers, Dorothy L (1928) The Vindictive Story of the Footsteps that Ran. In: *Lord Peter Views the Body*. Gollancz, London, 1979, 317 pp.; pp. 161–80 [p. 6, pp. 111–12].

Schneiderman LJ (1972) *Sea Nymphs by the Hour*. Authors' Guild Backinprint.-Com, Lincoln, NE, 2000, 176 pp.; p. 11, pp. 16–18, p. 36, pp. 55–8, p. 174 [pp. 107–8, p. 207, p. 223].

Schnitzler, Arthur (1912) *Professor Bernhardi*. Translated by Landstone, Hetty. Faber and Gwyer, London, 1927, 160 pp.; pp. 36–45, p. 136 [p. 247].

Scott, Walter (1831) *The Abbot*. Adam and Charles Black, London, 1893, p. 280 [p. 46].

Scott, Walter (1831) *The Surgeon's Daughter*. Adam and Charles Black, London, 1892, pp. 56–9 [p. 8].

Segal, Erich (1988) *Doctors*. Bantam Books, New York, 1989, 678 pp.; pp. 579–81 [p. 8, p. 24].

Seifert, Elizabeth (1941) *Bright Scalpel*. Aeonian Press Inc., New York, 1973, 224 pp.; pp. 7–8, p. 10 [p. 67, p. 134].

Seifert, Elizabeth (1969) *Bachelor Doctor*. Collins, London, 1971, 224 pp.; p. 68 [p. 149].

Selzer, Richard (1972) The Consultation. In: Selzer, Richard. *Rituals of Surgery*. Harpers Magazine Press, New York, 1974, 193 pp.; pp. 18–23 [p. 32].

Selzer, Richard (1979) In Praise of Senescence. In: Selzer, Richard. *Confessions of a Knife*. Simon and Schuster, New York, 223 pp.; pp. 100–10 [pp. 77–8].

Selzer, Richard (1985) My Brother Shaman. In: Jones, Anne Hudson (ed.) *Literature and Medicine*. Johns Hopkins University Press, Baltimore, vol. 2, pp. 41–4 [p. 110].

Sexton, Anne (1975) Doctors. In: Sexton, Anne. *The Complete Poems*. Houghton Mifflin, Boston, MA, 1981, 622 pp.; pp. 465–6 [p. 194].

Sexton, Anne (1962) The Operation. In: Sexton, Anne. *All My Pretty Ones.* Houghton Mifflin, Boston, MA, 68 pp.; p. 13 [p. 194].

Sexton, Anne (1960) Unknown Girl in the Maternity Ward. In: Sexton, Anne. *To Bedlam and Part Way Back.* Houghton Mifflin, Boston, MA, 67 pp.; p. 34 [p. 7, p. 102].

Shakespeare, William (1606) *The Tragedy of Macbeth.* Wright LB and La Mar VA (eds). Washington Square Press, New York, 1969, 93 pp.; Act V, Scene I, pp. 77–8, Act V, Scene III, p. 84 [p. 3, p. 24].

Shaw, George Bernard (1906) The Doctor's Dilemma. In: *The Bodley Head Bernard Shaw's Collected Plays With Their Prefaces.* Max Reinhardt The Bodley Head, London, 1971, vol. 3, 914 pp.; pp. 228–43, pp. 295–6, pp. 335–40, p. 346, p. 375 [p. 26, p. 36, p. 44, p. 64, pp. 144–5, p. 162].

Sheed, Wilfrid (1973) *People Will Always Be Kind.* Weidenfeld and Nicolson, London, 374 pp.; pp. 27–37 [pp. 135–6].

Sheldon, Sidney (1994) *Nothing Lasts Forever.* HarperCollins, London, 293 pp.; pp. 43–5, pp. 50–1, p. 74, p. 78, p. 97 [p. 2, p. 42, p. 64, p. 225].

Shem, Samuel (Bergman, Steven) (1978) *The House of God.* Richard Marek, New York, 382 pp.; pp. 37–8, pp. 43–4, pp. 218–19 [p. 1, p. 71, p. 73, p. 150, p. 209, p. 225, p. 227].

Shute, Jenefer (1992) *Life Size.* Houghton Mifflin Company, Boston, MA, 231 pp. [p. 191].

Simenon, Georges (1941) The Country Doctor. In: Simenon, Georges. *The White Horse Inn and Other Novels.* Translated by Ellenbogen, Eileen. Hamish Hamilton, London, 1980, 330 pp.; pp. 198–205, pp. 227–36, pp. 323–5 [p. 80, p. 132, pp. 232–3, p. 241].

Simenon, Georges (1950) The Heart of a Man. In: *The Second Simenon Omnibus.* Translated by Varèse, Louise. Hamish Hamilton, London, 1974, 480 pp.; pp. 151–62 [p. 8, p. 60, pp. 87–8, p. 109].

Simenon, Georges (1963) *The Patient.* Translated by Stewart, Jean. Hamish Hamilton, London, 236 pp.; pp. 1–13, pp. 33–4, pp. 35–6, pp. 54–5, pp. 56–9, p. 66, pp. 90–3, p. 178 [p. 107, p. 124, pp. 180–2, pp. 207–8].

Slaughter, Frank G (1964) *A Savage Place.* Arrow Books, London, 1966, 256 pp.; p. 77 [p. 26].

Smollett, Tobias (1771) *The Expedition of Humphry Clinker.* Knapp, Lewis M (ed.). Oxford University Press, London, 1971, 375 pp.; p. 5 [p. 215].

Snow, CP (Charles Percy) (1958) The Conscience of the Rich. In: Snow CP. *Strangers and Brothers.* Charles Scribner's Sons, New York, 1972, vol. 1, 1071 pp.; p. 720 [p. 214].

Snow, CP (Charles Percy) (1970) Last Things. In: Snow CP. *Strangers and Brothers.* Charles Scribner's Sons, New York, 1972, vol. 3, 921 pp.; pp. 731–53 [pp. 214–15].

Snow, CP (Charles Percy) (1968) The Sleep of Reason. In: Snow CP. *Strangers and Brothers.* Charles Scribner's Sons, New York, 1972, vol. 3, 921 pp.; pp. 388–417 [pp. 214–15].

Sobel, Irwin Philip (1973) *The Hospital Makers.* Doubleday, Garden City, NY, 431 pp.; pp. 11–16, pp. 20–6, pp. 68–9, p. 325 [p. 3, pp. 34–5, p. 206, pp. 209–10].

Solzhenitsyn, Aleksandr Isaevich (1968) *Cancer Ward.* Translated by Bethell,

Nicholas and Burg, David. Bodley Head, London, 1971, 619 pp.; pp. 57–8 [p. 55, p. 218].

Sophocles (approx. 460 BC) *Ajax*. Translated by Storr F Loeb's Classical Library, Heinemann, London, 1961, vol. 2, 493 pp.; p. 51 [p. 164].

Soubiran, André (1947) *The Doctors*. Translated by Coburn, Oliver. WH Allen, London, 1954, 288 pp.; pp. 222–3 [p. 160].

Spark, Muriel (1959) *Memento Mori*. Reprint Society, London, 1965, 287 pp.; pp. 69–70 [p. 86].

Stafford, Jean (1953) *The Interior Castle*. Harcourt Brace and Company, New York, 496 pp.; p. 198, p. 202, p. 205, p. 206, 208–17 [pp. 59–60, pp. 74–5, p. 164, p. 165].

Sterne, Laurence (1759–67) *The Life and Opinions of Tristram Shandy, Gentleman*. Work, James Aiken (ed.). Odyssey Press, New York, 1940, 647 pp.; p. 168 [p. 5, p. 143].

Strindberg, August (1887) The Father. In: Strindberg, August. *Twelve Plays*. Translated by Sprigge, Elizabeth. Constable, London, 1962, 689 pp.; p. 20, p. 22, p. 31, p. 48, p. 56 [pp. 175–6].

Strong LAG (Leonard Alfred George) (1945) The White Cottage. In: Strong LAG. *Travellers: Thirty-One Selected Short Stories*. Methuen, London, 297 pp.; pp. 124–43 [p. 7].

Tate, James (1976) On the Subject of Doctors. In: *Viper Jazz*. Wesleyan University Press, Middletown, CT, 79 pp.; p. 36 [p. 32].

Tate, James (1976) Who Gets The Bitterroot. In: *Viper Jazz*. Wesleyan University Press, Middletown, CT, 79 pp.; p. 43 [p. 195].

Thompson, Morton (1949) *The Cry and the Covenant*. Pan Books, London, 1969, 474 pp.; p. 123 [p. 60, p. 72].

Thompson, Morton (1955) *Not as a Stranger*. Michael Joseph, London, 702 pp.; pp. 275–7, p. 335, pp. 353–5 [p. 75, p. 167, p. 227].

Tolstoy, Aleksey Konstantinovich (1865) The Death of Ivan the Terrible. In: Noyes, George Rapall (transl. and ed.) *Masterpieces of the Russian Drama*. Dover Publications, New York, 1961, 902 pp.; 2 vols, vol. 2, Act IV, Scene II, p. 514, Act V, Scene I, pp. 533–4 [pp. 217–18].

Tolstoy, Leo (1886) The Death of Ivan Illych. In: Simmons, Ernest Joseph (ed.) *Tolstoy, Leo, Short Novels*. Translated by Maude, Louise and Maude, Aylmer. Modern Library, Random House, New York, 1966, vol. 2, 575 pp.; pp. 47–9 [p. 105, p. 130, p. 191].

Tolstoy, Leo (1891) The Kreutzer Sonata. In: Simmons, Ernest Joseph (ed.) *Tolstoy, Leo, Short Novels*. Translated by Maude, Aylmer. Modern Library, Random House, New York, 1966, vol. 2, 575 pp.; pp. 148–9 [pp. 25–6, pp. 104–5].

Traver, Robert (1958) *Anatomy of a Murder*. Dell, New York, 1959, 512 pp.; pp. 263–71, pp. 352–7 [p. 240].

Trollope, Anthony (1858) *Doctor Thorne*. World's Classics, Oxford University Press, London, 1963, 569 pp.; p. 123, p. 302 [p. 5, p. 33].

Turgenev, Ivan (1852) The District Doctor. In: *The Novels of Ivan Turgenev*. Translated by Garnett, Constance. Heinemann, London, 1920, vol. 1, p. 56 [p. 30].

Turow, Scott (1990) *The Burden of Proof*. Warner Books, New York, 1991, 564 pp.; p. 180 [p. 103].

Updike, John (1963) The Doctor's Wife. In: Updike, John. *Pigeon Feathers and Other Stories*. Andre Deutsch, London, 278 pp.; pp. 197–210 [p. 37].

Updike, John (1963) The Persistence of Desire. In: Updike, John. *Pigeon Feathers and Other Stories*. Andre Deutsch, London, 278 pp.; pp. 12–26 [p. 156, p. 164].

Van Der Meersch, Maxence (1943) *Bodies and Souls*. Translated by Wilkins, Eithne. William Kimber, London, 1953, 463 pp.; pp. 9–11, p. 36, p. 152 [p. 5, p. 59, p. 65, p. 89].

Van Duyn, Mona (1971) In the Hospital for Tests. In: Van Duyn, M. *To See to Take*. Atheneum, New York, 1971, 94 pp.; pp. 45–7 [pp. 100–1].

Wadd, William (Unus Quorum, pseudonym) (1827) *Nugae Canorae: Or Epitaphian Mementos (in Stone Cutters' Verse) of the Medici Family of Modern Times*. JB Nichols, London, 70 pp.; p. 7 [p. 83].

Waltari, Mika (1945) *The Egyptian*. Translated by Walford N. Panther Books, London, 1960, 352 pp.; pp. 34–9, p. 194 [p. 40, pp. 158–9].

Wambaugh, Joseph (1985) *The Secrets of Harry Bright*. Sphere Books, London, 1987, 307 pp.; p. 93 [p. 60, pp. 81–2].

Warren, Robert Penn (1946) *All the King's Men*. Modern Library, New York, 1953, 464 pp.; p. 113, p. 257, pp. 269–75, p. 343, pp. 399–405, p. 420 [p. 24, p. 42, p. 152, p. 220].

Warren, Samuel (1832) Preparing for the House. In: Warren, Samuel. *Diary of a Late Physician*. Blackwood, Edinburgh, vol. 1, 388 pp.; pp. 86–95 [p. 138].

Warren, Samuel (1832) Rich and Poor. In: Warren, Samuel. *Diary of a Late Physician*. Blackwood, Edinburgh, vol. 2, 409 pp.; pp. 223–43 [p. 216].

Warren, Samuel (1832) A Slight Cold. In: Warren, Samuel. *Diary of a Late Physician*. Blackwood, Edinburgh, vol. 2, 409 pp.; pp. 201–22 [p. 99].

Webster, John (1623) The Duchess of Malfi. In: Brown, John Russell (ed.) *The Revels Plays Series*. Manchester University Press, Manchester, UK, 1976, 220 pp.; Act I, Scene 1, p. 22, Act III, Scene V, p. 98 [p. 24, p. 167].

Weldon F (1976) *Remember Me*. Coronet, London, 1983, 223 pp.; p. 168, p. 201 [p. 2, p. 159].

Wells, Herbert George (1909) Tono Bungay. In: *The Essex Edition of the Works of HG Wells*. Ernest Benn, London, 1926, vol. 7, 445 pp.; p. 409 [p. 123].

Wharton, William (1978) *Birdy*. Jonathan Cape, London, 1979, 310 pp.; pp. 24–5, p. 131 [p. 223].

Wharton, William (1981) *Dad*. Alfred A Knopf, New York, 449 pp.; pp. 46–7, p. 63, pp. 102–19, pp. 129–30, pp. 159–62, p. 237, p. 249, p. 346 [p. 3, p. 13, p. 41, p. 124, pp. 133–4, pp. 196–7].

White, Patrick (1961) *Riders in the Chariot*. Penguin, Harmondsworth, 1986, 492 pp.; pp. 348–56 [p. 3].

Williams, Maslyn (1974) *Florence Copley of Romney*. Collins, Sydney, 191 pp.; p. 39, p. 170 [pp. 229–30].

Williams, Tennessee (1958) Suddenly Last Summer. In: *The Theatre of Tennessee Williams*. New Directions, New York, 1971, vol. 3, 423 pp.; p. 343, p. 351, p. 365, p. 423 [pp. 38–9].

Williams, Tennessee (1948) Summer and Smoke. In: *The Theatre of Tennessee Williams*. New Directions, New York, 1971, vol. 2, 591 pp.; p. 142 [pp. 149–50].

Williams, William Carlos (1938) Dance Pseudomacabre. In: Williams, William Carlos. *The Doctor Stories*. New Directions, New York, 1984, 142 pp.; pp. 88–91 [pp. 90–1].

Williams, William Carlos (1938) A Face of Stone. In: Williams, William Carlos. *The Doctor Stories*. New Directions, New York, 1984, 142 pp.; pp. 78–87 [pp. 65–6].

Williams, William Carlos (1938) The Girl with a Pimply Face. In: Williams, William Carlos. *The Doctor Stories*. New Directions, New York, 1984, 142 pp.; pp. 49–53 [p. 25].

Williams, William Carlos (1934) Jean Beicke. In: Williams, William Carlos. *The Doctor Stories*. New Directions, New York, 1984, 142 pp.; pp. 69–77 [pp. 111–12].

Williams, William Carlos (1932) Old Doc Rivers. In: Williams, William Carlos. *The Doctor Stories*. New Directions, New York, 1984, 142 pp.; pp. 13–41 [p. 248].

Williams, William Carlos (1938) The Use of Force. In: Williams, William Carlos. *The Farmers' Daughters*. New Directions, Norfolk, CT, 1961, 374 pp.; pp. 131–5 [p. 227].

Williamson, David (1980) *Travelling North*. Currency Press, Sydney, 88 pp.; pp. 46–7, p. 51 [pp. 124–5].

Wolfe, Thomas (1939) *The Web and the Rock*. Heinemann, London, 1969, 642 pp.; pp. 624–8 [p. 155].

Woolf, Virginia (1925) *Mrs Dalloway*. Zodiac Press, London, 1947, 213 pp.; pp. 104–13, p. 203 [p. 27, p. 44, p. 109, pp. 165–6, p. 195].

Wouk, Herman (1962) *Youngblood Hawke*. Doubleday, Garden City, NY, 783 pp.; pp. 330–1 [p. 123].

Yglesias, Helen Bassine (1972) *How She Died*. Heinemann, London, 1973, 338 pp.; p. 14 [p. 152].

Young, Francis Brett (1938) *Dr Bradley Remembers*. Heinemann, London, 745 pp.; pp. 14–16, pp. 242–5 [p. 80, pp. 85–6, p. 89, p. 106, p. 111, p. 132, pp. 163–4, p. 213].

Young, Francis Brett (1928) *My Brother Jonathan*. Heinemann, London, 595 pp.; p. 221, pp. 227–8, pp. 322–32 [p. 31, p. 232].

Zola, Émile (1893) *Doctor Pascal*. Translated by Kean, Vladimir. Elek Books, London, 1957, 292 pp.; pp. 201–2 [p. 36].

Zola, Émile (1887) *The Earth*. Translated by Parmee, Douglas. Penguin, Harmondsworth, 1980, 500 pp.; pp. 395–6, p. 486 [p. 79].

Selected secondary sources

Amm, Marita (1996) Utterances of discontent: the physician in the œuvre of Thomas Bernhard, Wien. *Klin Wochenschr*. **108**: 478–82.

Amundsen DW (1977) Image of physicians in classical times. *J Popular Culture*. **11**: 643–55.

Aull, Felice (2001) Arts and Medicine. Database at New York University School of Medicine, http://endeavor.med.nyu.edu/lit-med/lit-med-db/descrips.html

Ballantyne, John (ed.) (1995) *Bedside Manners*. Virgin, London (Anthology), 266 pp.

Bamforth, Iain (ed.) (2003) *The Body in the Library*. Verso, London (Anthology), 418 pp.

Ceccio, Joseph (ed.) (1978) *Medicine in Literature*. Longman, New York (Anthology), 324 pp.

Charon R, Banks JT, Connelly JE, Hawkins AH, Hunter KM, Jones AH, Montello M and Poirer S (1995) Literature and medicine: contributions to clinical practice. *Ann Int Med*. **122**: 599–606.

Cole, Hubert (ed.) (1963) *Under the Doctor*. Heinemann, London (Anthology), 301 pp.

Cousins, Norman (ed.) (1982) *The Physician in Literature*. Saunders, Philadelphia (Anthology), 477 pp.

Dans, Peter E (2000) *Doctors in the Movies*. Medi-Ed Press, Bloomington, IL, 384 pp.

Dunn JJ, Lee TH, Percelay JM, Fitz JG and Goldman L (1987) Patient and house officer attitude on physician attire and etiquette. *JAMA*. **257**: 65–8.

Flannery MC (2001) The white coat: a symbol of science and medicine as a male pursuit. *Thyroid*. **11**: 947–51.

Gawande, Atul (2002) *Complications: A Surgeon's Notes on an Imperfect Science*. Profile Books, London, 2003, 269 pp.

Gledhill JA, Warner JP and King M (1997) Psychiatrists and their patients: views on forms of dress and address. *Brit J Psych*. **171**: 228–32.

Gordon, Richard (IFG Ostlere) (ed.) (1993) *The Literary Companion To Medicine*. St Martin's Press, New York (Anthology), 431 pp.

Hamman, Louis (1938) As others see us. *Transact Assoc Amer Physicians*. **53**: 22–45.

Hill J (1987) The doctor as hero in nineteenth century British fiction. *The Pharos of Alpha Omega Alpha*. **50**: 31–3.

Hoffman NY (1972) The doctor as a scapegoat. A study in ambivalence. *JAMA*. **220**: 58–61.

Hunter, Kathryn Montgomery (1991) *Doctors' Stories: the narrative structure of medical knowledge*. Princeton University Press, Princeton, NJ, 205 pp.

Huth, Edward J and Murray, T Jock (2000) *Medicine in Quotations*. American College of Physicians, Philadelphia, 524 pp.

Illich, Ivan (1976) *Limits to Medicine*. Penguin, Harmondsworth, 1990, 296 pp.

Ingelfinger FJ (1980) Arrogance. *N Engl J Med*. **303**: 1507–11.

Jones, Anne Hudson (1989) Medicine and The Physician. In: Inge, M Thomas (ed.) *Handbook of American Popular Culture* (2e). Greenwood Press, New York, vol. 2, pp. 721–43.

Kalisch, Philip A and Kalisch, Beatrice J (1987) *The Changing Image of the Nurse*. Addison Wesley, Menlo Park, CA, 259 pp.

Kim J (2001) Emotional detachment and involvement of physicians in literature. *The Pharos of Alpha Omega Alpha*, vol. 64, Spring: 32–8.

Konner, Melvin (1987) *Becoming a Doctor*. Viking, New York, 390 pp.

Lamont EB and Christakis NA (2001) Prognostic disclosure to patients with cancer near the end of life. *Ann Int Med*. **134**: 1096–105.

Le Fanu, James (1999) *The Rise and Fall of Modern Medicine*. Little Brown, London, 490 pp.

Lehmann LS, Brancati FL, Chen MC, Roter D and Dobs AS (1997) The effect of bedside case presentations on patients' perceptions of their medical care. *N Engl J Med.* **336**: 1150–5.

Malmsheimer, Richard (1988) 'Doctors Only': the evolving image of the American physician. *Contributions in Medical Studies*, Number 25, Greenwood Press, New York, 173 pp.

McDonald SF (1931) Medicine in fiction in the last hundred years. *Med J Aust.* **1**: 709–21.

McLay RN, Lutz B, Baden MM, Bray R and Griffies S (2000) Kind strangers? Physicians through the eyes of Tennessee Williams. *J Louisiana State Med Soc.* **152**: 405–9.

McLennan MF (1996) Images of physicians in literature: from quacks to heroes. *Lancet.* **348**: 458–60.

Miller CJ (1931) The doctors of fiction. *Surg Gynecol Obstet.* **52**: 493–7.

Mitchell, S Weir (1888) *Doctor and Patient*. Arno Press, New York, 1972, 177 pp.

Mohr JC (2000) American medical malpractice: litigation in historical perspective. *JAMA.* **283**: 1731–7.

Moynihan, Berkeley George Andrew (Lord Moynihan) (1936) *The Story of Those Who Deserted Medicine, Yet Triumphed*. University Press, Cambridge, 109 pp.; p. 108.

Mukand, Jon (ed.) (1990) *Vital Lines: contemporary fiction about medicine*. St Martin's Press, New York (Anthology), 436 pp.

Norris, Carolyn Brimley (1969) The Image of the Physician in Modern American Literature. PhD dissertation, University of Maryland, 434 pp.

Osler, William (1903–5) *Aphorisms*. Bean, Robert Bennett and Bean, William Bennett (eds). Charles C Thomas, Springfield, IL, 1961, 164 pp.

Osler, William (1893) Physic and Physicians as Depicted in Plato. In: Osler W. *Aequanimitas*. HK Lewis and Co., London, 1920, 474 pp.; pp. 47–76.

Paton, Alan (1994) Doctors in Literature. In: Walton, John N, Barondess, Jeremiah A and Lock, Stephen (eds) *Oxford Medical Companion*. Oxford University Press, Oxford, 1038 pp.; pp. 214–17.

Pedrotti, Louis (1981) Chekhov's Major Plays: A Doctor in the House. In: Barricelli, Jean Pierre. *Chekhov's Great Plays*. New York University Press, New York, 268 pp.; pp. 233–50.

Peschel ER (ed.) (1980) *Medicine and Literature*. Neale Watson Academic Publications, New York, 240 pp.

Petersen, Christine E (1938) *The Doctor in French Drama, 1700–1775*. Columbia University Press, New York, 142 pp.

Posen S (1992) The portrayal of the physician in non-medical literature: 1. The physician and his fee. *J Roy Soc Med.* **85**: 5–7.

Poynter FNL (1968) Doctors in the human comedy. *JAMA.* **204**: 105–8.

Reynolds, Richard and Stone, John (1991) *On Doctoring: stories, poems, essays*. Simon and Schuster, New York (Anthology), 428 pp.

Rothfield, Lawrence (1992) *Vital Signs: medical realism in nineteenth century fiction*. Princeton University Press, Princeton, NJ, 235 pp.

Silvette H (1967) *The Doctor on the Stage: medicine and medical men in seventeenth century England*. University of Tennessee Press, Knoxville, TN, 291 pp.

Snow CP (1973) Human care. *JAMA*. **225**: 617–21.

Stoeckle, John D (1987) *Encounters Between Patients and Doctors*. MIT Press, Cambridge, MA, 440 pp.

Strauss, Maurice Benjamin (1968) *Familiar Medical Quotations*. Little Brown and Company, Boston, 968 pp.

Trautmann, Joanne and Pollard, Carol (1982) *Literature and Medicine: an annotated bibliography*. University of Pittsburgh Press, Pittsburgh, PA, 228 pp.

Turow, Joseph (1989) *Playing Doctor*. Oxford University Press, New York, 315 pp.

Vogel, Morris J (1980) *The Invention of the Modern Hospital (Boston 1870–1930)*. University of Chicago Press, Chicago, 171 pp.

Walter G (1992) The psychiatrist in American cartoons, 1941–1990. *Acta Psychiatr Scand*. **85**: 167–72.

Walter G (1989) The stereotype of the mad psychiatrist. *Aust NZ J Psychiatry*. **23**: 547–54.

Wilbanks ER (1958) The physician in the American novel, 1870–1955. *Bull Bibliogr*. **22**: 164–8 (Bibliography).

Winick C (1963) The psychiatrist in fiction. *J Nerv Ment Dis*. **136**: 43–57.

Young, Francis Brett (1936) The Doctor in Literature. In: Walpole H (ed.) *Essays by Divers Hands*. H Mulford, Oxford University Press, London, vol. 15, pp. 17–35.

Name index

List of major and minor works of fiction cited in this book. Also listed are a few non-fictional works, some place names and fictional characters. Unless otherwise indicated, untitled individuals are patients, patients' relatives or friends. The numbers indicate the pages where the relevant doctors, patients or literary works are mentioned in this book.

Subject index